CW00591362

Neurophysiology
—the essentials

Neurophysiology
—the essentials

George G. Somjen, M.D.

Professor
Department of Physiology
Duke University Medical Center
Durham, North Carolina

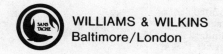

WILLIAMS & WILKINS
Baltimore/London

Copyright ©, 1983
Williams & Wilkins
428 East Preston Street
Baltimore, MD 21202, U.S.A.

All rights reserved. This book is protected by copyright. No part of this book may
be reproduced in any form or by any means, including photocopying, or utilized by
any information storage and retrieval system without written permission from the
copyright owner.

Made in the United States of America

Library of Congress Cataloging in Publication Data

Somjen, George G.
  Neurophysiology: the essentials.

  Includes index.
    1. Neurophysiology. I. Title. [DNLM: 1. Nervous system—Physiology. WL 102
S697n]
QP361.S65 1983   612′.8   83-5801
ISBN 0-683-07856-9

Composed and printed at the
Waverly Press, Inc.
Mt. Royal and Guilford Aves.
Baltimore, MD 21202, U.S.A.

Preface

The life is being squeezed out of physiology courses in medical schools. This text is an attempt to explain in writing what I should have taught my students, if we had the time. Anyone who compiles an introductory text must decide again and again what it is that the reader really must know. This text is written in the first place for medical students, but I hope that it will remain useful in the years of resident training in neurology, psychiatry and medicine. Of course the requirements of these groups are not identical. Moreover, "the essentials" cannot always be presented without some less essential background material. Those parts of the text that may be less essential than others have been printed in smaller type.

A difficult decision concerned the quotation of original sources. After much deliberation, references to original investigations have been deleted. To give credit to all would have made the text too long and ponderous; to select a few would have been arbitrary. Only a few pioneers and their classical contributions are mentioned. Exceptions were made in one or two cases where a still active investigator's name has become so closely associated with an idea that it customarily is referred to by his name (e.g. Hodgkin-Huxley equations; Henneman's size principle). Key reviews and selected research papers are listed at the end of each chapter and the names of the authors on whose discoveries this text is based and details of their investigations that could not be described here may be found in these sources.

Another problem perennially faced by teachers of introductory courses is how much to mention ideas that are interesting but not firmly established. Not long ago neurophysiology was short on facts, shorter yet on theory, but long on hypotheses. Today we face a mountain of data, but we still have too few cogent theories, and there is still plenty of loose conjecture. It is thus easy to get lost in a desert of fact or in a morass of speculation. It has been my intention to select as many of the facts known about normal function as are needed to understand disease states, and to add just enough of the currently widely discussed hypotheses to make these facts interesting and comprehensible in a wider context. Where there is controversy, I tried to summarize both sides of the argument, deleting only that which seemed unnecessary detail.

Neurophysiology can effectively be learned only in conjunction with its sister disciplines. I have assumed that the student will have at his or her disposal texts on other aspects of physiology, as well as on neuroanatomy and neurochemistry. For those who are using the companion volumes of this series, references are made to specific pages and illustrations in the following works:

Carpenter MB: *Core Text of Neuroanatomy*, ed 2. Baltimore, Williams & Wilkins, 1978.

Sernka T, Jacobson E: *Gastrointestinal Physiology: The Essentials.* Baltimore, Williams & Wilkins, 1979.

Smith JJ, Kampine JP: *Circulatory Physiology: The Essentials,* Baltimore, Williams & Wilkins, 1980.

West JB: *Respiratory Physiology: The Essentials,* ed 2. Baltimore, Williams & Wilkins, 1979.

Needless to say, many other texts can be used with equal profit.

I have been greatly helped by several people, to whom I am much indebted. Mrs. Marjorie Andrews typed most of the manuscript and helped with editing. Mrs. Joan Jones gave a professional touch to the illustrations. Dr. Barry Allen, at the time Mr. Barry Allen, read and criticized the draft manuscript from the student's point of view and also helped remove the foreign accent that could be heard when reading the draft. The following colleagues read parts of the draft and offered constructive criticism: Drs. Nels Anderson, John Casseday, Helen Cserr, Sid Gilman, James Houk, James McNamara, Elliott Mills, Edward Perl and Donald Sanders. Any remaining errors or shortcomings are, of course, my own. I would be glad to hear from readers who might wish to comment on the text.

Durham, North Carolina
April 1982

Contents

chapter 1

Introduction

The reader is introduced to the concepts, terms, and methods of investigation used in neurophysiology.

1.1. General Remarks and Some Important Early Discoveries

It is likely that the original vertebrate animal evolved from a segmented creature distantly reminiscent of an earthworm or a leech, though evidently it must have been different from any species living now. Its nervous system probably consisted of a chain of ganglia, or perhaps two chains of symmetrically paired ganglia, with an enlarged head ganglion at the front end. The head ganglion may have dominated other members of the chain; it may have made the "decisions" which required the cooperation of the entire neuronal assembly. But even so, each segmental ganglion probably enjoyed considerable autonomy of action, each knowing, so to speak, what it was doing. When cut to pieces, such a creature, like its modern descendants, may have been able to regenerate several complete new individuals.

The great transition from a segmented organism to a protovertebrate animal may have occurred by the fusion of the paired chains of ganglia into a tube-like structure of nervous tissue. From this primitive central nervous system paired nerve roots emerged, similar to the spinal roots of today's vertebrates. Through nerve fibers contained in these roots the central nervous system received information from sense organs and sent commands to muscles and glands. In the successive stages of vertebrate evolution, the head end of the neural tube, deriving from the original head ganglion, increased in size and in functional importance until it gained virtually complete domination over most functions of the nervous system. This evolutionary process was termed the *encephalization* of neural functions by the English neurologist Hughlings Jackson. Jackson, who worked in the 19th century, gave us many of the basic concepts not only of clinical neurology, but of neuroscience in general.

Even to this day, however, encephalization and centralization of the functions of the nervous systems of mammals are not complete. The paravertebral chains of sympathetic ganglia of vertebrates resembles the ganglion chains of invertebrates. Moreover, a measure of autonomy is retained by the intramural nervous system of the intestines, which is able to do its job even when disconnected from the central nervous system. We shall describe these in Chapter 17 (Section 17.3).

In the spirit of evolutionary theory it is customary to speak of "higher" and "lower" levels of organization in the nervous system, and of phylogenetically new and old component parts of the nervous system. This manner of speaking evokes the picture of the nervous system as a building to which successive generations have added story on story and wings tacked to the sides. Like most metaphors, this one can be quite misleading. Perhaps it would be a little closer to the truth to liken the evolution of the vertebrate central nervous system to those cathedrals that have entirely been rebuilt several times through the ages. To make way for each new structure, most of what preceded it has always been razed. In other words, any time evolution added a new element to a nervous system, all that was there already had to be redesigned. The brain of a mouse would be quite useless if grafted on the spinal cord of a goldfish.

As long as these reservations are kept in mind, it still is useful to distinguish between the more primitive, older parts of the central nervous system and its newer, more advanced parts. Man's cortex is, without a doubt, larger and more complex than that of any other mammal. By contrast, the spinal cords of different mammals are more similar, one to another, than are other parts of their central nervous systems—similar, but not identical.

Indeed, if there were no similarities in the structure, composition and functioning of the nervous systems of different organisms, it would be futile to study the nervous system of lower animals and hope to understand our own. Most closely related are the basic biochemical and biophysical processes. Thus similar chemical compounds have been found to perform similar functions in the nervous systems of all classes of animals that inhabit this planet. The conduction and the transmission of nervous signals differs only in minor details among species. The component units from which the systems are built are also quite similar in structure. It is the wiring diagram of their interconnections that differs vastly. In that respect, the closer the kinship, the more related the blueprint. So, we can learn much from studying the brains of cats or, better, of monkeys and apes, as long as we remain on guard against unwarranted generalizations.

Complete study of the nervous system requires the tools of morphology, biochemistry, physiology and psychology. This text must, by necessity, be limited to the third of these four disciplines. The others will not be ignored, but will not be discussed in any detail.

The first neurophysiological experiment happened by chance on a day late in the 18th century during a demonstration given by Luigi Galvani to a group of students. Galvani was dissecting a frog. In the back of the laboratory stood an electrostatic generator, one of those contraptions with a large spinning disc, brushes, and metal balls which discharge electric sparks. A bored student in the last row was playing with this machine, and each time he drew a spark, the frog's leg, held in a forceps by the Master, twitched. Intrigued, Galvani began to study the excitability of frogs' nerves and muscles, which resulted in his treatise on animal electricity published in 1791.

Galvani's principal thesis was that animal tissues generated electricity and that this "animal electricity" was the stuff of the excitation of nerves and of the contraction of muscles. In the history of science this is one of the most striking examples of a correct conclusion drawn from faulty experiments and incorrect reasoning. As was pointed out by Galvani's contemporary and countryman, Volta, none of the experiments performed by Galvani proved that the tissues either *made* or contained electricity, only that they *responded* to the electricity generated by an outside source. Only after the death of Galvani did his followers demonstrate that animal tissues indeed generate their own electric current. The decisive experiment demonstrated that "contraction without metal" was possible.

A leg nerve of a frog was dissected partially free but left in continuity with the muscles it innervated. The nerve was then laid in contact with a muscle from another frog the end of which had been sliced off. Part of the nerve touched the intact surface of the muscle, part the cut surface. If the (injured) muscle of the second frog was made to twitch, that of the first frog twitched also. In today's parlance, the action potential of the injured muscle stimulated the motor fibers in the nerve. In a variant of this experiment, a nerve of one frog was placed in contact with the beating heart of another. With each contraction of the heart, the muscle twitched. The electric current we now record as the electrocardiogram stimulated the motor nerve fibers.

The velocity with which nerve impulses are conducted was first measured by Helmholtz in 1850, long before electronic instruments were invented. The nerve was stimulated alternately at two different points. The stimulation caused a contraction of the muscle innervated by the nerve. The contraction was traced with the aid of a rapidly revolving smoked drum on which the time between stimulation and the onset of contraction could be measured. The interval was longer when the stimulated point was farther from the muscle. This difference in the time of onset of the contractions had to equal the time taken by the nerve impulse to travel from the farther to the nearer stimulating point, i.e. the *conduction time*. Dividing the distance between the two stimulating electrodes (the *conduction distance*) by the *conduction time* gave the *conduction velocity*. This principle is still used today to estimate conduction velocity of motor nerves of neurological patients; only the smoked drum has been replaced by electronic recording instruments (Fig. 1.1).

That nerves conduct impulses was at that time only an inference. Nerve impulses were proven to be brief variations of electric potential by Bernstein in the last decade of the 19th century. Bernstein achieved this with the aid of a rapidly spinning disc on which metal contacts made and broke electric circuits at variable, predetermined intervals. His device was, in essence, a mechanically operated analog computer. With it he plotted the time course of what we today call the *compound action potential* of a nerve. Bernstein correctly estimated the duration of the action potential to be 1 msec or slightly less.

The direct visualization of nerve impulses had to wait for the invention of vacuum tube amplifiers and the cathode ray oscilloscope, first used for electrophysiological investigation by Gasser and Erlanger in the 1920s.

1.2. Methods of Study in Neurophysiology

Since the signals of nerve cells and fibers are electrical, electronic instruments have become the principal tools of neurophysiology. The equipment of an electrophysiological laboratory includes a stimulator, designed to deliver electric current pulses to excite nervous tissue; amplifying and recording devices to register the electric response to the stimulus; and, most recently, computing circuits to aid in the analysis of the results.

In order to perform a neurophysiological experiment, access must be gained to the nervous system. The "preparations" studied range from a

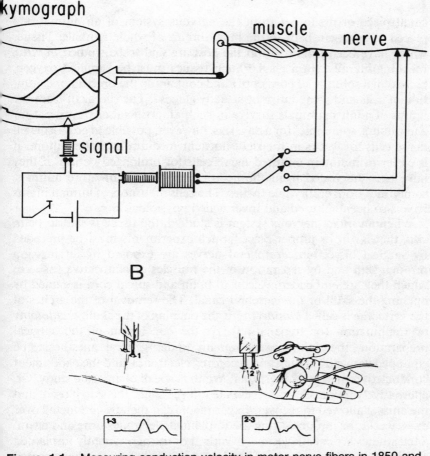

Figure 1.1. Measuring conduction velocity in motor nerve fibers in 1850 and today. *A*, the experimental arrangement used by Helmholtz. The nerve of an *in vitro* frog nerve-muscle preparation was stimulated through the secondary coil of an inductorium. When the switch in the primary circuit was either closed or opened, a brief current surged in the secondary circuit. The contraction of the muscle was recorded on the revolving smoked drum of a kymograph together with a time marker signaling the closing and opening of the switch. The muscle contracted later when the nerve was stimulated farther from the muscle (see text for calculation of conduction velocity). (Modified and redrawn after C. L. Evans: *Starling's Principles of Human Physiology,* ed 12. London, Churchill, 1956.) *B*, measuring motor nerve conduction velocity in the diagnostic electrophysiology laboratory. The nerve is stimulated through one of two electrode pairs (*1* or *2*). The compound muscle action potential is recorded through the small disc electrodes (*3*). The large electrode in the palm is connected to ground potential. Sample records *1–3* and *2–3* show the muscle action potentials recorded when either electrode *1* or electrode *2* is used to deliver the stimulus. (Modified and reprinted with permission from H. L. Cohen and J. Brumlik: *Manual of Electroneuromyography*, ed 2. New York, Harper & Row, 1976.)

5

small piece of tissue cut from the nervous system of an animal and placed in an organ bath to the intact brains of whole animals. Tissues which have been isolated from the host are said to be studied *in vitro*, meaning literally "in a glass." Such tissues must be supplied oxygen, bathed in a solution of correct pH and containing the proper concentration of salts and some nutrient, usually glucose. The slices cut from the brains of adult mammals survive in such an artificial environment for a few hours, sometimes for a day. It is, however, possible to grow isolated nerve cells for weeks in the right nutrient medium in tissue culture. It is easier to maintain cultured nerve cells for prolonged periods if they have been harvested from the nervous system of immature animals, sometimes from embryonic tissues. The cells of tumors of human brains have also been cultured and investigated physiologically.

When an intact nervous system is studied, the tissue is said to be *in situ*, that is "in its proper place." Such experiments must be preceded by surgical dissection. Peripheral nerves are exposed by an incision through skin and by separation of the muscles or connective tissue in which they are embedded. Access to brain and spinal cord is gained by opening the skull or the vertebral canal. The removal of the arches of the vertebrae is called *laminectomy*; the opening of the skull, *craniotomy* or trephination (or trepanation). At the conclusion of the surgical preparation, the animal may remain under general anesthesia, be equipped with stimulating and recording electrodes, and the experiment conducted immediately thereafter. We then speak of an *acute* study. Or, alternatively, electrodes may be sealed in the skull, the skin closed, and the animal allowed to recover. Experiments can then be conducted over days, weeks, or months, using the implanted electrodes time and again. Such studies are called *chronic*. A variant of the permanently implanted electrode is a device fastened to the skull which enables the repeated insertion and withdrawal of needle electrodes in the brain of conscious animals, sometimes by remote control. All physiological experiments are conducted *in vivo* ("in the living"), in contrast to morphological studies which may be performed *post mortem* ("after death").

Needle electrodes are needed to stimulate, or to record, the electric potentials deep in the brain. Such an electrode may be a simple straight wire, insulated except at its tip; or it may have an electric "shield" which is connected to ground potential. The purpose of the shield is to screen electric interference that might contaminate bioelectric signals. Such a "concentric" electrode may be constructed from a fine-gauge hypodermic needle, through which is threaded a thin, insulated wire (or pair of wires) with its (their) uninsulated tip exposed. The hypodermic needle acts as the shield.

The finest needle electrodes have tips small enough to record the signals generated by individual neurons. The giant neurons of some invertebrate organsms can be stripped of surrounding tissue under a dissecting microscope. The neurons of mammalian brains and spinal cords must be approached by an essentially blind search, like fishing in a murky pond. One inserts the electrode in a brain region presumed to be inhabited by the type of cell one is interested in. Then, as one listens to the audio monitor and watches the oscilloscope screen, the electrode is moved a few microns at a time into the tissue, until a cell "bites."

The action potentials of individual neurons can be recorded if a microelectrode is moved close to the cell, but to study the biophysics of cell membranes, the electrode must actually pierce the membrane. The potential difference between the inside of the cell and its environment can then be recorded. Glass capillary micropipettes, with tips between 0.2 and 1.0 μm in diameter, are used for this purpose. These pipettes are filled with a strong electrolyte to make them electrically conductive, and their glass wall serves as an insulator. By means of wire dipped into the electrolyte, the capillary is connected to the recording equipment (Figs. 1.2 and 2.12). Strictly speaking, the wire is the electrode and the pipette a salt bridge. But, in the loose jargon of the laboratory, the pipette itself is often called a microelectrode.

Through the efforts of several generations of investigators, the main masses of gray matter in the central nervous system (CNS) and the fiber tracts that connect them have been charted and named. Brain atlases are available for all the animal species commonly used in laboratory experiments. Current investigations seek to define the functions of these cell assemblies. To this end, the more intimate details of their interconnections must be discovered; and the electric signals these cells emit must be recorded during well-defined behaviors. To make these kinds of observations, electrodes must be inserted in specified *nuclei* (see Section 1.3) or neuron groups. Regions of the cerebral or cerebellar cortex can be identified by using the visible landmarks of gyri and sulci, but to aim an electrode into a deeper nucleus, a *stereotactic frame* must be used. (Fig. 1.3). Invented by Horsley and Clarke, a neurosurgeon-neuroanatomist team, it consists of parallel bars and orthogonally attached cross-pieces with millimeter scales. A clamp accurately fixes the animal's head in relation to the bars. Electrode carriers with fine movement and micrometer scales are rigidly attached to the frame at

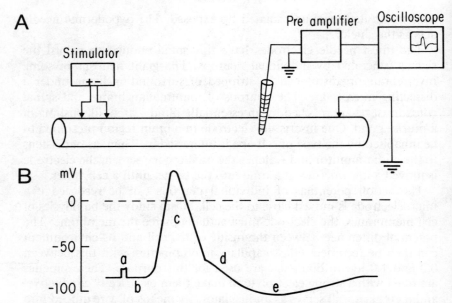

Figure 1.2.   Recording the membrane potential and action potential of a nerve or a muscle fiber with an intracellular micropipette electrode. *A*, schema of the recording arrangement. The tip of the micropipette has pierced the surface membrane and is recording the intracellular potential with reference to ground. The extracellular fluid is at ground potential. *B*, a generalized action potential; *a*, the stimulus artefact (trace of the pulse delivered by the stimulator at a distance from the recording point); *b*, resting potential; *c*, spike; *d*, after-depolarization; *e*, after-hyperpolarization. During the *latent time* elapsing between stimulus and the onset of the spike, the impulse travels from the stimulating cathode to the recording electrode.

predetermined angles. Special atlases have been compiled which show serial sections of brains, with stereotactic coordinates marked. With their aid, one can determine the angle of inclination and the distance of travel required to move the electrode to a given nucleus in the gray matter.

Neurosurgeons have adapted the stereotactic procedure to the conditions of the operating theater (see, for example, Section 18.2c). The human stereotactic instruments attach to the skull at predetermined points. In the operating room, the placement of needle electrodes is controlled using either conventional x-ray examination or, more recently, computer-assisted tomography. The usual purpose of stereotactic surgery is the destruction of a neuron mass that is believed to malfunction. This can be done by electric current, by heat, or by cold. The tissue can be heated by high-frequency alternating current passed through the electrode tip, or cooled by circulating cold liquid through a fine-tipped cryoprobe. Less often, direct current is applied which acts electrolytically.

At the close of animal experiments it is customary to verify the position of the stereotactically placed electrodes by histological examination of brain specimens *post mortem*. This is necessary because animals' heads do not come in precisely standardized sizes and shapes, and error is possible even with the most careful stereotactic technique.

A cornerstone of neurological diagnosis is the idea that disease or destruction of particular parts of the central nervous system cause specific and recognizable signs and symptoms. In this text we shall meet several examples; many more will be learned during clinical training. The same basic assumption, i.e. that specific lesions cause specific malfunctions, has guided much animal experimentation for at least a hundred years. In these experiments, either a fiber tract is cut or a part of the gray matter destroyed, and then the animal is examined for specific deficits. The examination may be electrophysiological, for example, to ascertain whether a certain stimulus evokes the same electric signal after the lesion as it had before. Or, the animal's overt behavior may be examined, for example, his ability to learn specific tasks.

1.3. Definitions

Nervous tissue consists of two types of cells, *neurons* and *satellite cells*. In the central nervous system, the satellite cells are called *neuroglia*, in the peripheral nerves, *Schwann cells*, but in the ganglia of the peripheral autonomic nervous system they have no universally accepted name; some authors call them *glia*, others simply *satellites*. Neuroglia has been regarded as the supporting tissue of the nervous system, but many investigators feel that its functions are more important than mere support. These questions will briefly be discussed in Chapter 5.

It is customary to divide the nervous system into the peripheral and the central part. The CNS of vertebrates consists of the brain, the brain stem (including the cerebellum) and the spinal cord. The peripheral nervous system consists of the peripheral nerves and the ganglia of the autonomic nervous system.

A *nucleus* is a compact region of gray matter of homogeneous cytoarchitecture and recognizable boundaries. A *center* is an assembly of

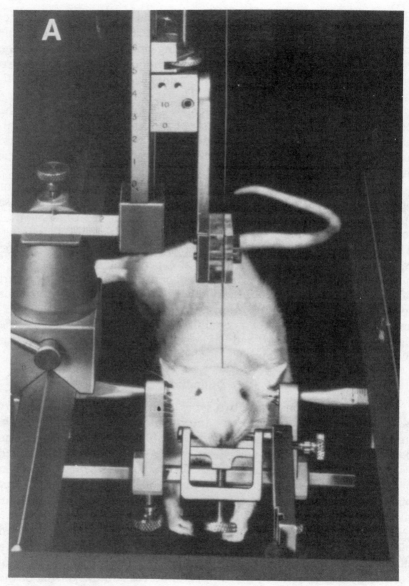

Figure 1.3.   The stereotactic method. *A*, a rat in a partially assembled stereotactic frame, with one electrode in electrode holder. (Courtesy of Trent Wells, Inc., South Gate, Calif.) *B*, stereotactic instrument used in surgery of human patients. (Courtesy of Radionics, Inc., Burlington, Mass.)

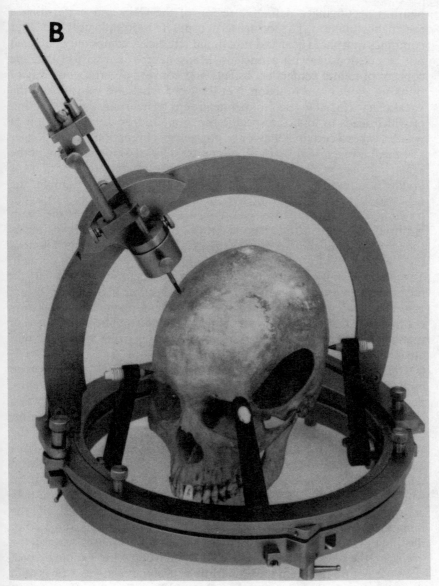

Figure 1.3*B*.

neurons occupying a definable region of the CNS and performing a specifiable function. The former term is purely morphological, the latter combines morphological and functional criteria. A center may but need not be coextensive with a nucleus. Many neuroscientists feel that the concept of neural centers is obsolete and conveys an erroneous way of thinking about brain function. Yet the word refuses to vanish from the vocabulary. It is now used to denote groups of neurons, the destruction of which leads to loss of a specific function, and/or the stimulation of which evokes a certain behavior or physiological function. We no longer assume, however, that brain functions are divided among centers in the same way as, for instance, the work of a large organization or plant is divided amongst its various offices and workshops. For example, the satiety center is located in the hypothalamus (see Section 17.5) and got its name from two experimental observations. If this part of the brain is stimulated in an animal having a meal, the animal will stop eating as though it has had enough. If the same structure is destroyed by a lesion, the animal eats too much and gets fat, as though it never has enough. These observations justify the conclusion that neurons in this part do have some essential role in evoking the sensation of satiety. No one assumes, however, that the feeding behavior is regulated in just one compact area of the brain; rather it is the result of the interaction of many neuron circuits in different regions. Thus the word "center" should always be read as in quotation marks.

The parts of a neuron are the *dendrites*, the *cell body* or *perikaryon* and the *axon* which is also referred to as nerve fiber. Cell bodies, dendrites and axons can be arranged in a variety of distinctive ways; examples are shown in Figure 1.4. Peripheral nerves consist of axons, Schwann cells and connective tissue sheaths. The fiber tracts of the *white matter* of the CNS are similar, except that glial cells replace Schwann cells and there is no connective tissue. The fibers in peripheral nerves conduct impulses either toward the central nervous system, in which case they are called *afferent*, or away from it, in which case they are *efferent*. The signals conducted by these fibers are, respectively, the *input* and the *output* of the central nervous system. In the spinal cord, the fiber tracts of the white matter conducting impulses toward the brain are the ones called afferent, and those from brain to spinal cord, efferent. Within the brain these definitions become relative. A fiber tract that connects nucleus A to nucleus B could be called the efferent tract of A conveying the output of A, but also the afferent tract of B, since it conveys input to B.

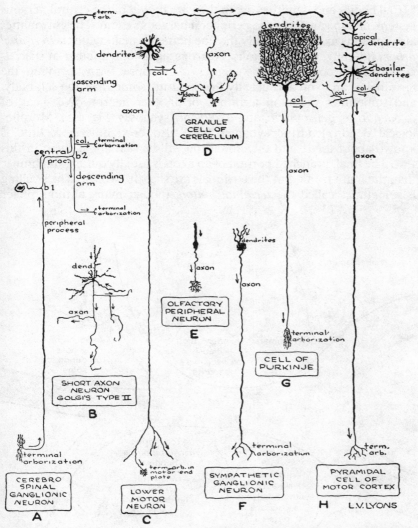

Figure 1.4. Types of neurons in the mammalian nervous system. The cerebrospinal ganglion cell (*A*) is also called a primary afferent neuron; the lower motor neuron (*C*) an alpha motor neuron. (Reprinted with permission from W. M. Copenhaver, D. E. Kelly and R. L. Wood (eds): *Bailey's Textbook of Histology*, ed 17. Baltimore, Williams & Wilkins, 1978.)

Cell bodies and dendrites are in the *gray matter* of the central nervous system, and in ganglia in the peripheral nervous system. The gray matter also contains axons, especially the fine branches making up the *terminal arbors* (literally, trees) of axons. Neurons signal one another at specialized contact points called *synapses.* A synapse forms between the terminal of an axon and usually the dendrite, sometimes the cell body, and sometimes the axon terminal, of another neuron. We speak of *axodendritic, axosomatic,* and *axoaxonic* synapses (Fig. 1.5). Morphological dendrodendritic synapses have also been described; little is known about these, and therefore little will be said about them in this text. The final, branched portion of an axon is usually quite thin, thinner than the main trunk, but the terminals are slightly swollen. The swelling is sometimes called the *terminal button,* though many authors prefer

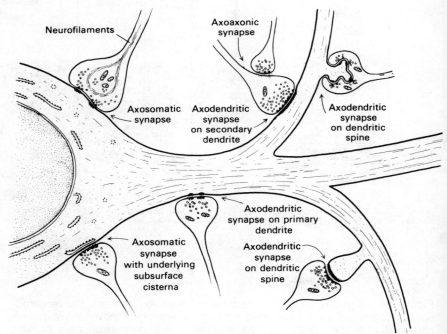

Figure 1.5.   Types of synapses in mammalian nervous systems as revealed by electron microscopy. (Reprinted with permission from W. M. Copenhaver, D. E. Kelly and R. L. Wood (eds): *Bailey's Textbook of Histology,* ed 17. Baltimore, Williams & Wilkins, 1978.)

the French equivalent, *bouton terminal*. Some axons have multiple swellings, as a string of beads, each bead forming a synapse; these synaptic beads are called *boutons en passage*. The axon terminals belong to the *presynaptic* neuron; the receiving cell is the *postsynaptic* neuron. Synapses may be *excitatory* or *inhibitory*. The latter act to prevent excitation.

Neurons are called *multipolar* if they have several dendrites and one axon. They are called *bipolar* if there are only two processes attached to the cell body, even if these processes branch profusely at some distance from the cell body. There are also unipolar cells that have but one process issuing from the cell body. It would be better to call these pseudo-unipolar, for the single process forms during embryonic development by the fusion of a dendrite with an axon. In the adult this process bifurcates at a short distance from the cell body, one branch derived from the original dendrite and the other derived from the original axon (Figs. 1.4*A* and 1.6*A*).

Afferent nerve fibers in peripheral nerves are the peripheral processes of bipolar or of pseudo-unipolar cells. Their cell bodies are located in sensory ganglia. These fibers conduct impulses toward the cell body in the ganglion. The other process conducts the signals from ganglion to the central nervous system. These cells are called *primary afferent neurons.*

Dendrites used to be defined as the processes that conducted signals toward the cell body; axons, as fibers that conducted signals away from the cell body. The difficulty is that the process of bipolar and of pseudo-unipolar cells which conducts toward the perikaryon looks and behaves as an axon, except for its branches near its peripheral receiving end. For this reason it has more recently become customary to call all structures axons that conduct action potentials and have certain ultrastructural features characteristic of axons. This leaves a certain ambiguity concerning the peripheral processes of bipolar cells and the peripheral branch of unipolar cells, which could be termed either dendrite or axon, depending on definition. The ambiguity can be circumvented by using the noncommittal term "nerve fiber."

A man-made electric stimulus can excite an axon anywhere. If such a pulse is applied to the middle of the axon, impulses will be conducted both toward the cell body and toward the axon terminal. Normal physiological processes, however, initiate impulses always at one end of the axon, so that normal impulse traffic in any nerve fiber is strictly one way. In the multipolar cells of the central nervous system, impulses are

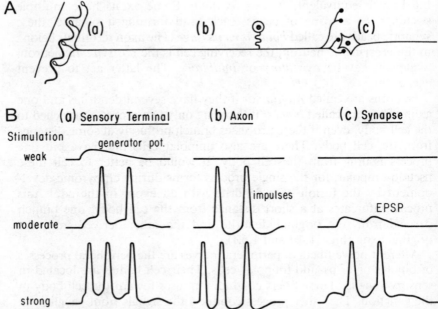

Figure 1.6. Potential signals generated by different parts of neurons. The sensory terminal (*a*) of a primary afferent neuron when stimulated produces the generator potential which remains localized in the terminal. If the generator potential is sufficiently strong, it triggers action potentials (impulses) which are conducted in the axon (*b*). When the impulses arrive in the presynaptic terminals, they cause the liberation of transmitter substance which evoke synaptic potentials in the postsynaptic neuron (*c*) and these in turn, if sufficiently strong, trigger impulses in the axon of the postsynaptic neuron.

born where the axon attaches to the cell body, the *initial segment* or axon hillock. To initiate an impulse, the neuron must normally be excited through its synapses. The latter are located on the dendrites and cell body, and their effect must be conveyed by *electrotonus* (see Sections 2.2, 2.5a, and 3.1b) to the initial segment of the axon.

In the fibers of primary afferent neurons the impulses start at the peripheral end of the fiber. In order that an impulse should be initiated in them, an appropriate stimulus must act on the sensory nerve terminal (e.g. see Fig. 1.6 and Section 6.1).

Conduction of an impulse in the normal direction is *orthodromic*. If, in an experiment, or as a consequence of a pathological process, impulses are conducted in the wrong direction, we speak of *antidromic* conduction.

The efferent fibers in peripheral nerves are the axons of *motor neurons* (often spelled motoneurons) or of secretomotor neurons. The peripheral terminals of motor axons form junctions with muscle fibers. These neuromuscular junctions are also called *motor endplates.* Through them the motor nerve fiber excites the muscle fiber. The arrangement of secretomotor autonomic fibers will be described in Chapter 17.

The term *internuncial* cell or *interneuron* was originally applied to all neurons that were neither afferent nor efferent, but connecting the two. The word grew from the idea that all actions of the central nervous system may be thought of as a *reflex*. The nature of simple and complex reflexes will be discussed in Chapter 4 (Section 4.2).

In today's language the word interneuron is used by most writers in a more limited sense to mean small neurons with short axons. Cells whose axons connect one part of the gray matter to another are referred to as *projection neurons*. Nerve cells with relatively long axons, afferent, efferent and projection neurons together fall in the general category described as Golgi's type I. Golgi's type II cells are the short-axon interneurons, the axons of which do not leave the nucleus in which the cell bodies are located. Speaking in general terms, Golgi's type I cells are conductor or connector elements. Golgi's type II cells are the logic elements that transact the most important businesses of the central nervous tissue. For technical reasons we know today more about the properties and behavior of type I than of type II cells. Until we find ways to study the latter, we will not understand the workings of the brain.

1.4. Bioelectric Signals and Their Recordings

The cytoplasm of virtually every living cell is electrically negative with respect to the fluid surrounding the cell. This includes, for example, algae, amebae, hepatocytes and erythrocytes. Because this potential difference is developed across the plasma membrane of the cells, it is called the *membrane potential.* Generally speaking, the resting membrane potential is larger in cells that are excitable than in those that are not (glial cells are exceptions; see Section 5.9). In the vertebrate organism neurons, muscle fibers and certain gland cells are excitable. Why nonexcitable cells have a membrane potential is not clear, but excitable cells could not do their job without it. The very processes of excitation consist of temporary changes of the membrane potential. In neurons, the resting membrane potential is between 60 and 85 mV, in skeletal muscle fibers around 90 mV.

Primary afferent neurons are the ones which gather information and send signals to the central nervous system. The membrane potential of the sensory ending of these afferent neurons is modulated by the stimuli acting on it. The various types of sensory nerve endings and their functions will be described in later chapters. For the time being we should consider the general case. In most sensory terminals, stimulation causes a *decrease* of the potential difference between inside and outside. This means that the inside becomes less negative or, if you will, relatively positive, compared to the "resting" state. A decrease of membrane potential is referred to as *depolarization.* The depolarization of sensory nerve terminals, caused by a sensory stimulus, is the *generator potential.* The stronger the stimulus, the greater the amplitude of the generator potential. The generator potential affects the membrane of the stimulated terminal and its immediate vicinity. If stimulation is of sufficient intensity, the generator potential triggers a nerve *impulse,* which then is *conducted without decrement* toward the central nervous system (Fig. 1.6). Of generator potentials as such, the brain knows nothing. Only if an impulse has been fired is the central nervous system informed of what happens at a sense organ. The stimulus that is just strong enough to cause the firing of an impulse is said to be of *threshold* or *liminal* intensity, anything less is *subthreshold* or *subliminal.* A neuron that is very excitable has a *low threshold*; one that is less excitable, a *high threshold.*

A nerve impulse is also known as an *action potential.* Action potentials consist of a brief "*spike*" potential, followed by smaller but more prolonged *afterpotentials* (Fig. 1.2). During the spike, the cytoplasm turns for a brief moment positive instead of negative. The magnitude of this positive "overshooting" varies from 5 to 35 mV in different nerve and muscle fibers. The duration of the spike is between 0.5 and 1.5 msec in nerve fibers and nerve cell bodies and around 2.0 msec in skeletal muscle. Since the conduction velocity of nerve fibers of mammals varies from 0.5 to 120 m/sec, the wavelength of the spike works out to be roughly between 0.1 and 6.0 cm.

The shape and magnitude of afterpotentials varies more between different fibers than does the spike. Typically, the spike is followed by a small "heel" called the *after-depolarization*; the potential "undershoots" the resting level: this is the *after-hyperpolarization* (Fig. 1.2).

At sensory afferent nerve terminals impulses are initiated by a sensory stimulus, through the mediation of the generator potential. In all other cases, impulses are started by the action of one excitable cell on another through synaptic junctions. Between motor nerve terminal and skeletal muscle the synapse has a special name, the *motor endplate*. Impulses are triggered in a muscle fiber after the arrival of a nerve impulse in the motor nerve fiber followed by an electric response in the endplate membrane, called the *endplate potential* (EPP). The EPP triggers the muscle's action potential. At neuron-to-neuron junctions the initial postsynaptic response is the *excitatory postsynaptic potential (EPSP)*. Like generator potentials, EPPs and EPSPs are localized depolarizations of the membrane that have the function to trigger the action potentials which then are conducted along the muscle or nerve fiber without any decrement. Further details of all these will follow (Chapters 2 and 3).

The reader may have noticed that in physiology the word "potential" is used more loosely than in physics. The membrane potential is the difference in potential between the inside and outside of a cell. Action potential, synaptic potential and generator potential all refer to transient variations of this potential difference.

Before the invention of intracellular recording, electrophysiological recordings were made from the extracellular medium close to, but outside of, nerve fibers. The mean potential of the extracellular fluid of the body is conventionally defined as zero, and all measurements are expressed relative to it. When a nerve or a muscle fiber is excited, current flows in the interstitial fluid around it, and the extracellular potential is briefly perturbed. The voltage transients recorded outside a fiber tend to be opposite in sign and smaller in magnitude than those on the inside. Thus at the height of the spike potential, while the inside potential turns positive, the extracellular phase shows a brief wave of potential that is negative relative to the resting level (Fig. 1.7).

Certain conventions have survived as a legacy of the extracellular era of electrophysiology. For example, on electroencephalographic (EEG) tracings, negative potential changes are usually plotted as upward deflections. On recordings made with intracellular electrodes, however, the convention is always to show "positive upward." In this text we shall plot positive deflections up in most illustrations of both intra- and extracellular potentials, except some which have been borrowed from other sources, and which will be appropriately labeled.

The traditions of the extracellular recording also survive in certain terms. Thus after-depolarization may be referred to also as the *negative afterpotential*, and after-hyperpolarization as the *positive afterpotential*.

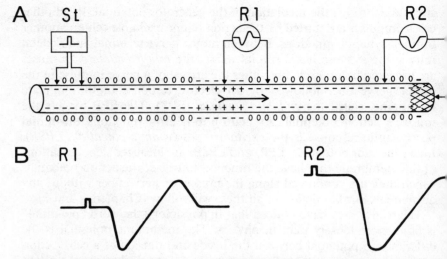

Figure 1.7.   Biphasic (*R1*) and monophasic (*R2*) extracellular recording of the impulse of a nerve fiber. *A*, experimental arrangement; *B*, the recording obtained as shown in *A*. In the resting state the inside of the fiber is electronegative with respect to the outside which is defined as zero potential. At the height of the impulse the inside turns positive (see Fig. 1.2) and the outside negative. For further description see text.

Similarly, blockade of nerve conduction by deliberate hyperpolarization of a nerve fiber is often called *anodal block*, and by depolarization as *cathodal block*.

1.4a. COMPOUND ACTION POTENTIALS

In many clinical and experimental applications it is neither desirable nor possible to record signals generated by individual neurons or nerve fibers. One then resorts to the usually simpler method of recording the discharge of many such unitary potentials together. The voltage deflection generated by the synchronized impulses of the many fibers contained in a nerve or a muscle is called a *compound action potential.*

The simplest electrodes used to stimulate nerves, or to record their action potentials, are wires bent around a nerve. In clinical applications electrodes are often in contact with the surface of the skin (Figs. 1.1*B* and 3.14). Pairs of electrodes are always needed for both stimulation and recording, or the electric circuits would not be complete. If a stimulating pulse of sufficient magnitude and duration is delivered to the nerve, it will excite some or all the fibers contained in the nerve. With brief pulses (0.05–1.0 msec), nerve impulses start only at the wire connected to the negative pole of the stimulator, that is, at the *cathode*. This is because an *external cathode* causes depolarization of the membrane, an *external anode* hyperpolarization. This will be explained in Section 3.1c and in Figure 3.6. If rather long and strong stimulating pulses are used, then a second nerve impulse may be started at the break of the current, now at the anode. This *"anode-break"* excitation occurs when the membrane potential which had been hyperpolarized by the anode returns to the resting level (Fig. 3.10).

Recording electrodes are best placed a few centimeters from the stimulating electrodes, with perhaps 1 cm spacing between the members of each pair. Of the two stimulating electrodes, the cathode should be the one nearer to the recording electrodes, and the anode farther (Fig. 1.2). The reason is that the anode may extinguish conduction by hyperpolarizing the nerve fibers. This need not always happen, for *"anodal blockade"* requires current pulses stronger in intensity and longer in duration than what is needed to stimulate the fibers.

A frog's nerve remains alive *in vitro* (cf. Section 1.2) for a few hours, if kept moist with a salt solution of appropriate composition (*Ringer's solution*). A mammalian nerve requires vigorous oxygenation, a temperature near to that which is normal in the body, and some glucose in the bathing solution. Assume that such a nerve is in contact with stimulating and recording electrodes, as shown in Figure 1.7. As impulses sweep past the pair of recording electrodes at the middle of the nerve they will make first the nearer, then the farther of the two recording wires negative. Our recording instrument will, therefore, register a *biphasic* potential wave. If we would like to see the waveform of the action potential as it is registered by one of the electrodes without interference by the other, we must prevent the impulse from reaching the farther one of the two recording electrodes. This is achieved the simplest way by crushing the nerve near its cut end with a forceps, and placing the farther recording electrode on the crushed part. The wire on the intact portion of the nerve is now the "active lead," the one on the crushed end the "reference" or "indifferent" electrode. Another method is to dip a few millimeters of the end of the nerve in a solution of 0.15 M (isotonic) KCl, and connect the indifferent electrode also in the KCl. Recording conditions are improved if a barrier made of non-conducting material such as vaseline or paraffin, or a pool of sucrose solution is erected between "active" and "indifferent" electrodes.

Crushing the end of a nerve or dipping it into isotonic KCl abolishes the membrane potential of the cut end so that inside and outside come to the same potential. This means that in the "resting" state electric current flows between the intact, polarized part of the nerve and the killed, depolarized end. This is called the *demarcation current*, or *current of injury*. Consequently, a standing potential exists between the "active" and the "indifferent" electrode. The monophasically recorded action potentials is, in fact, a decrease in the injury potential. So-called condenser-coupled (or AC coupled) amplifiers record fast transients such as action potentials, but not constant or slowly changing voltages such as the injury potential. Condenser-coupled amplifiers are generally used more than direct coupled (or DC) amplifiers.

1.4b. FOCAL RECORDING AND STIMULATION

We have already mentioned the use of needle electrodes to stimulate or to record from deep nuclei of the brain or spinal cord. We speak of focal *monopolar* stimulation or recording when the electrode consists of a simple needle or straight wire, insulated except at its tip. To be sure, there always must be a second pole somewhere in or on the body of the animal in order to close the electric circuit. This second distant (or indifferent or reference) electrode is usually placed in contact with an electrically quiet and non-excitable tissue outside the CNS, often an earlobe. When bipolar focal stimulating electrodes (paired instead of single wires) are used, there is no need for an indifferent pole. This has the advantage that the volume of tissue through which the stimulating current is dispersed remains limited to the vicinity of the exposed tips, but they may cause more tissue damage because of their larger diameter.

Both focal recording and focal stimulation have found use in clinical practice. Recordings are made of electroencephalographic activity and of evoked potential waves (see Sections 2.2, 7.7, and 10.7) in deep-lying brain structures, usually as part of diagnostic work-up in preparation of surgical treatment. The placement of depth electrodes requires a stereotactic procedure. Sometimes the electrodes are left in place for several days, allowing repeated and detailed examination. Focal stimulation is an experimental therapy, used for example in cases of intractable pain, and as a pacemaker for the urinary bladder of paraplegic patients. These will be described later (see Sections 7.9b, 17.3d). The permanent implantation of electrodes in the central nervous system of human patients has technological problems, not all of which have been solved. These concern the reaction of tissue to the presence of a metallic foreign body.

When action potentials are recorded with a monopolar focal depth electrode in the gray matter, they rarely appear as simple negative waves like the monophasic action potentials described above. If the tip of a needle electrode lies in a tract of axons, and a compound action potential approaches, sweeps by, and then recedes from the electrode tip, the tracing has the form of a triphasic, positive-negative-positive wave. The middle negative component is the largest and represents the arrival of the spike potential in the immediate vicinity of the electrode. The reason for the positive phases (*sources*) that precede and follow the passing of the spike may be understood from the manner in which current flows in the extracellular environment of partially depolarized cable-like structures (see Section 2.2 and Fig. 2.4). If the recording electrode tip is among the nerve cells near the point where impulses are sent on their journey, then the waveform is biphasic, negative-positive. If the electrode is near terminals where impulses arrive, the waveform is also biphasic, but now the sequence is positive-negative. If a positive phase precedes the negative spike, it means that the impulse is approaching the electrode; a positive phase after the negative spike indicates that it is moving away from the electrode.

1.5. Chapter Summary and Study Guide

This chapter contains definitions of the following terms:
action potential (nerve impulse)
conduction velocity of nerve impulses and its measurement
compound action potential
afferent fiber and afferent neuron
efferent fiber, efferent neuron, motor fiber and motor neuron
internuncial neuron (interneuron)
projection fiber and projection neuron
membrane potential, depolarization, hyperpolarization
afterpotential; after-depolarization (negative afterpotential, post-spike depolarization); after-hyperpolarization (positive afterpotential, post-spike hyperpolarization)
anode, cathode
anodal block, cathodal block, anode-break excitation
orthodromic conduction, antidromic conduction
generator potential
synapse, synaptic bouton, bouton terminal, *bouton en passage*
excitatory postsynaptic potential (EPSP), inhibitory postsynaptic potential (IPSP)
endplate, endplate potential (EPP)
electrotonus
experimentation *in situ*, *in vitro*, *in vivo* and *post mortem* studies
threshold (limen); subthreshold

nerve center, nerve nucleus
the stereotactic method and the use of implanted electrodes

Reading List

See at end of Chapter 3.

Electric Potentials
of Excitable Cells: I

This chapter deals with the mechanisms of the resting membrane potential, generator potentials and synaptic potentials. A brief summary of the laws of electric potentials, currents, and diffusion potentials introduces the chapter.

2.1. Electricity in Electrolyte Solutions

The next few pages briefly review aspects of electricity needed to understand nerve potentials, the topic of the bulk of this chapter and the next. This review is designed for those who had this material in an earlier course but have forgotten it. If you still remember the discussion of electricity from a course in physics or physical chemistry, then you may omit this section and skip to Section 2.2. However, if you never had physics at an upper high school or college level, then you should consult an appropriate physics textbook.

2.1a. CHARGE, POTENTIAL AND CURRENT

Charge is the fundamental quantity of electricity. It is measured in *coulombs*. Like heat or matter, it can be thought of as occupying a place and moving through space. Two kinds of charge exist: positive and negative. To generate one, the other must be generated at the same time.

Electric potential, like chemical potential, is a concept related to energy. To achieve a potential difference, positive and negative charge must be separated, and to do that work has to be done. Once a potential difference has been created, it can do work; in other words, it can return part of the invested energy. In practice one does not measure absolute potentials, only potential differences. Their unit of measurement is the *volt*.

A potential difference between two points can cause charge to flow. Moving electric charge is electric *current* and it is measured in *amperes*. An ampere equals a flow of 1 coulomb/sec. Current intensity is determined by the potential difference between two points and by the *resistance* of the conductor between them. If one unit of resistance (1 *ohm*) connects one unit of potential difference, one unit of current (*ampere*) will flow. This is Ohm's law:

$$I = V/R \tag{2.1}$$

The reciprocal of resistance is *conductance*. The proper name for the unit of conductance is the *siemens*, but it also is referred to as the *mho*.

Electric charge can be stored. The unit of storage capacity is the *farad*. Practical capacitors are called condensers. A simple condenser consists of two conducting plates separated by insulating material (that could be air), the dielectric. When a condenser is charged, its one plate is positive, the other negative. The capacity of a condenser increases with the surface of the plates and decreases with the distance between them. The capacity is also influenced by the properties of the material separating the plates, expressed mathematically by the dielectric constant.

The charge stored in a condenser equals the product of voltage times capacity; 1 farad stores 1 coulomb at 1 volt.

$$Q = VC \tag{2.2}$$

When the plates of a charged condenser are connected to each other through a resistor, current flows. The current carries charge away from the plates, and thus the voltage will diminish; with the voltage, the current will diminish also. Therefore, as a condenser is discharged through a resistor, its voltage decays exponentially. If two condensers, one of larger capacity than the other, carried equal charges and were made to discharge through two equal resistors, the current delivered by the larger condenser (which had the smaller voltage; see Equation 2.2) would initially be less intense but would flow for a longer time. The total energy dissipated by the two would be the same.

The *time constant* of a resistance-capacitance (RC) circuit is the time in which the voltage drops to $1/e$ of its initial value (e = base of natural logarithms). If R is given in ohms, C in farads, then the time constant in seconds is equal to their product, $R \times C$. The time constant is independent of the charge.

By a *battery* we mean a device in which the energy of a chemical reaction is converted into electrical energy. In an ideal battery the voltage remains constant until the substrates of the chemical reaction are depleted, so that they deliver a constant current into a constant resistance (*load*), or none at all. Few practical batteries behave ideally, but ideal behavior is assumed when electric symbols are used in diagrams representing biolectric processes.

If the two poles of a battery are connected to the plates of a condenser through resistors, current will flow and the voltage on the condenser will increase; when the voltage on the condenser becomes equal to that of the battery, the current will stop (Fig. 2.1*A*). The charging of a condenser follows an exponential course just like its discharge; charging and discharging have the same time constant.

If a resistor and a condenser are connected not to a battery, but to a source of alternating current (AC), then the plates of the condenser will in turn be charged positively, then discharged, then charged negatively, so that current will surge back and forth in the circuit. Even though charge does not flow through the dielectric of the condenser, the circuit will behave as though it admitted alternating current. The *resistance* (to direct current, DC) of such a circuit is said to be infinite, but its *impedance* (to AC) is finite, and is a complex function of the magnitudes of the resistor, the capacitor and also of the frequency of the AC. The current flowing at any moment in such an RC circuit depends on the rate of change of voltage, as follows:

$$I = \frac{dv}{dt} \frac{C}{R} \tag{2.3}$$

2.1b. ELECTRONS AND IONS: CURRENT FLOW IN SOLUTIONS

Electric charge is either an excess or a lack of electrons. For historic reasons, the former has been defined as negative, the latter as positive charge. In metal wires current is always carried by electrons; hence it is in fact negative charge that moves.

Aqueous solutions of electrolytes contain both positively charged ions (cations) and negative ones (anions). In an electrolyte solution there are, for all practical purposes, always equal numbers of cations and anions. When a potential difference exists between two points in a solution, current will be carried by two-way flux of both kinds of ions. It should be noted: that the *negative* electrode is the *cathode*, which attracts *positive* ions, the *cations*; the anode is the positive pole attracting the anions. Nevertheless it is the convention to indicate the direction of the current as flowing from the positive to the negative pole (Fig. 2.2). Also, in order to maintain an electrolytic current, at each electrode chemical reactions must take place to take care of the arriving ions, which lose their own charge as they accept charge from the electrode. Cations become electrically neutral as they accept electrons from the cathode, anions as they donate them to the anode.

When current flows between two electrodes in a solution of uniform composition, the greatest current density is near a straight line connecting the two poles. Some current will, however, flow everywhere, filling the entire volume of the solution (Fig. 2.2). It is this very fact, that any potential difference in a *volume conductor* sets up a current field that fills the entire volume, that makes electrocardiography, electroencephalography and electromyography possible. In the situation illustrated in Figure 2.2, a potential difference exists between any two points except those lying on any surface at right angles to the current lines.

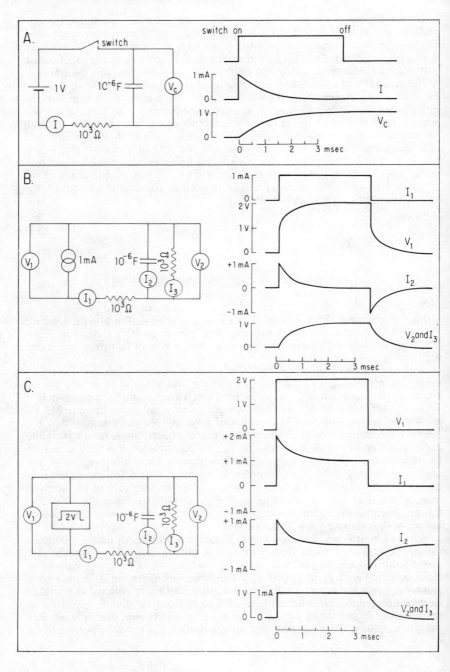

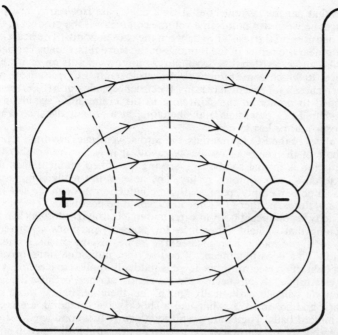

Figure 2.2. Current flow in a volume conductor. *Arrows* indicate the direction of the current; *broken lines* the isoelectric surfaces.

Figure 2.1. Voltages and currents in simple RC circuits. *A,* if a battery is connected to a condenser and a resistor in series, current (I) will flow until the voltage on the condenser plates (V_c) is equal to the voltage of the battery. Note that 1 μf capacity and 1 kilohm (kΩ) of resistance produce a time constant of 1 msec. *B,* the circuit of *A* is modified as follows: instead of a battery (constant voltage), we use a constant current generator; we inserted an additional resistance in parallel with the condenser. Note that current I_2 flows into the condenser when the current generator (I_1) is turned on, and that I_2 flows in the reverse direction after I_1 has been turned off and the condenser discharges through the resistor in parallel with it. Current I_3 and voltage V_2 are plotted in one graph because their time courses are identical. Note also that $I_1 = I_2 + I_3$. Note finally that when the current is turned on, part of it flows at first into the condenser, but once the condenser is fully charged, all the current must flow through both resistors in series; at that time 2 V are required (V_1) to drive 1 mA through 2 kΩ. *C,* a circuit similar to *B,* except that 2 V constant voltage are generated, instead of 1 mA constant current. Note that here, as in *B,* $I_1 = I_2 + I_3$.

Surfaces that cut the current lines at right angles are *isoelectric*. The potential differences between two points in a volume conductor is the product of the local current density and the resistance between the chosen points. The heart occupies a position near the center of the thorax, but the currents set up by cardiac action potentials can be registered between almost any two points on or in the body. The places to which conventional electrocardiograph (ECG) leads are attached have been chosen for practical reasons. Electroencephalograph (EEG) leads must be fastened to points on the skin close to the brain. EEG signals are much smaller than ECG potentials and, therefore, at a greater distance from their generator would be lost in noise.

In analyses of the ECG potentials, the cardiac ventricles are often represented as a dipole in the center of an empty cavity. It is well to remember that this representation is formal symbolism, serving simplified mathematical approximation to an all too complex reality. The heart is not really comparable to a magnetic dipole in empty space. Without conduction through the salt solutions of the body fluids, neither ECG nor EEG would be possible.

Electricity is conducted both in wires and in electrolyte solutions at a velocity approaching that of light. Therefore, for practical purposes, a current pulse applied to a conductor is registered the same instant at all points of the conductor. This does not mean, of course, that individual ions travel at the speed of light. If an electromotive force is suddenly applied to electrodes dipping into an electrolyte, all ions begin to move almost at once, because the ions near the electrode will electrostatically "push" on their neighbors, those on their neighbors, and so on, somewhat like a shock wave spreading among closely packed billiard balls. Therefore, even though current is conducted with almost infinite speed, for any particular ion to travel a measurable distance in an electric field takes a finite amount of time. This becomes a practical consideration in the so-called iontophoretic administration of drugs. In *iontophoresis* an electric current is used to speed up the delivery of an ionized compound into a target tissue. Iontophoresis can be much faster than diffusion, but certainly not infinitely faster.

2.2. The Generation of EEG and Evoked Potential Waves

In 1929 Hans Berger fastened electrodes to the head of his son, connected these to a new model double-coil mirror galvanometer, and recorded the voltage fluctuations on photographic film. This was the first electroencephalogram. Inevitably, Berger's claim of having recorded "brain waves" met with some skepticism. Some have pointed out that if two wires are dipped in a jelly made with salt and gelatin, and if the jelly is gently shaken, potential waves rather like an EEG tracing can be created. But before long it became clear to all that EEG potentials are truly produced by live brain cells. It took much longer to get a clear idea how these potentials are generated, and even now we still do not completely understand them. The pages that follow will introduce the reader to the basic principles of current flow around neurons which make EEG recordings possible. The neural interactions underlying EEG activity will be the topic of later chapters (see Sections 4.8 and 19.2).

If part of an excitable cell is depolarized, for example by an excitatory postsynaptic potential (EPSP) or by an impulse, and the remainder is not, then current will flow between the normally polarized and the depolarized regions. Since depolarization means that the cytoplasmic potential becomes more positive, i.e. less negative than at rest, current will flow inside the cell from the depolarized to the non-depolarized region. The circuit will be completed by current flowing in the reverse direction in the extracellular medium—from the nondepolarized toward the depolarized region. If part of a cell is hyperpolarized, for example by an inhibitory postsynaptic potential (IPSP), then similar currents will flow, but of course the direction will be reversed (see Figs. 2.4, 2.5, 2.6 and 2.13).

It is easy to see that during depolarization the intracellular potential of the depolarized region moves in a positive direction and the extracellular potential becomes negative. It is intuitively not so obvious, yet it is a fact that the extracellular medium near non-depolarized parts of a locally depolarized membrane becomes positive at one or several points. Not just positive relative to the depolarized part, but positive relative to its own resting level. Figure 2.4 is an attempt to make clear how this comes about. Readers not familiar with the flow of current in networks of resistors may find it helpful to first consider the simpler examples shown in Figure 2.3. Before we discuss Figure 2.4, consider also a few definitions. As already mentioned, the mean extracellular potential in the resting state is conventionally taken to be the zero potential, and all others are measured relative to it. An electrically positive point in extracellular medium is called a "source," and a negative point a "sink." Current flows from source to sink.

In Figure 2.4A, the voltages for the batteries symbolizing the electromotive force of the membrane potential (V_m) and the ohmic value of all resistive elements have arbitrarily been chosen. The resultant currents and voltages plotted in Figure 2.4B were computed, assuming only that Ohm's laws are valid.

To simplify the model, the excitable fiber is shown as a one-dimensional structure embedded in a two-dimensional plane. Instead of a very large number of infinitesimal elements, the components of the system are shown as a small number of discrete parts. The lowest row of resistors (r_c) in Figure 2.4A represents the cytoplasm of our fiber; the orthogonal network of resistors (r_e) in the upper part of the figure the interstitial plane; the batteries and resistors connecting the cytoplasm with the extracellular space stand for the membrane potential and the membrane resistance. The capacitance of the membrane was neglected; this is permissible as long as the model represents constant voltages or events that change slowly compared to the membrane time constant. In one place in the "membrane" the battery was deleted and the membrane resistance decreased. This (r_{EPSP}) represents the depolarized point. It is in fact known that, where an

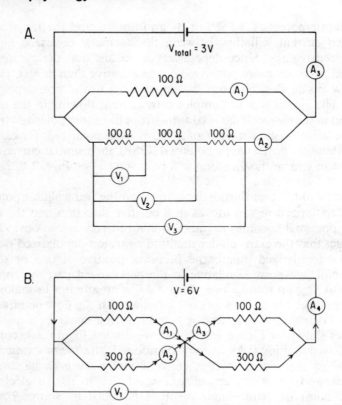

Figure 2.3. Currents and voltages in voltage dividers. For exercise, solve the values for the currents (*A*) and voltages (*V*), given the size of the battery and the value of the resistors. For answers turn to the end of this chapter.

endplate potential (EPP), EPSP or generator potential act, the membrane resistance usually is decreased (see Section 2.5).

The important point to note is that where the membrane is depolarized, a sink occurs just outside the membrane (marked by the open circle with minus sign); and near to it two sources (open circle with plus sign) are found. At the source the potential rose above the zero level.

Earlier it was mentioned that traveling impulses recorded with microelectrodes within the central nervous system (CNS) appear as bi- or triphasic waves (see Section 1.4b). Figure 2.4 is the model of a standing depolarization, not a traveling one. To properly represent a conducted impulse, the model would have to incorporate the membrane capacitance and take account of the time course of ionic currents across the membrane. Even though these features are absent in Figure 2.4, it nevertheless should help to appreciate why the traveling sinks of a nerve impulse are preceded and followed by sources.

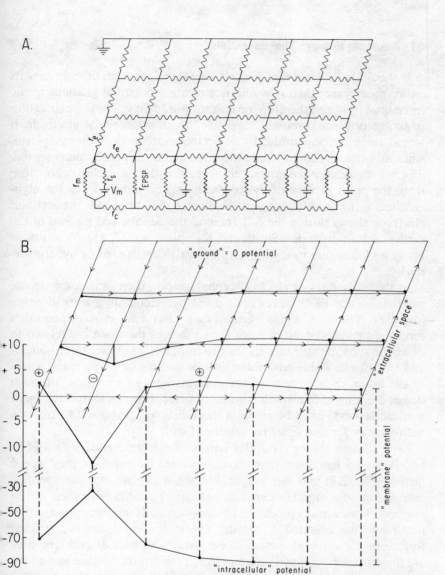

Figure 2.4. Model of the voltages and current flow in and around a locally depolarized fiber (neuronal dendrite or muscle fiber). *A*, the network representing the "fiber" and its extracellular environment: r_e, interstitial resistance; r_m, membrane resistance; V_m, electromotive force of the membrane potential; r_s, resistance in series with the membrane potential generator; r_{EPSP}, reduced membrane resistance at the site where the excitatory synaptic (or endplate) transmitter is acting; r_c, cytoplasmic (intracellular) resistances. *B*, the voltages in the network represented in *A*, plotted relative to the mean extracellular (ground) potential. Note different scales for extracellular and intracellular potentials. *Arrows* show direction of current flow in the resistors r_e of diagram *A*. For further explanation see text. (Based on computations by Dr. Michael Hines.)

It should be realized that if a cell were depolarized uniformly over its entire membrane, then it would not create a potential gradient in the interstitial fluid and therefore no current would flow. The depolarization of such a cell would remain "invisible" to an extracellular electrode; it would, however, be recorded by an electrode inserted into the cytoplasm, since an intracellular electrode measures the transmembrane potential. The S-T segment of the normal electrocardiogram is isoelectric, because from the point of view of the conventional Einthoven leads the myocardium is uniformly depolarized during that time. An intracellular electrode shows during the S-T interval the depolarized plateau of the cardiac action potential (Smith and Kampine, pp. 77, 86). Neurons, so far as we know, are rarely if ever uniformly depolarized or hyperpolarized.

In the early days of electroencephalography there was some debate whether or not EEG waves are caused by electrically summed nerve impulses. Today it seems certain that EEG and evoked potentials recorded from the scalp or from the surface of the brain are related to dendritic synaptic currents and not to impulses. Impulses in cell bodies and in axons probably contribute little or nothing to the potential waves of the brain surface, because the current fields of impulses, although dense, are limited to a small volume of tissue. For this reason the tip of a microelectrode must be within a short distance, perhaps 0.1 mm, of a neuron in order to register its impulse (Figure 2.5).

Even though the extracellular current fields associated with EPSPs and IPSPs are less dense than those generated by impulses, they spread farther (Fig. 2.5) and last longer. For these two reasons the synaptic currents of adjacent cells can summate more readily than their action currents. The currents produced by many neurons reinforce one another if the cells are oriented in parallel. Geometric regularity is a striking feature in the cerebral cortex, where pyramidal cells of different sizes are lined up with dendritic trees pointing toward the surface and axons pointing toward the white matter below. EEG waves recorded from the scalp are generated by cortical pyramidal cells. If cells or fibers are arranged in a geometrically regular pattern, we speak of an electrically anisotropic tissue. If cells and fibers are randomly intertwined, the tissue is electrically isotropic. Other tissues with conspicuously anisotropic cytoarchitecture include the olfactory bulb and the hippocampal cortex. Both generate typical wave activity, which, however, is too far from the

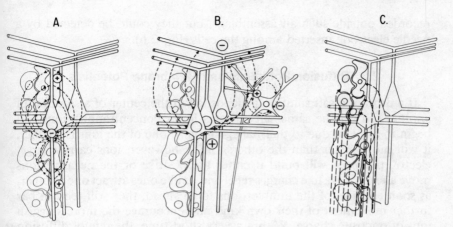

Figure 2.5. Extracellular currents generated by various cellular processes in gray matter of the CNS. *A*, an impulse that started at the initial segment of the axon of a neuron and is conducted along its axon generates current which is quite dense near the membrane but the density of which falls off rapidly with distance. *B*, synchronized synaptic potentials generate less dense fields which, however, spread in a wider volume since they flow between cell body and dendritic tree. *C*, currents associated with the sustained potential shifts generated by glial cells (see Section 5.9b and Figs. 5.4 and 5.5). (Reprinted with permission from G. Somjen: *Progress in Neurobiology* 1:201–237, 1973.)

surface to be recorded from the scalp. In principle, if activated neurons are oriented entirely at random (isotropy), then the currents they generate cancel and yield no recordable signal in extracellular space. If, however, any significant fraction of the cell population that is activated in synchrony shows any kind of geometric regularity, its electric signals become detectable even in a histologically isotropic tissue. In the thalamic nuclei, for example, the projection cells are oriented with axons turned toward the cortex among smaller cells not arranged in any particular pattern. The currents generated by the projection cells are the probable generators of evoked potentials and spontaneous EEG-type activity in the thalamus.

So-called closed fields are a special case. Neurons oriented in radial symmetry, with dendritic trees pointing either inward toward a center or radially outward, present an isoelectric surface to the outside. Potential waves generated by synapses on their dendritic tree could not be recorded outside such an assemblage, but they could be detected by a needle electrode inserted among the cells (Fig. 2.6).

2.3. Diffusion Potentials and Membrane Potentials

If a drop of a salt solution is deposited in the center of a solution of another salt (or the same salt but at a lower concentration), ions will begin to disperse due to thermal agitation. If one of the ions is smaller, it will move faster than the others. Since, however, ions carry charge, electric potential will build if either the positive or the negative ions move ahead. Since like charges repel and unlike ones attract one another, as soon as a few of the nimbler ions forge ahead, they will tend to bar further movement of their own kind and encourage the more sluggish ions of opposite charge. Within a very short time, the rate of diffusion of both ions will be equal, and it will be a compromise between the flux rates which would be achieved by uncharged particles of similar sizes. In this way ions of unequal size are forced into lockstep by the voltage known as the *diffusion potential* (Fig. 2.7).

The magnitude of a diffusion potential depends on (1) the gradient of concentration; (2) the difference in the mobilities of the ions; (3) the absolute temperature; and (4) certain constants (Equation 2.4). In most practical cases more than two ions must be considered; in the example of a drop of a solution of one salt deposited into a larger volume of

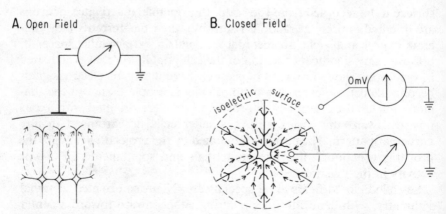

A. Open Field   **B.** Closed Field

Figure 2.6. Current flow in an "open field" (A) and in a "closed field" (B). For further description see text. (Modified and redrawn after Lorente de Nó: *Journal of Cellular and Comparative Physiology* 29:207–287, 1947.)

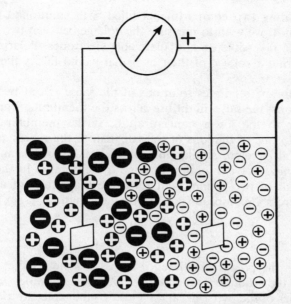

Figure 2.7. Representation of a diffusion potential. The left side of the vessel is supposed to have been filled with a salt solution composed of a large anion and a small cation; the right side with a salt of ions of equal size. The smaller cations tend to move from left to right faster than the larger anions do in the same direction; this difference establishes the diffusion potential which slows the small cations and speeds the large anions so that in fact both diffuse at the same rate. As the concentration gradients diminish, the diffusion potential declines also and, when all ingredients will be thoroughly mixed, it will cease altogether.

another, not only do ions move out of the drop, but the others also diffuse from the surrounding solution into it. Calculations of diffusion potentials in cases of several salts must take into account the mobilities and the concentration gradients of all the ions in the solution.

The mobility of an ion in a solution depends on its size and its interactions with the solvent. Other things being equal, mobility is inversely proportional to the square root of the molecular weight. With ions in aqueous solution the hydration of the particles must, however, also be taken into account. The larger the hydrated ion radius, the lower the mobility.

Obstacles may be placed in the way of diffusing solutes which can alter their mobilities; for example, a membrane of differential permeability separating two compartments filled with solutions of different composition. If we wish to measure the voltage between two solutions, we must use reversible or nonpolarizable electrodes. Polarizable electrodes generate a voltage of their own that would falsify the measurement.

If a membrane separates solutions of the same salt at two different concentrations, the salt will diffuse across the membrane from the side with higher to the lower concentration. If the membrane is more permeable to one of the ions of the salt than to the others, a diffusion potential will develop, similar to that in bulk solution, as discussed above. *Permeability* is mobility through a membrane. In the simplest case of a salt of two monovalent ions, the magnitude of a diffusion potential across a membrane is given by the equation:

$$E_m = \frac{RT}{F} \ln \frac{u - v}{u + v} \frac{C_1}{C_2} \tag{2.4}$$

where E_m is the potential difference across the membrane; R the gas constant; T the absolute temperature; F Faraday's number; u and v are the mobilities of the two ions; and C_1 and C_2 the concentrations on the two sides of the membrane. The gas constant and the absolute temperature enter into this equation because diffusion depends on the kinetic energy of the thermal agitation of the ions. Divalent ions contribute only half the voltage of monovalent ions, and trivalent ions only one-third. This may be confusing at first, since intuitively one might feel that the ion with the larger charge should add more voltage. However, it should be remembered that the diffusion potential is the voltage that *slows down* the fast ion and *speeds up* the slow ion until their velocities are equal (see above). The ion that carries the larger charge is the one that requires the lesser voltage to modify its velocity.

The limiting case of a diffusion potential across a membrane is when the membrane is permeable to some degree to one member of an ion pair, and not at all to the other. This situation was analyzed first by Gibbs and by Donnan, and it bears their name. Suppose that such a membrane separates two fluids, one containing a higher concentration of the salt in question than the other. Suppose, also, that the cation is permeant and the anion is not. Then, as cations move from the higher to the lower concentration, they leave a deficit of positive charge, a negativity behind, and carry excess positive charge into the solution of lower concentration. The general rule is that the *mobile* ion imposes *its* own *sign* on the solution of *lower* concentration. The movement of ions will stop altogether when the *chemical concentration* difference is *balanced* by the *electrical potential* difference. The voltage at which this is achieved is the *equilibrium potential* and it can be calculated by the *Nernst equation* as follows:

$$E_{eq} = \frac{RT}{zF} \ln \frac{C_1}{C_2} \qquad (2.5)$$

where z is the valence and the meaning of other symbols is as in Equation 2.4.

Notice that Equation 2.5 is similar to Equation 2.4, except that the term relating to mobilities has disappeared, since the mobility of one of the ions is zero. Furthermore, while a diffusion potential tends to dissipate to zero, an equilibrium potential remains, in theory, stable forever, without any expenditure of energy.

With each new class of students, a difficulty must be cleared up when we arrive at this point. We must reconcile the ideas that in an electrolyte solution the number of anions always equals the number of cations (the requirement of electroneutrality), but nevertheless diffusion potentials are generated by one ion species moving away from the others. Although seemingly contradictory, both propositions are true. For the membranes of nerve and muscle cells, it has been calculated that about 10^{-12} moles of ions/cm^2 of surface area would create a voltage of about 100 mV. The surface area of individual cells is far less than 1 cm^2, and therefore the amount of ions involved is also less. An excess or deficit of so few ions compared to the total amount present could not be detected by any chemical analysis, nor need it be taken into account in any theoretical calculation.

Two more points must be raised concerning Gibbs-Donnan equilibria. In such systems an osmotic pressure difference usually exists. In the simplified example described above, this would be the case because a solution of high concentration is separated from one of low concentration by a membrane that is permeable to water. The cytoplasm of live cells is, however, at osmotic equilibrium (but not at electrochemical equilibrium) with the fluid that surrounds them. But, then, living cells are not Gibbs-Donnan systems, as we shall soon see.

The last point concerns the definition of "equilibrium." If an ion is at equilibrium, then there is no *net flux* of that ion in any direction. This does not mean, however, that there is no movement whatsoever. Thermal agitation still moves particles about, but, statistically, for each ion moving in one direction, another of the same species will move in the opposite direction. Such *exchange diffusion* does not result in a net transfer of material, nor in a change of free energy. The magnitude of exchange diffusion can be estimated if a radioactive isotope of the ion in question is added to the solution on one side of the membrane. The rate at which the tracer appears on the other side is a measure of the exchange. Its magnitude, like that of simple diffusion, is influenced by temperature and by the permeability of the membrane. It should also be kept in mind that a system at equilibrium does no work.

Let us now consider a slightly more complicated Donnan system. On one side of a membrane, let us say the left side, we place a solution containing an impermeant anion that we shall call I^-, a permeant anion, call it P^-, and a permeant cation C^+. On the right side we put only C^+ and P^-. We then allow the system to come to equilibrium. Since both C^+ and P^+ are able to cross the membrane they would, in the absence of I^-, diffuse until equal concentrations would be reached on both sides of the membrane. Since, however, there is also I^- on the left side, the concentration of P^- must be lower there. The concentration of $[C^+]$ on the left side must equal $[P^-] + [I^-]$ in order to obtain electroneutrality; whereas on the right $[C^+] = [P^-]$, since no I^- is present. When such a system comes to equilibrium, $[C^+]$ will be higher in the solution on the left than on the right side and there will be less $[P^-]$ on the left than on the right side. Moreover:

$$\frac{[C^+] \text{ left}}{[C^+] \text{ right}} = \frac{[P^-] \text{ right}}{[P^-] \text{ left}}$$

The solution of the left side will furthermore be electrically negative relative to the right; and there will be an osmotic pressure difference owing to the higher total osmolarity of the left solution. Living cells contain impermeant anions in the form of large charged organic molecules. The special problem they represent for cell function will be discussed in Section 2.4b.

2.4. The Resting Membrane Potential of Living Cells

Living systems are not at equilibrium. The membranes of living cells nevertheless sustain a potential difference that remains steady as long as the cell is at rest. What constitutes "rest" and "activity" will become clear presently.

The steady *resting membrane potential* of living cells is maintained by a steady diffusion of ions of different permeabilities. Diffusion at a constant rate presupposes a constant concentration gradient. This, indeed, is demonstrably present. This means that ions that have diffused away must constantly be replaced. This is accomplished by *active transport* processes, also called "ion pumps," which will be explained later.

The great majority of the cells in animal tissues, and certainly all nerve and muscle cells, contain a solution richer in potassium and poorer in sodium than the fluid that surrounds them. There also are differences in the concentrations of calcium, magnesium, chloride, hydrogen, and a host of other less interesting ions (Tables 2.1 and 2.2). We will first discuss the roles played by Na^+ and by K^+.

The permeability of the resting membrane is greater for K^+ than for Na^+. If Na^+ and K^+ particles would not be electrically charged, then at any given moment more K^+ would diffuse from the inside of the cell into the surrounding fluid than would Na^+ ions in the reverse direction. Both K^+ and Na^+ are, however, positively charged. If more positive charges leave the cell than enter it, a deficit is created and the inside grows negative with respect to the outside. Such a potential difference retards the outflow of K^+ and accelerates the inflow of Na^+ until the two fluxes are equal. The voltage which equalizes the Na^+ and K^+ fluxes in spite of their unequal permeabilities is the *resting membrane potential*.

Table 2.1.
Free Ion Concentrations and Equilibrium Potentials in Mammals

Ion	Plasma	CSF and CNS Interstitium	Cytoplasm Muscle	Cytoplasm Central Neuron	Muscle	Central Neuron
	(mM)				(mV)	
K^+	4.4		140.0		−92	
		3.2		130.0		−98
Na^+	140.0		15.0		+59	
		148.0		25.0		+47
Ca^{2+}	1.1		0.0005		+102	
		1.2		0.0005		+103
Cl^-	105.0		4 to 7		−72 to −87	
		130.0		4.0		−92
				25 to 35*		−43 to −35*

Free Ion Concentration columns: Plasma, CSF and CNS Interstitium, Cytoplasm (Muscle, Central Neuron). Equilibrium Potential at 37.5°C columns: Muscle, Central Neuron.

*The two $[Cl^-]_i$ values given are the presumed levels in "low-chloride" and "high-chloride" cells; the former are hyperpolarized, the latter are depolarized when g_{Cl} increases. The motor neurons of the spinal cord, the large projection neurons of the brain stem diencephalon and cerebral cortex seem to be low-Cl cells, the primary afferent neurons of the somatic sensory system high-Cl cells.

Sources of values of extracellular ion concentrations: R. Katzman and H. M. Pappius: *Brain Electrolytes and Fluid Metabolism.* Baltimore, Williams & Wilkins, 1973; Federation of the American Society of Experimental Biology: *Biological Data Book*, 1973; and measurements of Ca^{2+} and K^+ in CNS tissue and in circulating arterial blood of cats made in the author's laboratory. Intracellular concentrations, taken from miscellaneous sources, have been indirectly derived and are subject to error.

Table 2.2.
Resting and Reversal Potentials

	Muscle	Central Neuron
	(mV)	
Resting membrane potential	−80 to −90	−65 to −90
EPP reversal potential	−15 (frog) 0 to −5 (man)	
IPSP reversal potential		−80 to −90

Values taken from miscellaneous sources.

It is between 50 and 100 mV in excitable cells, different in different tissues, but constant during rest for any one of them.

2.4a. ACTIVE TRANSPORT OF IONS

If cells were lifeless, then as K^+ would leave and Na^+ enter, the concentration gradients would diminish and with them the magnitude of the membrane voltage. In living cells, however the K^+ ions that are lost due to diffusion are constantly replaced from the surrounding fluid, and the Na^+ ions that are gained are extruded again.

The active transport processes that maintain the concentration gradients of ions across cell membranes are akin to those which secrete salts through the epithelia of the kidneys and of the intestines (see Sernka and Jacobson, Chapter 12). Active transport of ions means, of course, the transfer of charge and as such it also can generate a voltage. If it does, it is referred to as a *secretory potential* or as an *electrogenic ion pump*. No voltage is generated if *either* an equivalent number of oppositely charged particles are transported in the same direction *or* an equivalent number of identically charged particles are transported in opposite directions. Such non-electrogenic transport does not perform electric work, but it does perform chemical work and requires metabolic energy.

If in nerve and muscle membranes the rate of outward transport of Na^+ equaled the inward transport of K^+, then the pumping of the two ions would neither add to nor subtract from the membrane potential generated by the diffusion of the two ions. Opinions differ whether or not the transport of these two ions is neutral or electrogenic. The prevalent view today is that the outward transport of Na^+ and the inward transport of K^+ are coupled, but not exactly in a one-to-one ratio. With each "revolution" of the ion pump, more Na^+ ions are believed transported out than K^+ ions transported in. This adds a small extra negative potential to the resting potential, which in turn speeds up the inflow of K^+ and thereby ultimately equalizes ion fluxes. This contribution of the ion pump to the membrane potential is, however, small compared to the diffusion potential, and it is often neglected in theoretical calculations.

The physical mechanism of the ion transport is not known. The pumps are believed to be protein molecules incorporated in the membrane structure (Figs. 2.8 and 2.9). Moving ions against their concentration gradient is work, and it requires energy. Energy for membrane transport is supplied by an enzyme, a *membrane-bound adenosine triphosphatase (ATPase)*, that splits the high energy bond of adenosine triphosphate (ATP). It has been shown that membrane-bound ATPase is stimulated when the activity of Na^+ ions in the cytoplasm and that of K^+ ions in the environment of the cell rise above the resting level. Thus the supply of energy increases whenever the need to pump ions increases. The ATPase of the membrane is, for this reason, also called *Na/K-activated ATPase.*

To do their job, the ion pumps of the membrane must continuously be supplied with fresh fuel, that is with ATP. ATP is being replenished by the oxidative metabolism of the respiratory chain in the mitochondria. As phosphate is split from ATP, adenosine diphosphate (ADP) is produced, which reaches the mitochondria and stimulates the electron transport chain of the cytochrome system. ATP is then regenerated from ADP by the action of the respiratory chain. Newly formed ATP is then made available to energy-demanding cellular processes, including the membrane transport of ions. The chemical work required to regenerate ATP is fueled by the oxidation to water of hydrogen donated by nutrient metabolic substrates. The oxygen is taken in molecular form from the cytoplasmic solution (Fig. 2.9).

2.4b. THE ROLES OF IONS IN THE RESTING POTENTIAL

If the membrane were permeable only to K^+ and to no other ion, then the system would come to equilibrium, and the membrane potential would equal the quilibrium potential for K^+, given by the Nernst equation (equation 2.5). For the constant temperature of the mammalian body (37.5°C), and the specific case of K^+ ions Equation 2.5 may be simplified to:

$$E_K = 61 \log_{10} \frac{[K^+]_o}{[K^+]_i} \qquad (2.6)$$

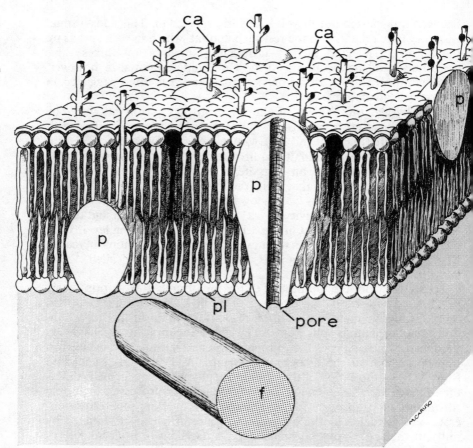

Figure 2.8. General model of the surface membrane (plasma membrane) of cells. The membrane is formed by a bilayer of lipoproteins with their hydrophilic polar protein heads (*pl*) turned outward, and their hydrophobic lipid tails turned toward each other. Carbohydrates (*ca*) are seen protruding from the outer surface of the membrane; cytoplasmic filaments (*f*) are numerous near its inner surface. The specialized functions of the membrane are performed by proteins (*p*) embedded in the membrane, some nearer to the outer and some to the inner surface. Some proteins span the entire thickness of the membrane, and some are believed to be hollow, forming the channels ('pore') through which ions pass. (Reprinted with permission from W. M. Copenhaver, D. E. Kelly and R. L. Wood (eds): *Bailey's Textbook of Histology*, ed 17. Baltimore, Williams & Wilkins, 1978.)

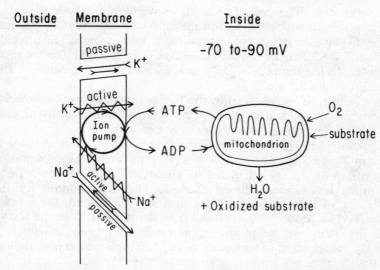

Figure 2.9. Diagram of active and passive K⁺ and Na⁺ transport through resting cell membranes. Active movement is shown as uphill, passive as downhill. Passive outward movement of K⁺ is favored by its chemical gradient and by the high permeability for K⁺ of the membrane, but it is retarded by the resting membrane potential (negative inside). Passive inward movement of Na⁺ is favored by both the chemical and electric gradients, but it is hindered by the low permeability for Na⁺ of the resting membrane. See text for further description. (Modified and redrawn after J. C. Eccles: *The Physiology of Nerve Cells*. Baltimore, The Johns Hopkins University Press, 1957, and other sources.)

Notice, that the natural logarithms have been replaced by logarithms to the base 10. The bracketed symbols $[K^+]_o$ and $[K^+]_i$ denote the concentration* of K^+ outside and inside the cell, respectively. Notice also that the ratio $[K^+]_o:[K^+]_i$ is less than one, so that E_K appears as a

*Instead of concentration, the relevant quantity is *ion activity*. Ion activity is that fraction of the ions present that is available for participation in physicochemical reaction; in other words, is not screened by other ions in the solution. Unfortunately, two difinitions of activity coefficient are used: (1) activity coefficient = activity/free ion concentration; (2) activity coefficient = activity/total ion concentration (where total = free + bound). By the first definition, the activity coefficient of K^+ in extracellular fluids of mammals is about 0.74; for Ca^{2+} it is about 0.32. Calcium is present in plasma in four forms: (1) bound to macromolecules (non-ultrafiltrable); (2) bound (chelated) to smaller molecules (ultrafiltrable but not ionized); (3) free but screened (ionized but not active); (4) free and active. Equations of the form of Equations 2.5, 2.6 and 2.7 may be expressed in terms of either free ion concentration or activity if and *only if* the activity coefficients in- and outside the cell are equal. This is assumed but not proven to be the case for K^+.

negative number. This conforms to the convention to equate the extra-cellular potential with zero, and to measure transmembrane potentials relative to the external (zero) level. Finally, notice that if $[K^+]_o$ would be 0.1 of $[K^+]_i$, then E_K would be -61 mV. In fact $[K^+]_o$ is for most excitable cells less than 0.1 of $[K^+]_i$, and E_K is usually between -85 and -98 mV (Tables 2.1 and 2.2).

Now, in fact, K^+ is not the only ion that permeates nerve and muscle membranes, although it is the one that does so most readily. Consequently, the membrane potential does not exactly behave as predicted by Equation 2.6. How much it deviates from the predicted value is shown in Figure 2.10. At high levels of $[K^+]_o$ the membrane potential is very close to the values calculated by Equation 2.6, but at lower $[K^+]_o$ it is much less sensitive to its changes. This is important for the functioning of nerve cells. In the central nervous system, the average resting $[K^+]_o$ is around 3.0 mM and it is about 4.5 mM in the rest of the body. Thus, in the physiological range, membrane potential is relatively independent of variations of $[K^+]_o$. This is not so in pathological conditions as will become apparent later (see Section 3.4a).

How do the effects of different ions combine to determine the membrane potential? The mathematical solution to this problem is *Goldman's constant field equation*. Although Goldman's derivation has recently been criticized because it is based on certain simplifying assumptions, it remains useful for its very simplicity, and it may be accepted as a first approximation of the effect of different ions on the resting potential:

$$E_m = 61 \, \log_{10} \frac{P_K[K^+]_o + P_{Na}[Na^+]_o + P_{Cl}[Cl^-]_i}{P_K[K^+]_i + P_{Na}[Na^+]_i + P_{Cl}[Cl^-]_o} \qquad (2.7)$$

P in this expression is the permeability of each ion. There are, of course, other ions to be considered, such as Ca^{2+}, Mg^{2+}, HCO_3^-, and even H^+, but to illustrate the principle, K^+, Na^+ and Cl^- are sufficient.

Some assumptions implicit in the Goldman equation are, that the contribution of each ion to the membrane potential is (1) independent from that of the other ions; (2) in proportion to both the concentration gradient and the permeability of the ion; and (3) that permeabilities are independent of membrane potential.

The following properties of this equation should be noted. First, $[Cl^-]_i$ appears in the numerator and $[Cl^-]_o$ in the denominator, whereas K^+ and Na^+ are the other way around. This is, of course, because Cl^- has a negative charge. Second, in the case of sodium, $[Na^+]_o > [Na^+]_i$, whereas $[K^+]_o < [K^+]_i$. Thus, if Na^+ ions had free reign over the membrane potential, the cell would be positive inside. Since, however, at rest $P_K \gg P_{Na}$, the membrane potential is closer to E_K than to E_{Na}. It is because P_{Na} is not negligible, that the membrane potential is not exactly equal to the equilibrium potential of K^+, but deviates from it to the extent shown in Figure 2.10.

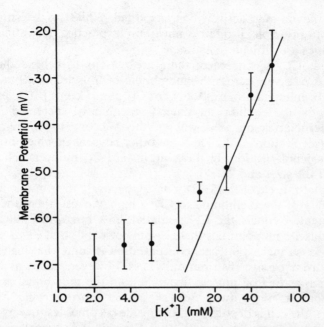

Figure 2.10.   The resting membrane potential of rat dorsal root ganglion cells bathed in solutions containing various concentrations of K^+. The diagonal straight line shows the Nernst function (Equation 2.6) assuming constant $[K^+]_i$; the points show mean values (in 4–9 cells per point), and the standard errors of the measurements. Normal $[K^+]_o$ is 4.5 mM in dorsal root ganglia and about 3.0 mM in the CNS. (Reprinted with permission from G. Somjen, R. Dingledine, B. Connors, and B. Allen: Extracellular potassium and calcium activities in the mammalian spinal cord, and the effect of changing ion levels on mammalian neural tissues. In *Ion-Selective Microelectrodes and Their Uses in Excitable Tissues*, edited by E. Sykova, P. Hnik and L. Vyklicky. New York, Plenum Press, 1981.)

Of the numerous other ions in and around cells some may and others need not be transported actively. Those that are not, distribute themselves by diffusion so that in the "resting" state their concentration gradients across the membrane conform to the equilibrium prescribed by the prevailing membrane potential. Whether a particular ion is "passively" distributed or actively transported can be determined if its inside and outside concentrations (rather, activities) and the membrane potential are known. If the concentrations of a particular ion are not those the Nernst equation (Equation 2.5) would predict for that potential, then the ion must actively be transported. While this determination is simple in principle, it often is uncertain in practice, for intracellular ion activities are difficult to estimate.

As far as Cl^- is concerned, there are reasons to believe that it is distributed passively across the membrane of muscle cells, but not of neurons. In many neurons an outward Cl^- pump keeps $[Cl^-]_i$ less than predicted for the equilibrium state. Consequently, increased P_{Cl} can cause hyperpolarization, as we will see when we come to the mechanism of IPSPs (see Section 2.5d). There are other neurons in which increased P_{Cl} causes depolarization. In these, an inward Cl^- pump is believed to operate (Tables 2.1 and 2.2).

In skeletal muscle of frogs Cl^- ions are passively distributed, and the permeability of the membrane to Cl^- is high. At rest, then, the membrane potential equals the Cl^- potential, E_{Cl}. For some but not all skeletal muscles in mammals there is some evidence that Cl^- is actively transported, so that its internal concentration is somewhat higher than expected from passive distribution. P_{Cl} is, however, about as high in mammalian as in frog muscle fibers. Should the membrane potential change, that is, move away from E_{Cl}, a Cl^- current will flow. For example, if the cell is depolarized, the inside becomes less negative than E_{Cl} and this will attract more Cl^-; if the cell is hyperpolarized, the increased negativity will expel Cl^-. Such Cl^- currents will continue until enough Cl^- either entered or left the cell to reach new equilibrium. As long as the Cl^- current flows, however, it will tend to partially counteract the membrane potential change. A given depolarizing current will therefore cause a more rapid voltage change in a membrane with low P_{Cl}, than one with high P_{Cl}. Abnormally low permeability to Cl^- is the membrane defect causing some forms of myotonia (see Section 3.4d). More in general, all passively distributed ions act as "inertial brakes" slowing transient changes of membrane potential, but they do not influence the level at which the membrane potential eventually settles. The degree of braking action by any ion depends on its permeability and on its concentration relative to other permeant ions.

Most of the other ions have been studied less intensively than K^+, Na^+ and Cl^-. Ca^{2+} plays an important part in the generation of the signals in certain nerve and muscle cells (cf. Section 3.11) but it probably has little direct effect on the resting potential. The transmembrane gradient of Ca^{2+} is very steep, possibly the steepest of all ions. In extracellular fluid, its activity is around 10^{-3} M, in intracellular fluid 10^{-6} M or less (Tables 2.1 and 2.2). If it contributes little to the resting potential, then its permeability across the resting membrane must be very low.

Before concluding this discussion, something must be said about the large organic anions in cytoplasm to which the membrane is impermeable. Since these are impermeant, their term P in the Goldman equation (Equation 2.7) is zero, and they do not directly contribute to the membrane potential. By their presence in intracellular fluid, they must, however, displace a number of permeant anions (cf. Section 2.3), and therefore influence the concentration gradient of these permeant anions. Moreover, the impermeant ions contribute an osmotic force. Besides, there also are compounds that are electrically active (have free charges) but not osmotically active (if they are not in solution, but built into structural proteins). Other compounds may be osmotically active (dissolved) but electrically neutral (chelated or altogether uncharged). Since we do not have a complete inventory of cell contents, our understanding of cell osmolarity, and therefore of the regulation of the water content and of the volume of cells, is far from complete.

Two facts stand out. (1) Healthy cells are in osmotic equilibrium (but not in electrochemical equilibrium) with their environment. (There are exceptions, for example in the renal collecting ducts, which do not concern us here.) (2) Cells gain water, Na^+ and Cl^-, and they swell whenever they are deprived of oxygen and when their energy metabolism is impaired. This indicates that normally the osmotic pressures inside and outside the cell are equalized by the active transport of solutes out of the cell. How the transport that regulates osmolarity (and thus also cell volume) is related to ion transport is unclear at present.

Cell swelling in hypoxic tissue is especially important in the brain, and will be discussed when we arrive to the pathophysiology of cerebral edema (see Section 5.6).

2.5. The Ionic Mechanism of Receptor Potentials and Synaptic Potentials

In the preceding pages, we have learned that the membrane potential of nerve and muscle cells is determined by (1) the concentration (activity) gradients of various ions across the membrane; (2) the relative permeability of the membrane to those ions, and (3) to a lesser degree the electrogenic active transport of ions. We also took notice of the fact that the signals of nerve and muscle cells are transient variations of the membrane potential. As a general rule, the *physiological*, normal responses of membrane potential are brought about by transient *changes of membrane permeability* to one or more ions. *Pathological* changes of membrane potential are more often caused by changes of *ion concentrations*, either in intracellular or extracellular fluids (e.g., see Section 3.4a). As it is generally with general rules, there are exceptions to both these points.

Before proceeding it is necessary to introduce another term. In biophysical texts *ion conductance* is often used instead of ion permeability. The difference is in the units of measurement. The conductance of an ion (expressed in siemens or mhos) is the number of amperes carried by that ion under a volt of potential difference. Its permeability is the number of moles moved per unit time in a unit concentration gradient. Needless to say, in the case of uncharged compounds such as sugars, one can speak of permeability but not of conductance.

The symbol of total membrane conductance is G_m, capitalized if it refers to the specific conductance (i.e. conductance per unit surface area of membrane), and written lower case (g_m) if it refers to actually measured conductance (for example, of a cell under a particular experimental condition). If the conductance of one particular ion is referred to, then the symbol of the ion becomes the subscript (e.g. G_{Na} or g_{Na}). The same convention applies to the use of R_m for the resistance of unit surface area of membrane and r_m for total resistance. A similar distinction is made between C_m and c_m for specific and total capacitance. It will be remembered that with increasing surface area capacitance and conductance grow and resistance decreases. It shall be noted that not all writers adhere to the distinction between capital and lower case notation.

The fraction of the membrane current carried by a particular ion is denoted by I with that ion's symbol as subscript. The magnitude of the ion current is determined by a modification of Ohm's law (Equation 2.1). For Na^+, for example, we write:

$$I_{Na} = (E_m - E_{eqNa})G_{Na} \qquad (2.8)$$

The difference between membrane potential and equilibrium potential ($E_m - E_{eq}$) is known as the *driving potential* of the ion in question. If $E_m = E_{eq}$, then there is no reason for that ion to move, and its current will be 0.

For the membrane potential to remain constant, the total outward current of all ions must equal the total inward current so that the net membrane current is 0. If the membrane current is not 0, then the membrane potential will change. A net inward ion current will depolarize, and an outward ion current hyperpolarize the membrane. At the risk of repeating the obvious, I should add, that an inward electric current could be carried by either an influx of positive ions or an outflux of negative ions. It is also important to remember that the membrane potential may change by the movement of only a small quantity of ions.

In excitable cells in the resting state g_K exceeds g_{Na} by a factor somewhere between 50 and 100, depending on cell types. In astrocytes, which are inexcitable, the g_K/g_{Na} ratio is even higher. We shall consider the functions of glial cells in Chapter 5.

As mentioned earlier and illustrated in Figure 1.6, when a stimulus acts on a sensory nerve terminal the membrane becomes locally depolarized. This is the *generator potential*. The mechanism that produces the generator potential is not known for all sensory terminals, but where satisfactory experiments have been conducted it usually is caused by an increase of g_{Na}, reducing the ratio g_K/g_{Na} and moving the membrane potential closer to E_{Na}, therefore making it less negative inside.

In receptor cells similar ion conductance changes generate *receptor potentials*. At excitatory synapses, also, similar changes in ion conductance operate, which will be discussed in the net two sections.

2.5a. ENDPLATE POTENTIALS

The stimulus changing the ion conductance of postsynaptic membranes is the transmitter substances released by presynaptic nerve terminals. At the junctions between the motor nerve terminal and the endplate membrane of skeletal muscle (Fig. 2.11), the transmitter is acetylcholine. Under its influence both g_{Na} and g_K increase above resting level, but g_{Na} rises more than g_K, so that their ratio approaches unity. Thus, while at rest $g_K \gg g_{Na}$ and the membrane potential is near E_K and therefore internally negative; under the influence of acetylcholine g_{Na} approaches g_K, which moves the membrane potential toward E_{Na} in the positive direction, resulting in strong depolarization, which then triggers a muscle action potential.

The normal function of the neuromuscular junction is of course to initiate the muscle action potential, but to a researcher interested in the mechanism of the endplate potential, impulses are unwanted interference. One method to suppress the action potential and observe uncontaminated endplate potentials is to poison the muscle with tetrodotoxin (TTX), which blocks the so-called voltage-gated Na channels required to generate impulses (see Section 3.1a). Another is provided by nature in the form of the electric organ of Torpedo. This organ is a modified muscle without contractile protein and without a mechanism to generate

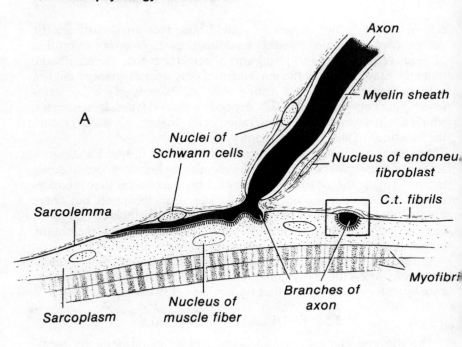

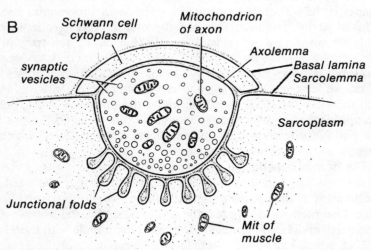

Figure 2.11. Diagram of a motor endplate. *B* shows framed portion of *A*, enlarged. (Reprinted with permission from W. M. Copenhaver, D. E. Kelly and R. L. Wood (eds): *Bailey's Textbook of Histology*, ed 17. Baltimore, Williams & Wilkins, 1978.)

an action potential, as if it were a tissue composed of hypertrophied endplate membranes. Acetylcholine causes depolarization of endplate membranes, moving from the resting level of −90 mV toward a value near −15 mV in frog, nearer to 0 mV in human muscle (Table 2.2).

The membrane potential does not actually reach these levels for several reasons. Normally acetylcholine is rapidly broken down by acetylcholinesterase, and therefore has no time to achieve full effect. Also, under normal conditions the endplate potential is interrupted by the muscle impulse before the endplate potential reaches its maximum. Furthermore, the endplate membrane occupies but a small part of the surface of the muscle fiber, and acetylcholine has an effect only at the endplate (except denervated muscle: see Section 3.4f). Since the cytoplasm of muscle fibers has a low resistance, the membrane potential of the endplate region is influenced by that of adjacent parts of the fiber. With the endplate moving the potential toward −15 mV under the influence of acetylcholine, but the surrounding non-acetylcholine-sensitive membrane pulling it toward the resting level of −90 mV, the actual measured potential takes a value somewhere in between these two values.

How do we know to what potential the endplate tends under the influence of acetylcholine, if that potential is never actually attained? The limiting level may be determined as follows (Fig. 2.12). Two micropipette electrodes are inserted into a muscle fiber, one to deliver current, the other to measure potential. A third pipette filled with acetylcholine chloride is placed in an extracellular position near the endplate to deliver small "puffs" of acetylcholine. The preparation is treated with TTX to eliminate muscle impulses. With the aid of one of the electrodes, constant direct current (polarizing current) can be passed through the membrane to force its potential to voltages specified by the experimental design. At each of these artificially induced membrane potentials, the effect of a puff of acetylcholine on the membrane can be tested. The magnitude of the transient potential changes evoked by pulses of acetylcholine (artificial EPPs) can then be plotted as a function of membrane potential.

As shown in Figure 2.12, the more negative inside is the prevailing membrane potential, the larger is the amplitude of the artificial EPP evoked by acetylcholine. At levels less negative (that is more positive) than −15 mV, the acetylcholine causes transient hyperpolarization instead of depolarization. At −15 mV, acetylcholine has no effect on the membrane potential, presumably because the currents of Na⁺ and

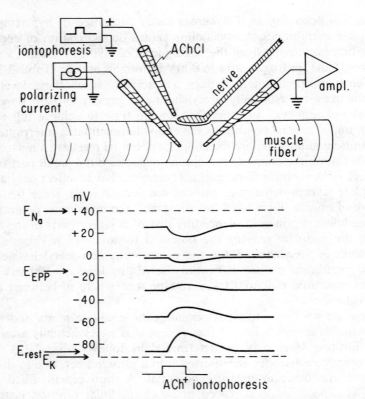

Figure 2.12. Diagram of an experiment designed to determine the reversal potential of the EPP (E_{EPP}) of a frog neuromuscular junction. The preparation is bathed in a solution containing TTX to abolish action potentials. Acetylcholine is delivered from a micropipette containing acetylcholine chloride (*AChCl*) by iontophoretic current, ACh^+ being ejected from the pipette if the solution is made electrically positive. The membrane potential of the cell is influenced by electric (polarizing) current passed through the membrane. E_{Na} = equilibrium potential of Na; E_{rest} = resting membrane potential. See text for further description.

of K^+ are equal and opposite, so that their effects cancel. This is known as the *reversal potential* of the EPP, expressing the fact that at this point the EPP changes from a depolarizing response to a hyperpolarizing one. Although acetylcholine does not cause a change of potential if the membrane potential is at the reversal level, it does cause the resistance of the endplate membrane to decrease, as g_{Na} and g_K are increased.

The time has come to introduce the concept of an *electrotonic spread of potential*. It will be discussed more fully when we come to consider the conditions of stimulating nerve and muscle fibers (see Section 3.1b). For the moment we must note the following. Even though only the endplate membrane is sensitive to acetylcholine, the change of potential it causes (that is, the endplate potential) can be recorded outside the endplate region. But the farther a recording microelectrode is moved from the endplate, the smaller the recorded amplitude of the EPP. Its amplitude decays exponentially with distance. At the endplate the membrane potential change is said to be active, because it involves a change of the membrane resistance (and of the membrane current). Outside the endplate region the membrane potential is changed passively. This means that the change is imposed on the resting membrane by a current for which the generator is located elsewhere, namely, at the endplate. Such passive spread of potential is said to be electrotonic.

In the normal condition, in the absence of TTX, the endplate potential triggers an action potential. Unlike the passive electrotonic spread of the EPP, the action potential involves active changes along the entire fiber. It is precisely to overcome the inevitable loss of signal, typical of passive electrotonic spread of potential, that nerve and muscle fibers need nerve impulses for signal transmission (see Chapter 3).

2.5b. EXCITATORY POSTSYNAPTIC POTENTIALS OF NEURONS

The mechanism of the many different types of excitatory synapses is not identical in all cases. None of them has been investigated as thoroughly as the vertebrate neuromuscular junction. In many but not in all, the ionic mechanism of the excitatory postsynaptic potentials of neurons appears to be similar to that of the endplate potential.

If a micropipette electrode is inserted into a large neuron in the central nervous system, and an excitatory afferent pathway, for example, a peripheral nerve or a central fiber tract, is stimulated by an electric pulse, a brief depolarization is recorded. This transient depolarization is the EPSP, which may or may not trigger an action potential. The form of these EPSPs is rather similar to EPPs of muscle fibers. The membrane potential of neurons can be altered experimentally in ways similar in principle to the method shown in Figure 2.10 for muscle fibers. In some cases, the reversal potential of EPSPs of central neurons has been shown to be around −5 mV; in others it was technically not possible to demonstrate a reversal point.

Skeletal muscle fibers are usually innervated by a single branch of a motor axon. Each muscle fiber thus has but one endplate. Exceptions are the very long fibers of large muscles, which may have two. The important point is, however, that a single action potential in a motor axon normally evokes an impulse (and therefore a contraction) in all the muscle fibers its branches innervate. Central neurons differ from muscle fibers in that they usually are the targets of many excitatory axon terminals, spread over the surface of their dendrites and parts of the cell body. The effect of one action potential arriving at any of these presynaptic terminals is but a small EPSP which, by itself, does not trigger an action potential in the (postsynaptic) neuron. To depolarize a central neuron sufficiently to fire postsynaptic impulses, the effects of several synapses must be summed (see also Chapter 4).

Acetylcholine is a transmitter at a few central synapses. Glutamic acid is believed to be the excitatory transmitter in many others. The transmitter of many central synapses is unknown. More will be said about transmitter substances a little later.

"Conventional" EPSPs, with the characteristics just described, have been recorded from numerous central neurons, for example, from the motor cells of the ventral horns of the spinal cord and of the motor nuclei of the cranial nerves; from pyramidal cells of the motor area of the cerebral neocortex, and hippocampal cortex; from neurons in some of the thalamic nuclei, and from others. In these the depolarization is believed to be due either to an increase of g_{Na} alone or to a simultaneous increase of both g_{Na} and g_K.

Since the membrane potential is maintained at its resting level by the ratio of g_K/g_{Na}, the membrane could be depolarized not only by an increase of g_{Na} but also by a decrease of g_K. In fact slow decline of g_K is responsible for the pacemaker potential of the sinoatrial node of the heart (see Smith and Kampine, pp. 79–90). A similar lowering of g_K is the most likely explanation of EPSPs transmitted by acetylcholine to some neurons in the cerebral cortex. These potentials are slower in onset and longer in duration than the conventional EPSPs, and they are mediated by muscarinic receptors (see Section 2.5e and Table 17.1). The decrease of g_K caused by acetylcholine in many central neurons is considered by some to be an example of a *modulatory action*, in that it alters the responsiveness of the cell to other excitatory transmitters (see also Section 19.4).

2.5c. ELECTRICAL SYNAPSES

Over a hundred years ago Du Bois Reymond stated that, hypothetically, excitation may be transmitted from motor nerves to skeletal muscles either by the "current of action" generated by the nerve or by an irritant chemical substance secreted by it. With that began a protracted debate between two camps of investigators, one favoring the theory of chemical transmission, the other of electrical transmission. The former idea became known as the theory of the "soup," the latter, appropriately, as the theory of the "spark." The fortunes of battle favored now the one camp, then the other, until the war ended, not long ago, in a draw. It turned out that some nerve junctions transmit by electric current and others (the majority) transmit by chemical transmitter substances.

The key to one cell being able to excite another by means of electricity is the ability to inject enough current into the cytoplasm of the postsynaptic cell to depolarize its membrane sufficiently. Without special low-resistance junctions between the cytoplasm of two cells, the current generated by one of two adjacent cells disperses in the interstitial fluid, and only a small fraction penetrates the relatively high resistance membrane of the other. The specialized junctions that make electrotonic spread between certain cells possible have been recognized to be *gap junctions.*

Electric excitatory synapses, with anatomical gap junctions, have been found in many invertebrate nervous systems and also in some cold-blooded vertebrates. In mammals, they join smooth muscle cells of "unitary" or "quasi-syncytial" organization (cf. Section 14.3). In the intercalated discs of cardiac muscle, similar junctions serve a similar purpose. In the central nervous system of mammals there is good, but not yet conclusive, evidence for electric transmission from dendrite to dendrite of neurons in, for example, Deiters' nucleus and in the inferior olives. Gap junctions have been found at these sites between the dendritic spines of adjacent neurons. The gap junctions linking glial cells will be discussed in Chapter 5.

2.5d. INHIBITORY POSTSYNAPTIC POTENTIALS

Synapses in the central nervous system and autonomic division of the peripheral nervous system may have either excitatory or inhibitory functions. Inhibitory synaptic action may be presynaptic or postsynaptic. Presynaptic inhibition is mediated by axoaxonic synapses (Figs. 1.5 and 3.13), located at or near axon terminals, and it operates by preventing the release of excitatory synaptic transmitter. These will be described in the next chapter (Section 3.2c).

Inhibitory postsynaptic potentials consist of a transient hyperpolarization of the membrane (Figs. 2.13 and 2.14). The membrane could in principle be hyperpolarized either by an outflow of K^+ ions (due to increased g_K moving the membrane potential closer to E_K than it is at

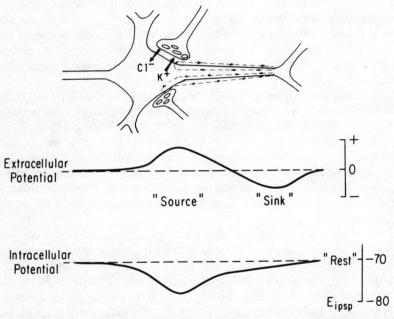

Figure 2.13. Ion currents of an IPSP. The *top* diagram shows the inhibitory synapse on the cell body, and the current flowing between subsynaptic membrane and a dendrite. The *center* and *bottom* diagrams show the distribution of potentials along cell body and dendritic membrane during action of an IPSP. Either an outflow of K^+ or an inflow of Cl^- causes hyperpolarization of the membrane; in neurons of the mammalian CNS the latter is the predominant mechanism of IPSPs. Near the activated inhibitory terminals is an extracellular current source, at some distance from it a sink (more probably, several sinks). (Compare with Fig. 2.4 which shows the current flows associated with locally depolarizing potentials.) The extracellular and intracellular potential changes are not drawn to the same scale.

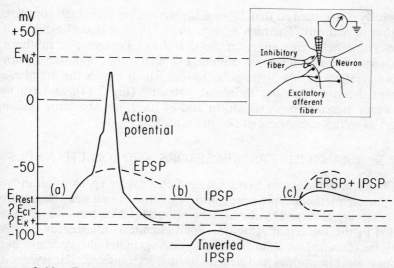

Figure 2.14. Equilibrium potentials of ions and potential changes of a central neuron. The inset shows the recording conditions: a micropipette electrode has been inserted into a neuron. An inhibitory and an excitatory pathway are available for stimulation. E_{Na}, E_{Cl}, and E_K are the equilibrium potentials of the ions; E_{rest} is the resting membrane potential. In a an excitatory volley evoked an EPSP, which then triggered an action potential. In b an inhibitory volley evoked an IPSP. In c both excitatory and inhibitory volleys arrived simultaneously; the resulting curtailed EPSP was too small to trigger an impulse. To produce an "inverted IPSP," first a hyperpolarizing current must pass through the membrane, in an experiment similar in principle to the one illustrated in Figure 2.12. (In practice it is not possible to insert two separate electrodes into the same neuron, but double-barreled pipettes can be used, one barrel for recording and the other for passing current.) The reversal potential of the IPSP is near either to E_{Cl} or to E_K, depending on which ion's conductance is most increased by the inhibitory transmitter.

rest) or by an inflow of Cl$^-$ ions (due to increased g_{Cl}). The inhibitory effect of the vagus on the pacemaker of the heart is caused by an increase of g_K. So far as it is known the IPSPs of central neurons are mediated by an increase of g_{Cl} with a possible lesser contribution by g_K. Chloride ions can have a hyperpolarizing effect only if chloride is actively transported out of the cell (see Section 2.4b) so that the chloride equilibrium potential, E_{Cl}, is more negative inside than is the resting poential (Tables 2.1 and 2.2).

We have seen that in most muscle cells, unlike neurons, Cl$^-$ is passively distributed so that $E_{Cl} = E_{rest}$, but resting g_{Cl} is high compared to that in neurons. The high g_{Cl} acts as an "inertial brake" against any transient depolarizing effect (cf. Section 2.4b). Postsynaptic inhibitory synapses of central neurons combine two effects that oppose excitatory depolarization: (1) the hyperpolarization, which moves the membrane potential away from the threshold potential (Fig 2.14); and (2) the transient increase in g_{Cl} which, in and of itself, has the same braking effect as in the membrane of skeletal muscle.

2.5e. TRANSMITTERS, RECEPTORS AND ION CHANNELS

Chemical reactions of living tissues fall, broadly speaking, into two categories: metabolic processes and regulatory processes. Regulatory processes are governed by chemical compounds which carry information coded in the molecular structure. Such chemical information carriers may be classified as follows: genetic coding materials; systemic hormones; local hormones and neuro-modulators*; intercellular (synaptic) transmitter substances; and intracellular ("second") messenger substances.

The boundaries between these categories are not always sharp. The materials released by the neurosecretory cells of the hypothalamo-pituitary system may be called "transmitters" while they are contained in the nerve terminal, and "hormones" once they have entered the bloodstream. Even more blurred is the dividing line between neuro-modulator and synaptic transmitter substances. The structural features of synapses of the mammalian central nervous system have been described in great detail. There are, however, nerve terminals in the gray matter which do not form junctions of such specialized and readily recognizable structure. Instead, they seem to end in a string of varicosities without specialized junctions and in no special relationship of selected postjunctional neurons. It is believed that these nerve endings release their transmitter (or neuromodulator substance) into interstitial fluid and influence the activity of many neurons in a region. The substances released by such multiply beaded unspecialized nerve endings are believed to be catecholamines (noradrenaline or dopamine). It takes

---

* The word "neuro-modulator" has been used to denote two different concepts. Some writers mean by it a substance which when released from a cell or from a nerve fiber is able to reach and act on a whole group of other cells diffusely and uniformly. Its other meaning is a substance which, although having no effect by itself, influences the effect of some other synaptic transmitter substance. Both definitions may be applicable to one and the same chemical agent (see e.g. Section 19.4).

only a moderately audacious leap of the imagination to suppose that their function may be the general regulation of excitability in neuron populations, such as may be required for the setting of a "mood" or for the alerting of the brain.

Concerning synaptic transmitter substances, the following rules are worth remembering:

1. Any one neuron releases the same one transmitter substance at all the presynaptic terminals formed by branches of its axon. Known as *Dale's principle*, this rule seemed valid for all neurons until quite recently. Reports that some nerve terminals contain both a peptide and an amine have now appeared. Until it is proven that both these substances indeed function as transmitters at these junctions, Dale's principle cannot be considered refuted, only to be liable of possible future revision.

2. Most neurons of the central nervous system are innervated by numerous axon terminals originating from neurons of various functions and releasing different transmitters which have differing effects.

3. One and the same transmitter can have different effects on different target neurons. The best known examples are acetylcholine and noradrenaline. Acetylcholine inhibits the cardiac pacemaker and excites the smooth muscle of the intestines. Noradrenaline has the reverse effect in both cases (see also Chapter 17). It has been shown that suspected transmitter substances have different effects on different neurons in the central nervous system. This makes it likely, but does not prove, that these substances act as synaptic transmitters of differing function on these cells.

What enables the same transmitter molecule to exert such various and often opposite effects on different cells? The difference must be in the receiving cells. As we now see it, a transmitter molecule combines with a component of the postsynaptic membrane for which it has a specific chemical affinity. This component is the *receptor molecule* for that transmitter. The transmitter-receptor complex then causes a change in a specific ion channel. It either opens the channel, or, less often, closes it. This causes a change in membrane current and, therefore, in membrane potential (Figs. 2.13 and 2.15). The whole chain of effects may be represented as follows:

Transmitter + receptor $\rightleftharpoons$ transmitter-receptor complex $\rightarrow$

$$\text{ion channel} \rightarrow \Delta g_{ion} \rightarrow \Delta i_{ion} \rightarrow \Delta E_m$$

Note that the combination of transmitter and receptor is shown as a reversible chemical bond. The more transmitter there is in the vicinity of the membrane, the more binds to the receptor. If the concentration of transmitter decreases, then the reaction reverses and the transmitter effect ceases.

Different receptor molecules may exist for the same transmitter. At least three types are known for acetylcholine: two kinds of "nicotinic" and one "muscarinic" receptor. Representative examples of these three acetylcholine receptors are found in the skeletal muscle endplate (nicotinic) (see Section 2.5a); the postganglionic neurons of the autonomic ganglia (nicotinic) (see Section 17.3a); and various visceral target tissues (muscarinic) (see Section 17.3). There are two known receptors for noradrenaline (α and β; see Table 17.1). Probably there are more than one for dopamine, and for histamine as well. The action of a transmitter is, however, not determined by the receptor molecule either but by the ion channel it controls. Acetylcholine bound to the muscarinic receptor of the cardiac pacemaker opens channels for potassium ions and so inhibits the pacemaker. The excitatory effect mediated by again a muscarinic receptor of the intestines is probably due to the opening of sodium channels.

What is the physical nature of ion channels? It has been debated for some time whether or not ions move through the membrane by first being captured by a side chain of a membrane molecule, perhaps a protein, and then transferred from one side to the other by a conformational change of the carrier molecule. Such a mechanism could in some cases be passive and thermodynamically downhill, and in other active and uphill, fueled by ATP. Such a mechanism could also account for the specificity of the channel, if the affinity of the membrane molecule would be limited to one species of ion only. More recently, however, the weight of evidence seems to shift in favor of the idea that the channels are, what the name implies, real holes in the membrane, which may or may not be filled with water molecules. These holes could either be at the center of one giant macromolecule, or they could be formed by several similar molecules (Figs. 2.8 and 2.15). Conformational changes of the macromolecule(s) might open and close the channel and could be controlled by nearby transmitter-receptor complexes.

Identification of receptors has depended on pharmacological methods. For each receptor a list can be drawn of the various drugs that mimic the transmitter; these are called *agonist* substances. Other drugs oppose the natural transmitter and its agonists; these are pharmacological

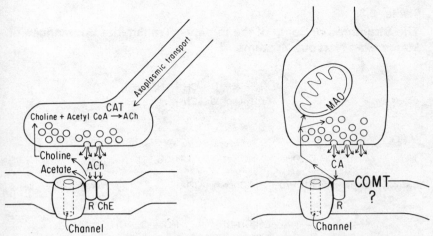

Figure 2.15. Diagrams of a cholinergic and a catecholaminergic junction. Choline acetyltransferase (CAT) is delivered by axoplasmic transport to the presynaptic terminal; it synthesizes acetylcholine (ACh) already as it moves down the axon. ACh is then packaged in presynaptic vesicles. When a nerve impulse arrives, a large number of these vesicles fuses with the membrane and empties its contents into the synaptic cleft. ACh then reacts with the receptor (R) and the ACh-R complex opens the ion channel. Cholinesterase (ChE) breaks ACh into choline and acetate. Fresh Ach is made by CAT transferring acetate from acetyl-CoA to choline. Some of the choline comes from spent and recycled transmitter. Catecholamines (CA) are released by a similar mechanism. The action of CA is terminated by the whole CA molecule being taken back into the presynaptic terminal. Here part of it is repacked in vesicles, part oxidized by monoamine oxidase (MAO). Another enzyme inactivating CA is catechol-*o*-methyltransferase (COMT). Its exact cellular location and functional importance at various junctions are not definitely known.

antagonists. For example the α- and β-receptors of adrenergic substances were distinguished by pharmacological affinities of various drugs. Furthermore, atropine and related drugs block the effects of acetylcholine on muscarinic receptors; curare and related drugs block acetylcholine's effect at nicotinic receptors. The compounds which interact with synaptic receptors are dealt with in detail in pharmacological texts.

A complete catalog of all the compounds that investigators have proposed as transmitters in the mammalian nervous system would be out of place, but a few of the most discussed ones will be mentioned (Table 2.3).

Excitatory amino acids. These transmitter candidates belong to the

Table 2.3.
The Structures of Some of the Synaptic Transmitter Substances of Mammalian Nervous Systems

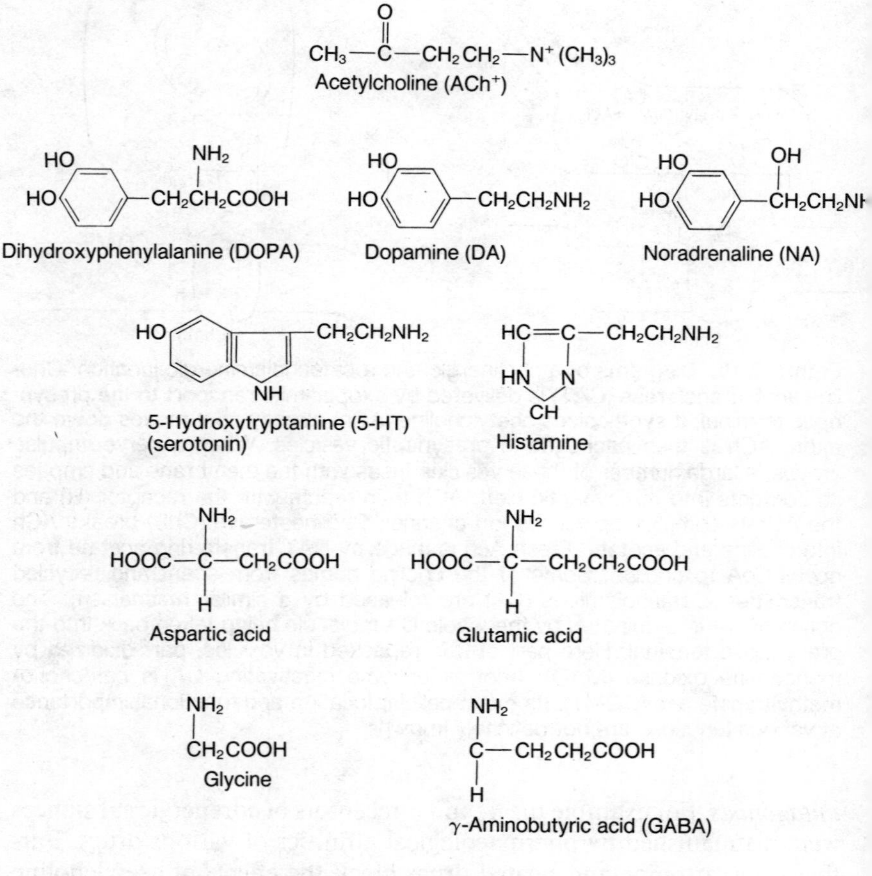

$$CH_3 - \overset{\overset{\displaystyle O}{\|}}{C} - CH_2 CH_2 - N^+ (CH_3)_3$$
Acetylcholine (ACh⁺)

Dihydroxyphenylalanine (DOPA)

Dopamine (DA)

Noradrenaline (NA)

5-Hydroxytryptamine (5-HT)
(serotonin)

Histamine

Aspartic acid

Glutamic acid

Glycine

γ-Aminobutyric acid (GABA)

Arg–Pro–Lys–Pro–Glu–Glu–Phe–Phe–Gly–Leu Met(NH₂)
Substance P

Tyr–Gly–Gly–Phe–Met–OH
Met-enkephalin

acidic (i.e. dicarboxylic) amino acids (though not all acidic amino acids are excitants). Best known are glutamic and aspartic acids. These compounds are capable of exciting almost all neurons in the mammalian CNS, which, however, does not necessarily mean that they are natural transmitters to all cells. In order to prove that they are, it is necessary to show that presynaptic terminals actually release the amino acid in the amount required for transmission. This proof is lacking in most cases.

Inhibitory amino acids. Several neutral amino acids exert strong inhibitory action on most neurons in the CNS. γ-Aminobutyric acid (GABA) and glycine are the best known two. GABA is almost certainly the postsynaptic inhibitory transmitter at several inhibitory junctions of the brain, including the hippocampus, the cerebellum and some brain stem nuclei. Glycine is the transmitter at several junctions of the spinal cord, especially those acting on motor neurons of the ventral horn. These glycinergic inhibitory junctions operate by a chloride conductance mechanism.

Acetylcholine. Conforming to Dale's rule, acetylcholine is the transmitter not only at the neuromuscular endplate, but also recurrent collaterals of motor axons which terminate in the gray matter of the spinal cord (see Section 15.3c). High concentrations of acetylcholine have also been found in the basal ganglia, the hippocampus, and some of the layers of the cerebral cortex. Many acetylcholine receptors in the brain seem to be muscarinic. Their effect is sometimes excitatory (see Section 2.5b and 19.4), sometimes inhibitory.

Monoamines. These include *serotonin* (also known as 5-hydroxytryptamine or 5-HT) as well as the *catecholamines*: adrenaline, noradrenaline, and dopamine. Adrenaline is a hormone secreted by the adrenal medulla and is probably not a neurotransmitter in mammals; noradrenaline is. In biosynthetic pathways dopamine is made from the amino acid, dihydroxyphenylalanine (DOPA); noradrenaline is made out of dopamine; and adrenaline from noradrenaline. In dopaminergic neurons the biosynthetic process stops at the first step, in noradrenergic neurons at the second, and in the adrenal medulla it can run to completion.

There are high concentrations of monoamine-containing neurons in specific nuclei in the brain stem. Serotonergic neurons are found in largest numbers in the raphe nuclei. Dopaminergic neurons are found in the substantia nigra. Noradrenergic neurons are concentrated in the locus coeruleus of the midbrain. The axons of these cells connect these nuclei to a variety of structures in brain and spinal cord. The best known of these connections are shown in Figure 2.16. The list given

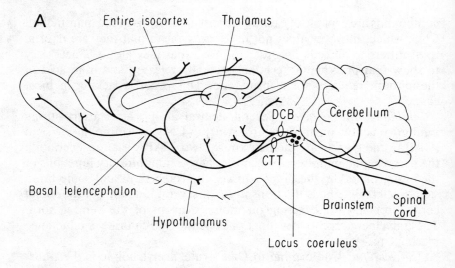

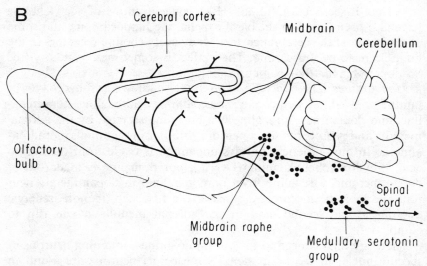

Figure 2.16. Some of the better known monoaminergic neuron groups and the most important target areas of their axons. *A*, noradrenergic neurons of the locus coeruleus; *DCB* = dorsal catecholaminergic bundle; *CTT* = central tegmental tract. *B*, serotonergic neurons of the raphe nuclei. (Modified and redrawn after J. B. Angevine and C. W. Cotman: *Principles of Neuroanatomy*. London, Oxford University Press, 1981.)

here and in Figure 2.16 do not show all the known anatomical locations of monoaminergic neurons of their connections, but include the systems that have been most studied so far.

Some of the functions of monoaminergic pathways will be mentioned later (e.g. Sections 7.3, 7.9b, 17.5, 18.2b, and 19.4). Disorders of monoaminergic neurons have been implicated in several psychiatric conditions, including the affective psychoses and schizophrenias, but the exact role of these substances in psychiatric cases is still uncertain.

Peptides. There is a steadily lengthening list of peptides, some simple and some quite complex in structure, that are suspected of being transmitters in the CNS. One of these, enkephalin, is described in Section 7.9c. Another much discussed peptide, substance P, may be the transmitter in some of the primary afferent nerve fibers of the spinal cord (see Section 7.3).

Chapter Summary and Reading List

See at end of Chapter 3.

Answers to Problems of Figure 2.3

A: $V_1 = 1$ V
   $V_2 = 2$ V
   $V_3 = 3$ V
   $A_1 = 30$ mA
   $A_2 = 10$ mA
   $A_3 = 40$ mA

Note that the total resistance is 75 Ω.

B: $V_1 = 3$ V
   $A_1 = 30$ mA
   $A_2 = 10$ mA
   $A_3 = 30$ mA
   $A_4 = 40$ mA

Note that the total resistance is 150 Ω.

Electric Potentials of Excitable Cells: II

How action potentials are generated and how they are conducted. Functional differences between nerve fibers. Disorders of excitability and conduction.

3.1. Ionic Mechanisms of Action Potentials

At the height of a spike potential the inside of nerve and muscle fibers changes from the resting level of between −65 and −90 mV to between +5 and +35 mV (see Figs. 1.2 and 2.14). How is this short-lived but quite substantial change achieved? In the resting state the membrane potential is closer to E_K than to E_{Na}; at the height of the action potential it comes closer to E_{Na} than to E_K (see Fig. 2.14). Many observations indicate that as the spike potential develops g_{Na} comes to exceed g_K and it is because of the high g_{Na} that the membrane potential approaches E_{Na}.

It will be recalled that sodium channels open during generator potentials, endplate potentials (EPPs) and excitatory postsynaptic potentials

(EPSPs). There is, however, an important difference between the Δg_{Na} relating to these local potentials and to action potentials.

The sodium channels of the sensory nerve terminals, postsynaptic membranes and endplate membranes are all opened by an outside agent, namely a physical stimulus or a chemical compound. By contrast, the sodium channels that generate spike potentials are opened by a change of membrane voltage. In laboratory parlance they are *voltage-gated*.

Sometimes the two kinds of channels are segregated to separate parts of the same membrane. For example, in skeletal muscle, chemically gated channels are found only in the endplate membrane, voltage-gated channels in the entire remainder of the surface membrane muscle fiber (but see Section 3.4f for pathological breakdown of this separation). In some other membranes channels of different types may mingle. Biophysicists have estimated channel density for some types of membranes and concluded that considerable distances—of the order of micrometers—separate one from another. In other words, there is enough surface area to accommodate all the ion transport mechanisms, with room to spare. The idea that the channels operated by outside stimuli and the voltage-gated ones are separate entities is confirmed by pharmacology. *Tetrodotoxin* (TTX) blocks the voltage-gated Na^+ channels but none of the others. For example, neither voltage-gated K^+ channels nor the Na^+ channels operated by chemical or physical stimuli are blocked by it.

The spike potential is generated in a rapidly evolving self-reinforcing cycle of events. Figure 3.1A shows that if an excitable membrane is depolarized by whatever means, the depolarization enhances sodium conductance, which in turn causes further depolarization which again increases sodium conductance, and so on. Such a cycle is a form of *positive feedback*. It could also be called a "vicious circle."

Now if the positive feedback mechanism represented in Figure 3.1A would be the only one operating, then the potential of the stimulated membrane would move from the resting level to near E_{Na} and then remain there forever. In fact, however, the membrane potential never quite reaches E_{Na} during an action potential, and it returns to the resting level within a short period of time. Two mechanisms ensure the return of the membrane potential from the summit of the spike to the negative level which follows the spike (the after-hyperpolarization: see Figs. 1.2 and 3.1B). The first is the *inactivation* of the sodium channels, and the second an increase of g_K. It is in the nature of the voltage-gated sodium channels to close automatically after having been opened. Both the

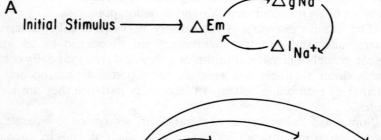

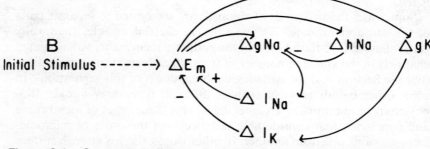

Figure 3.1. Causes and effects in the operation of voltage-gated membrane channels. *A*, an initial depolarization, for example by an EPP or an EPSP, causes voltage-gated Na channels to increase g_{Na}, which in turn increase I_{Na}, which then leads to further depolarization; this is positive feedback. (Modified and redrawn after B. Katz: *Nerve, Muscle and Synapse.* New York, McGraw-Hill, 1966). *B*, in normal excitable membranes depolarization causes not only increased g_{Na}, but also inactivation of the sodium channels (Δh_{Na}) and increased g_K. Both inactivation and g_K counteract the depolarization caused by increased g_{Na}; thus the membrane is first depolarized and then repolarized; it is this sequence that we call a spike potential. (See also Fig. 3.2 and text.) (Reprinted with permission from G. Somjen: *Sensory Coding in the Mammalian Nervous System*, New York, Plenum. 1975.)

opening (activation) and the closing (inactivation) are set in motion by the initial depolarization, but the inactivating mechanism works more slowly.

The second repolarizing mechanism, the increase of g_K, is also voltage-dependent. At rest $g_K > g_{Na}$. Then during the development of the spike, g_{Na} grows so that $g_{Na} \gg g_K$. Subsequently, however, g_K increases well over its resting level until it once more exceeds g_{Na}. These various changes are summarized in Figures 3.1*B* and 3.2. As depolarization sets in, both g_{Na} and g_K start to increase together, but the race is to the swift; the sudden steep upturn of g_{Na} enables it to get ahead of g_K (Fig. 3.2*C*). If activation of the sodium channels did not accelerate faster than either

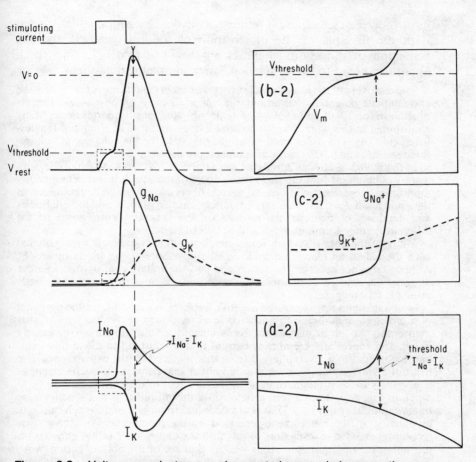

Figure 3.2. Voltage, conductance and current changes during an action potential. *a*, time course of the stimulating current; *b*, voltage changes; *b-2*, framed part of *b* enlarged; *c*, Na and K conductances during the action potential; *c-2*, framed portion of *c* enlarged; *d*, ion currents associated with the action potential, with part enlarged in *d-2*. Note: threshold is reached when $I_{Na} = I_K$ (*d-2*); furthermore, g_{Na} and g_K begin to change together but g_{Na} accelerates faster then g_K; and the summit of the action potential is reached when I_K once more equals, and subsequently exceeds, I_{Na} (*d*). (After works of Hodgkin, Huxley, Katz, and others.)

their own inactivation or the activation of the potassium channels, then an action potential could never happen. The enhancement of g_{Na} is *positive feedback,* because it reinforces the depolarization which caused it in the first place. The inactivation of sodium channels and the activation of potassium channels are *negative feedback,* since both oppose and tend to cancel the depolarization that caused them.

The discovery of the ion conductances involved in generating action potentials and endplate potentials was among the major advances in physiological investigation in the 1940s and 1950s—quite possibly the most important one. Many contributed to this work, but the greatest names are those of Hodgkin, Huxley, Katz and Cole. The differential equations that describe the behavior of voltage-gated sodium and potassium conductances (published in 1952) are often referred to as the Hodgkin-Huxley equations, or "H and H" for short. Much of the early work was conducted on the giant nerve fibers of the squid. It was subsequently found that nerve fibers and skeletal muscle fibers of vertebrates behave much as the squid axon does, but that smooth muscle, cardiac muscle, and the cell bodies and dendrites of neurons are variants on the general theme. Some of the differences among impulse types will be described below.

Many of the data on which ionic membrane theory is based were gathered with the aid of an electronic trick called the *voltage clamp* by its inventors. Although it is not necessary to understand how the voltage clamp works in order to grasp the essence of membrane ion currents, a brief summary of its basic principle follows here.

In voltage clamping electronic negative feedback is used to force the potential of a biological membrane to a desired level regardless of the reactions of that membrane. An electronic source feeds current to the membrane to exactly match and cancel any membrane current that would tend to move the membrane potential to a level different from that required by the experiments. The heart of a voltage clamp circuit is an amplifier that delivers as much current as is necessary to keep the membrane potential equal to the command voltage (*I ampl.* in Fig. 3.3). The current generated by this amplifier is recorded (*current monitor* amplifier of Fig. 3.3). It is always equal in magnitude, though opposite in polarity, to the ion current generated by the membrane. Analyzing such recordings enabled investigators to establish the dependence of ion currents on prevailing membrane potential as well as changes of membrane current with time and to deduce relationships such as the ones depicted in Figure 3.2*C* and *D.*

3.1a. THE CONDITIONS OF EXCITATION

Small depolarizations will not trigger an impulse. If they would, nerves and muscle fibers would be excited frequently for no good reason. This does happen in certain pathological conditions, for example in tetany (see Section 3.4b). In a healthy organism excitation occurs when an excitable membrane is depolarized by a certain minimum amount to the *threshold voltage* of excitation. For normal function the threshold should be high enough to ensure stability but not so high to prevent normal excitability.

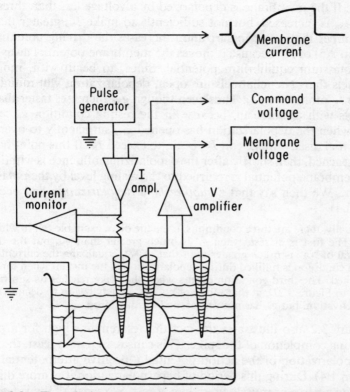

Figure 3.3. The principal components of a voltage clamp circuit. The voltage (V) amplifier measures the potential difference between the inside and the outside of the cell. A current (I) amplifier delivers current which passes through the membrane and then to ground. The current delivered by the I amplifier is just sufficient to keep the membrane potential clamped at the command voltage: it is equal and opposite to the net ion current that, in the absence of the voltage clamp, would move the membrane potential to a level different from the desired one.

The thresholds of different excitable cells are not always the same. We speak of a high threshold if much depolarization is needed to excite a cell, and a low threshold when less is enough. Clearly, high threshold is synonymous with low excitability, low threshold with a high degree of excitability.

Threshold is reached when a membrane is depolarized sufficiently for the (inward) Na^+ current to exceed the (outward) K^+ current (cf. Fig.

3.2*D*). If the membrane is depolarized by a voltage less than threshold, then g_{Na} is increased, but not sufficiently to make I_{Na} greater than I_K. Remember that any depolarization increases the driving potential (cf. Section 2.5) of K^+ because it moves the membrane potential away from the potassium equilibrium potential. Since, to begin with, more K^+ channels than Na^+ channels are open, depolarization will initially increase I_K more than I_{Na}. Thus even though g_{Na} increases faster than g_K, it starts with a handicap, because in the resting condition $g_K \gg g_{Na}$. Only when the depolarization has opened g_{Na} sufficiently to overcome this initial disadvantage can I_{Na} begin to exceed I_K. If this point has not been reached, then shortly after the depolarizing influence is withdrawn, the membrane potential is returned to the resting level by the potassium current. We then say that a *subthreshold depolarization* had occurred (Fig. 3.4).

Actually, there are three conditions in the life of an excitable cell in which I_{Na} = I_K. The first is at rest, when g_K is much greater than g_{Na} but the driving potential of Na^+ is much greater than that of K^+, equalizing the currents. The second condition is fulfilled during depolarization at the instant when threshold is reached. The third condition occurs when the spike reaches its summit. As shown in Figure 3.2*D*, at that moment g_{Na} has already begun to decline due to its inactivation, but g_K has not yet reached its maximum.

Figure 3.2 also illustrates the fact that g_K remains high for a period following completion of the spike. This causes, in part at least, the after-hyperpolarization of the action potential ("positive afterpotential": see Section 1.4). During this period of hyperpolarization it is more difficult to excite a nerve or muscle fiber than at rest. We speak of the *subnormal period.*

While the spike takes place, the membrane is inexcitable: no second new spike can be initiated as long as one is in progress. This is different from EPSPs, since successive EPSPs can be summed (see Section 4.2c). During a spike, the membrane is thus in the *absolute refractory period.* This is followed by the *relative refractory period*, when excitation is possible but only if stimulation is stronger than usual. The relative refractory period overlaps with the subnormal period of the after-hyperpolarization, and the two cannot always be clearly separated. There is a difference in mechanism, however. The refractory period is caused by residual inactivation of Na^+ channels, the subnormal period by high g_{K^+}.

So far the after-depolarization (negative afterpotential (see Section 1.4)) has not been mentioned. Its mechanism is different in different tissues and not

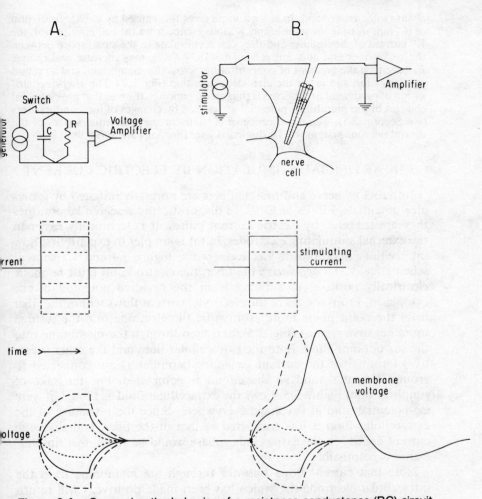

Figure 3.4. Comparing the behavior of a resistance-conductance (RC) circuit to that of a live neuron. *A*, the voltage changes caused by constant current pulses of varying polarity and intensity flowing in a circuit of a condenser and resistor in parallel (compare also with Fig. 2.1). *B*, the potential responses of a neuron, recorded through one barrel of a double-barreled electrode, to constant current pulses passed through the other barrel. Note that the hyperpolarizing currents cause voltage changes that are similar to those in the passive RC circuit shown in *A*. The responses to the depolarizing currents are very different: even the weakest one evokes a subthreshold yet non-linear response; the two stronger depolarizing pulses evoke all-or-none impulses.

always fully understood. In at least some cases it is caused by the accumulation of K^+ ions outside the membrane. K^+ ions escape from the cell interior with the K^+ current of the impulse and they can accumulate in the small space between the nerve fiber and adjacent cells. Thus $[K^+]_o/[K^+]_i$ may increase and change E_K (decrease the gradient of concentration across the membrane) and so retard repolarization and cause the after-depolarization (Fig. 1.2). The after-depolarization of peripheral nerve fibers is thus an exception to the rule that physiological changes of the membrane potential are caused by changes of ion conductances (see Section 2.5). The significance of K^+ ions in the interstitial spaces of the central nervous system will be discussed later (Sections 5.8 and 5.9b).

3.1b. ARTIFICIAL STIMULATION BY ELECTRIC CURRENT

Impulses of nerve and muscle fibers are normally initiated by generator potentials, EPSPs or EPPs. In diagnostic and research laboratories they are triggered by electric current pulses. It is technically easier to use external stimulating electrodes; but it is simpler to explain first how intracellular micropipette electrodes work. Figure 3.4 and 3.5 show it schematically. To *depolarize* the fiber, the electrode tip must be made electrically positive, to subtract from the negative potential of the cytoplasm. From the tip of the electrode, current flows within the fiber from the point made more positive by the electrode into the resting, more negative regions (Fig. 3.5), and then through the membrane into the surrounding fluid. Both the extracellular fluid and the other (negative) terminal of the current generator (stimulator) are connected to ground potential, and so the circuit is completed. For the sake of simplification, Figure 3.5 shows the extracellular fluid as though it were iso-potential, and at 0 voltage everywhere. Since the resistance of the extracellular fluid is low compared to that of the fiber, and since the current density in the extracellular phase would be small, this simplification is permissible.

Note that current flows *outward* through the membrane from the intracellular electrode tip, which has been made positive. I will return to this point presently. An *inwardly* directed current (with inside electrode negative) would *hyperpolarize* the cell membrane. Note also that the current density is greatest in the vicinity of the electrode and falls off with distance. Consequently the depolarization of the membrane falls off exponentially with distance. This is an example of *electrotonic spread*, with which we have met already (Section 2.5a).

Current from an intracellular point source (such as the electrode tip), is divided between the resistors formed by the cell's membrane and its cytoplasmic core. The higher the membrane resistance and the lower

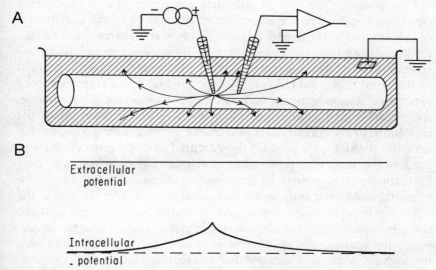

Figure 3.5. Electrotonic spread of a subthreshold depolarizing potential in a nerve or muscle fiber. *A*, diagram of experimental arrangement. The intracellular electrode shown to the left is delivering current and the one to the right records the potential with reference to ground. *B*, distribution of intracellular potenital change along the fiber. In practice such plots are obtained by inserting the recording electrode repeatedly into the same fiber at various distances from the point of current injection.

that of the core, the farther will the polarization spread. The *length constant* (or space constant) of a fiber is the distance over which a transmembrane electrotonic potential decays to $1/e$ of its original voltage. It is determined as follows:

$$\lambda = \sqrt{r_m/r_c} \qquad (3.1)$$

where r_c is the resistance of the fiber's core.

If two fibers have membranes with identical properties and contain similar cytoplasm but one has a larger diameter than the other, the larger fiber has the longer length constant. This is because the core resistance is inversely proportional to the square of the radius (i.e. to cross-sectional area), but the resistance of the surface membrane is inversely proportional to the radius itself (i.e. to the area of the mantle). Thus, other things being equal, the distribution of current and voltage is a matter of geometry.

Now consider the case of stimulating a nerve fiber with external electrodes. Figure 3.6 is a schematic representation of the distribution of current and voltage. Much larger voltages and currents are needed for stimulation from the outside than for intracellular stimulation. This is because much of the current delivered by external electrodes is shunted by the extracellular fluid (represented by r_e in Fig. 3.6). Excepting special experimental arrangements, such as the so-called sucrose gap technique, the extracellular medium has much lower resistance than either the membrane or the core of nerve and muscle fibers. Figure 3.6 shows that near the positive pole (anode) the potential in both extracellular and intracellular fluid rises to a more positive level than at rest, and near the cathode it is moved in the negative direction. The changes of potential inside and outside are not equal so that near the anode the *difference* between inside and outside potential increases, and near the cathode it decreases. This amounts to *hyperpolarization* near the *anode*, where the transmembrane current is *inward*, and *depolarization* near the *cathode*, where it is *outward*. For this reason with external stimulating electrodes it is always the *cathode* that stimulates, whereas with an intracellular stimulating electrode it is an anode.

3.1c. DEPOLARIZATION BY INWARD AND OUTWARD CURRENT

Attentive readers may be puzzled at this point. In Section 2.5 it was explained that depolarization is achieved by *inward* Na$^+$ current, and now it is stated that an *outward* stimulating current is required to depolarize nerve fibers. Here is the reason for this seeming contradiction.

If Na$^+$ ions move from the extracellular into the intracellular medium, depolarization is achieved by *redistributing* charge *within* the system. When we use man-made current we *add* charge to the system *from an extraneous source*. Placing either the cathode of the stimulator on the outside or the anode on the inside of the membrane "neutralizes" the existing charge. Whether the positive pole of the stimulator is inside or the negative pole outside, the direction of the current through the membrane will be outward.

3.1d. STIMULATING MULTIFIBER PREPARATIONS

Except when nerve or muscle fibers have been separated by microdissection, external stimulation is usually applied to whole nerves or muscles. This is

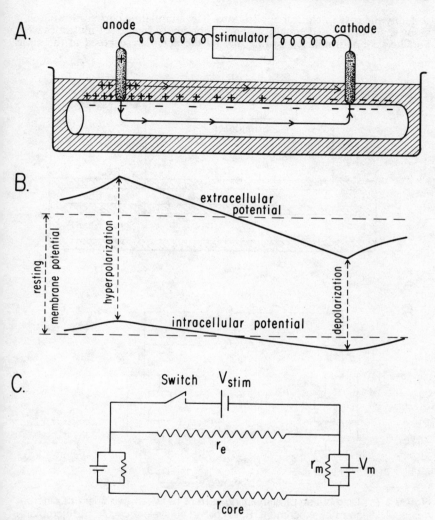

Figure 3.6. Passing a current through a fiber using a pair of extracellular electrodes. *A*, diagram of the experimental arrangement. *B*, the distribution of the changes of voltage along the fiber while a constant current flows between the electrodes. *C*, an electrical analog model: V_{stim}, stimulating voltage; r_e, resistance of the extracellular medium; r_{core}, cytoplasmic resistance; r_m, membrane resistance; V_m, membrane potential. Note that the externally applied anode adds to the difference across the membrane (hyperpolarization), whereas the external cathode subtracts from it (depolarization).

certainly the case in clinical applications. The stimulating current flowing in a tissue is not distributed equally among all the fibers. Figure 3.7 illustrates why. For the sake of simplicity assume that all the fibers are exposed to the same

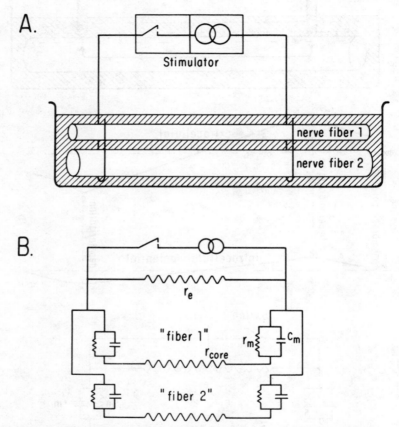

Figure 3.7. Distribution of stimulating current between two fibers of different radius. *A*, diagram of experiment. *B*, simplified equivalent circuit. c_m, membrane capacitance; other symbols as in Figure 3.6 (but with V_m deleted). If the radius of fiber 2 is twice that of fiber 1, then the core resistance of fiber 2, per unit length of fiber, will be ¼ of that of fiber 1; the membrane resistance of fiber 2 will be ½, its membrane capacitance twice that of fiber 1 per unit length. Consequently the membrane voltage change (ΔV_m) achieved by a given intensity of constant stimulating current shared by the two fibers will be in fiber 2 twice that achieved in fiber 1. Moreover, since the membrane time constant of fiber 2 will be ½ that of fiber 1, the voltage change will, at the onset of stimulation, reach its final steady value faster in fiber 2 than in fiber 1.

external voltage. This is not strictly true in a thick nerve, where the fibers in the center are exposed to a lower voltage than those at the surface, which are closer to the electrodes. These differences are, however, usually small, because the resistance of the interstitial fluid that separates the fibers is low. The share of the current that each fiber receives is, then, inversely proportional to the sum of its membrane resistance and core resistance. In fibers of large diameter both these resistances are lower than in small-diameter fibers. Now the magnitude of the depolarization of the membrane depends not on total current, but on membrane current density. In the large fibers the current is distributed over a larger surface. *But* the core resistance decreases in proportion to the square of the radius, and the surface area increases in direct proportion with the radius itself. Thus the larger fiber wins.

Thus for purely geometric reasons, larger nerve fibers are more easily stimulated by electric current than small fibers. This is both fortuitous and fortunate. Experimenters and clinicians alike often wish to stimulate larger fibers, leaving smaller ones undisturbed. One very good reason is that stimulation of smaller fibers is painful (see Section 6.7 and Fig. 6.4).

It often is said and written that large-caliber fibers have a lower threshold than small-caliber fibers. It should be understood that this rule applies *only* to artificial electric stimulation, and only because of the geometry. Sensitivity to natural stimuli is determined by the properties of sense organs or of excitatory synapses, which are independent of fiber size. The threshold voltage (critical depolarization (cf. Section 3.1a) does not depend on the size of cells or fibers.

3.1e. STIMULATION BY SHORT PULSES

Usually it is advisable to stimulate with brief pulses, not with prolonged currents. One reason is that prolonged currents can burn tissues, especially with transcutaneous stimulation. When a stimulating current is turned on, it takes some time before the membrane capacitance is fully charged: the voltage does not change instantly, but exponentially (see Fig. 2.1). If the stimulating pulse is short compared to the membrane time constant, then depolarization will not have reached its final value when the current ceases.

Figure 3.4 illustrates the time course of charging and discharging a "passive" circuit, compared to the "active" membrane of a nerve cell. The drawing illustrates intracellular stimulation of a neuron cell body, but the membrane capacity influences the time course of extracellular stimulation in a similar manner.

In using short pulses as stimuli, there is a tradeoff between pulse duration and intensity, because shorter but stronger current can bring the membrane potential to the same level as a longer, weaker one. This tradeoff is graphically represented in so-called *strength-duration curves* (Fig. 3.8), which show the current intensity that is just sufficient to stimulate a cell (or a nerve), as a function of pulse duration. *Rheobase* is the threshold intensity for prolonged constant current long enough to allow the membrane potential to reach a steady level. "*Chronaxie*" is a somewhat old-fashioned but still useful measure of the time dependence of excitation. It is the minimum duration of current that will just stimulate at an intensity twice that of the rheobase. Chronaxie depends on the time constant of the membrane of the stimulated fiber. It is however easier to determine the chronaxie than the membrane time constant.

Fibers of small caliber have longer time constants than large fibers. Time constants are a function of the product of membrane resistance and capacitance (see Section 2.1a). Because of their shorter time constants, larger fibers require shorter pulses for stimulation than small ones. Large fibers also have a lower rheobase than small-caliber fibers for reasons explained earlier (Fig. 3.7). In Figure 3.8 curve *a* is the

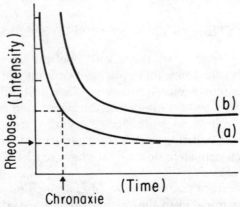

Figure 3.8. Strength duration curves of two (hypothetical) nerve fibers, *a* of large caliber than *b*. Rheobase is the threshold intensity for stimulation with prolonged constant current. Chronaxie is the minimum duration of a current pulse required for stimulating at twice rheobase intensity.

strength-duration curve of an hypothetical fiber of larger caliber than curve *b*.

3.1f. ACCOMMODATION

If a current is increased gradually, then it usually has to reach a higher intensity in order to stimulate than a sudden current would. The German literature of the 19th century spoke of a current "sneaking in" on the nerve—as though the nerve would then not "notice" the stimulus (*einschleichender Strom*). This property is referred to as *accommodation* to slowly rising stimuli.

Accommodation means that the threshold becomes higher if depolarization progresses slowly. The reason is that if g_{Na} is turned on slowly, I_K can keep ahead of I_{Na} and, meanwhile, inactivation of the Na channels also gets a chance to counteract activation (Fig. 3.9*A*). If depolarization is so slow that I_{Na} never exceeds I_K, then no impulse is fired, no matter how strong the depolarization eventually becomes. In this case the *rate* of depolarization is subliminal. One then can define a *minimal current gradient* of stimulation (Fig. 3.9*B*).

Not all excitable cells accommodate equally. The fibers in peripheral nerves usually cannot be stimulated by slowly increasing currents, but the sensory terminals of these same nerve fibers, and most neurons in the central nervous system, generally can be. Accommodation is then said to be incomplete or wholly absent. The degree of accommodation of an excitable membrane is related to its function. The stimuli acting on sensory terminals and the EPSPs of neurons in the central nervous system may have quite slow rates of rise and still must be effective. These structures could not accommodate as axons do. The only function of axons is to conduct impulses, so that they never need to be excited by "slowly sneaking" stimuli.

3.1g. ANODE-OFF (OR REBOUND) EXCITATION

As we have seen earlier (Section 3.1) inactivation of sodium channels is a function of depolarization. In some excitable cells sodium channels are partially inactivated even at the resting membrane potential. In these, hyperpolarization of the membrane extinguishes the inactivation present in the resting condition. The return of the membrane from the hyperpolarized to the resting state can then activate these channels and trigger an action potential. Since hyperpolarization is achieved by an external anode, this form of excitation is triggered at the anode, but after the current is turned off (Fig. 3.10).

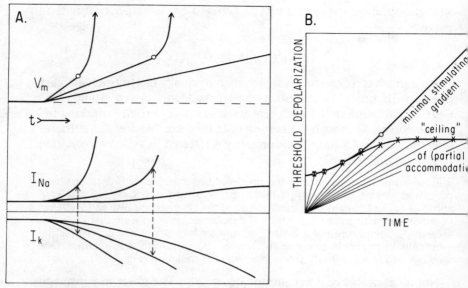

Figure 3.9.   Accommodation to gradually rising stimuli. *A*, membrane potential (V_m) and membrane ion currents, I_{Na} and I_K, during linearly increasing depolarization of three different gradients. *Open circles* on V_m curves mark the moment when threshold is reached (that is when I_{Na} becomes equal to I_K: see also Fig. 3.2). Note that the faster the depolarization the lower (less depolarized) is threshold V_m. Note also that the slowest depolarization fails altogether to reach threshold (it is rising at less than the minimal stimulating gradient) because I_K always remains greater than I_{Na}. *B*, plots of the thresholds of linearly increasing depolarization for two hypothetical excitable cells, one that has a minimum stimulus gradient requirement (*open circles*) and another that does not (*crosses*). The latter accommodates only partially: with stimuli of progressively decreasing slope the threshold rises somewhat and then comes to a ceiling.

It takes stronger and longer current pulses to cause anode-off excitation than the usual cathode-on excitation (Fig. 3.10).

3.1h. THE CONDUCTION OF IMPULSES

An action potential occupying any place in a nerve or muscle fiber is a stimulus that excites adjacent, resting portions of the fiber. Once that adjacent portion generated its action potential, it too will act as the stimulus for the next segment, and so on, until the end of the fiber is reached. Action potentials are conducted without decrement, because

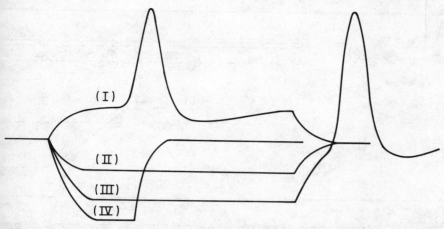

Figure 3.10. Impulses triggered by cessation of hyperpolarization: so-called anode-off (rebound) excitation. Curve *I* is the membrane potential response to depolarization of slightly above rheobase intensity (cf. Fig. 3.8). *II*, hyperpolarization equal in magnitude and duration to the depolarization of *I*; there is no active membrane response. In the wake of stronger hyperpolarization (*III*), an impulse is fired. Brief hyperpolarizations fail to stimulate even if quite strong (*IV*).

each portion of the fiber has the equipment to "make its own" impulse. Nerve fibers are not like telephone cables; they are more like an infinitesimal succession of repeater stations.

That an action potential can excite the resting membrane of an adjacent region is because both the core of the fiber and the interstitial fluid are electrically conductive. At the site of the action potential the inside of the fiber is positive relative to the resting fiber and the outside is electronegative compared to the resting regions (Fig. 3.11*A*). The potential gradients cause longitudinal current to flow both inside and outside, and the circuit is completed by current crossing the membrane. Note that the current that crosses the resting region of the membrane flows outward (Fig. 3.11*A-a*)! It is this outward current that depolarizes the resting region. To the resting portion of the nerve fiber, the action potential of the adjacent portion acts as though it were an "extraneous stimulator" (cf. Section 3.1c). Once the membrane has been depolarized sufficiently, it begins to generate its own sodium current, it thus converts from the "resting" to the "active" state, and the current turns inward.

Large-caliber fibers conduct impulses faster than small ones for two reasons. First, the larger the fiber, the shorter the time constant (see

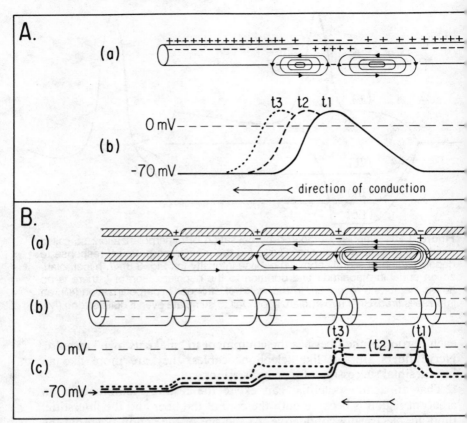

Figure 3.11. The conduction of impulses. *A*, in unmyelinated nerve fibers and in muscle fibers, *a* shows the currents flowing at time t1; *b*, the distribution of inside potential along the fiber at successive moments t1, t2 and t3. Note current flows inward through the membrane in the region occupied by the impulse, and outward ahead and behind the impulse. *B*, saltatory conduction in a myelinated nerve fiber. *a*, current flowing at time t1. Note that current crosses membrane only at the nodes of Ranvier. *b*, schematic representation of the fiber, not drawn to scale (internodal segments are shown too short). *c*, distribution of intracellular potential at successive times t1, t2 and t3. Note that impulses occur only at the nodes, internodal segments act as passive cables.

Section 2.1a). Second, the larger the fiber, the longer the length constant (see Section 3.1b). With a shorter time constant the resting portion ahead of the active region is depolarized more rapidly and the longer length constant ensures that the current generated by the spike potential spreads farther ahead of the advancing wavefront.

When an action potential is completed, it leaves the membrane refractory for a short period (see Section 3.1a). It is for this reason that a nerve impulse does not turn around and run backward (antidromically) after it has arrived at the fiber terminal. For the same reason, if in an experiment two impulses are started simultaneously at two points of the same nerve fiber, they *collide* and *extinguish* each other when they meet in the middle.

3.1i. SALTATORY CONDUCTION IN MYELINATED FIBERS

All nerve fibers are wrapped in an envelope formed by satellite cells. In the central nervous system the satellite cells of axons are called oligodendrocytes (see Fig. 5.3), in the peripheral nerves Schwann cells. Many of the fibers of vertebrate nervous systems have not one but many tightly wrapped layers. These are *myelinated* fibers.

The thick myelin sheath is interrupted at regular intervals by gaps called *nodes of Ranvier*. Myelin is a good electric insulator, so that current can pass through the membrane only at the nodes, and myelinated fibers generate impulses only at these nodes. The *internodal segments* serve as mere passive conductors of electricity. The impulse is said to leap from node to node; this is the meaning of *saltatory conduction*. The electric current generated by the action potential occupying one node flows through the internodal segment to the next node with a speed approaching that of light (see Section 2.1b). Significant time is lost only in charging the membrane capacitance of each successive node of Ranvier to raise the local membrane potential to threshold (Fig. 3.11B).

Since no time is consumed in conducting through the internodal segments, a myelinated fiber with a given axon diameter propagates impulses much faster than an unmyelinated fiber of the same caliber. Myelinated fibers vary in diameter from 2 to 20 μm (measured at the outside of the myelin sheath, not the axon). The thicker myelinated fibers conduct faster than the thinner ones. In part the time constant and length constant account for this difference, as explained in the preceding section for unmyelinated fibers. But, more importantly, the larger myelinated fibers have nodes of Ranvier spaced at longer intervals than do small-caliber myelinated fibers. Among afferent fibers in muscle nerves of cats internodal spacing varies from 0.3 to about 1.6 mm.

One may ask why nature could not have designed a nerve fiber with just two nodes, one at each end of the fiber. Would not conduction in such a fiber have been almost instantaneous? Unfortunately this would not work because the action potential could not drive enough current to depolarize to threshold a node so distant. The limiting factors are the resistance of the core, which increases with length, and the loss of current through the myelin sheath, which, although a good insulator, is not a perfect one. The internodal spacing of nerve fibers is a compromise between the requirement of fast conduction and the *safety factor of propagation*. The spacing can be greater in thicker fibers because (1) the core resistance is lower, and (2) the myelin sheath is thicker. In healthy mammalian myelinated fibers the action potential has enough power to excite not just the next node or the one thereafter, but the third one down the line.

For some time investigators were unsure whether the axon membrane beneath the myelin sheath does or does not have the usual complement of voltage-gated sodium and potassium channels. It is now known that the internodal axolemma has some of these, but they are few and far between and would not be able to conduct impulses.

The myelin sheath of nerve fibers degenerates in a number of pathological conditions. *Demyelination* in patches of tissue scattered over various locations of the central nervous system is the characteristic lesion of *multiple sclerosis*. The exotoxin of the *diphtheria* organism causes demyelination of peripheral nerves. If demyelination is incomplete and affects only a segment here and there, conduction is merely slowed, but if long stretches of fiber become completely demyelinated, conduction is blocked even if the axon seems intact.

Partial recovery of function in a demyelinating lesion may occur. Some axons may regain myelin, but the sheath is then abnormally thin, and the internodal distances too short. In other instances conductance may, however, be restored across a permanently demyelinated segment. This could be achieved by the formation of Na^+ channels in the axon membrane of the demyelinated, former internodal segments; or to a prolongation of the action potential by which the safety factor of propagation across the demyelinated segments would improve. In favorable cases victims of multiple sclerosis who have for a while been almost totally blind can regain enough vision to be able to read. Typically, in these cases the amplitude of the visual evoked potential (see Section 10.7) recovers but its latency remains abnormally long, indicating that demyelinated optic nerve fibers conduct again, but do so abnormally slowly.

3.1j. COMPOUND ACTION POTENTIALS

If one stimulates a nerve of mixed function at one point, and records the compound action potential monophasically at some distance (see Fig. 1.7), then the impulses of fibers of different caliber arrive at the recording sites at different times. The farther the recording point from the place of stimulation, the greater the difference in the arrival times, rather as the field of runners in the Boston Marathon spreads out as the race progresses. If conduction velocities were randomly distributed among nerve fibers, then the compound action potential would be symmetrical and bell-shaped, like the Gaussian curve. In that case the bell-shaped potential wave would simply widen at the base with increasing conduction distance. In fact, however, the statistical distribution of conduction velocities is *multimodal*, meaning that certain velocities occur more frequently than others. As a result, the compound spike has not one but several distinct peaks (Fig. 3.12) that become increasingly separated with conduction distance.

The separation of the compound spikes of myelinated and unmyelinated fibers is the most marked since the difference in conduction velocities is greatest between these two groups. Gasser and Erlanger, who were the first to record compound action potentials using a cathode ray oscilloscope, designated these A fibers and C fibers, respectively. B fibers are the small-caliber myelinated axons of preganglionic autonomic neurons (cf. Fig. 6.4 and Chapter 17), and are not found in the nerves of the limbs, where such recordings usually are made. The myelinated fibers of the A group were divided into the alpha, beta, gamma and delta subgroups.

About two decades after Gasser published his classification of nerve fibers, Lloyd found that conduction velocities of afferent nerve fibers of skeletal muscles cannot properly be separated into the groups defined by Gasser. Lloyd introduced his own classification using Roman numerals I through IV. Lloyd's groups are used today to designate afferent fibers of mammalian skeletal muscles, and Gasser's classification remains accepted for other nerve fibers. The relationships of fiber sizes and functional groups of axons are shown in Figure 6.4.

3.1k. THE ROLE OF DIVALENT CATIONS IN EXCITABILITY

An early observation on excitable tissues was that if Ca^{2+} is deleted from the Ringer's solution bathing a nerve or a muscle *in vitro*, the tissue becomes abnormally excitable. If left in a calcium-free medium for some time, skeletal muscle begins to twitch on its own accord, without any deliberate stimulation, and it becomes excitable by stretching. Stretch sensitivity is normal for mechanoreceptors and for some smooth muscles, but not for skeletal muscle. If too much Ca^{2+} is in the bathing fluid, all tissues become less excitable than normal.

A deficit of Ca^{2+} can be made up for adding Mg^{2+}, but more than the chemically equivalent amount of Mg^{2+} must be added to compensate

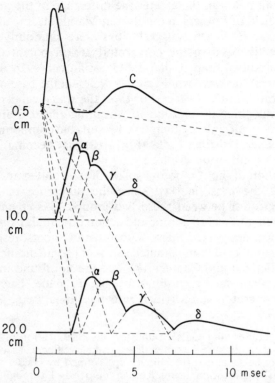

Figure 3.12. The compound action potential of a large nerve recorded at successively greater distances from the stimulated point. (Schematic representation based on the work of Erlanger and Gasser: *Electrical Signs of Nervous Activity*, University of Pennsylvania Press, Philadelphia, 1938.)

for a shortfall of Ca^{2+}. Adding extra Mg^{2+} to a bathing solution which already contained enough divalent cations makes excitable tissues less excitable than normal.

The effect of divalent cations on membrane excitability is sometimes described as *stabilizing* action. Neither Ca^{2+} nor Mg^{2+} contribute significantly to the resting membrane potential, because the permeability of the resting membrane to these two ions is very low. But the divalent cations seem to keep the voltage-gated sodium channels in the proper state of readiness to react when depolarized. If there are too many divalent cations, then the gates open in too sluggish a fashion; if there are too few, they open too easily; and if there are no divalent cations at all, the gates tend to fall open without stimulation.

Various biophysical models have been proposed to explain the stabilizing effect of divalent cations, but they must be considered hypothetical and we shall not discuss them. This much should, however, be remembered: the stabilizing effect is exerted by Ca^{2+} and Mg^{2+} in the extracellular fluid acting on the outside of the membrane. The intracellular activity of Ca^{2+} in resting excitable cells is very low. There is much more magnesium than calcium in cytoplasm but how much of it is ionized and how much is bound to proteins is not yet known. The activity of free Ca^{2+} in cytoplasm does increase in certain excitable cells under specific conditions. The intracellular functions of Ca^{2+} are very different from its extracellular membrane-stabilizing effect. Three groups of these functions have, so far, been clearly defined. (1) As an "internal messenger substance" Ca^{2+} serves excitation-contraction coupling in muscle cells (Chapter 14), and excitation-secretion coupling in some gland cells. It may perhaps have a somewhat similar role in coupling photochemical reaction and receptor potential of photoreceptor cells (see Section 9.2a). (2) Ca^{2+} ions entering presynaptic terminals with nerve impulses trigger the release of transmitter substance, described a little later in this chapter. This function could be regarded as a special case of excitation-secretion coupling. (3) Ca^{2+} entering the cytoplasm enhances g_K in some, but not all, excitable cells. Such an interaction, where one ion influences the permeability of another, has first been described in erthrocytes, and is known in those cells as the Gárdos effect. In excitable cells the Ca^{2+}-mediated increase of g_K acquires special significance, because it causes hyperpolarization and therefore a decrease of excitability. Several types of neurons in the central nervous system generate larger than average after hyperpolarizations, which seem, in part at least, to be mediated by Ca^{2+} entering the cytoplasm (cf. Section 4.5).

Skeletal muscle has Ca^{2+} ions sequestered in the sarcoplasmic reticulum (see Section 14.1b). In all other cells where it has an intracellular function, calcium must enter from the extracellular fluid. The mechanism of the influx of Ca^{2+} is the subject of the next section.

3.11. CA SPIKES

Several excitable cells have been found in which action potentials are generated partly or predominantly by calcium currents. The first discovered, and the most significant for medical practice, are the calcium-dependent action potentials of some smooth muscle cells, especially of the intestines and the blood vessels. If a skeletal muscle fiber or a nerve axon is placed in a Na^+-free solution or if it is poisoned by TTX (see Section 3.1), that fiber can no longer generate action potentials. Yet intestinal and vascular smooth muscle can, as long as Ca^{2+} remains present.

In those smooth muscle cells that operate by primarily calcium-dependent action potentials, excitation-contraction coupling depends on the entry of calcium into the cell from the surrounding medium (see Section 14.3). Therefore, if Ca^{2+} entry is prevented, the contractile mechanism cannot function. This is the mechanism by which Ca channel-blockers, recently introduced into clinical practice, exert their vasodilator effect.

Cardiac muscle is in many ways similar to skeletal muscle, but resembles smooth muscle in its dependence on environmental calcium for contracting. The action potentials of cardiac cells are generated by a succession of inward currents of Na^+, Ca^{2+} and outward current of K^+. The exact timing, and the proportions, of the currents carried by these three ions have not quite precisely been determined yet.

Lastly, one of the most recent discoveries has been that the dendritic membranes of some large neurons in the central nervous system also generate calcium-dependent action potentials. The evidence is strongest in the case of the Purkinje cells of the cerebellum, and there are reasons to believe that the pyramidal cells of the hippocampal cortex may also be among them and there may be others which have not yet been found. Dendritic calcium action potentials are of unusually long duration, 5–10 msec, and their exact role is not clear at present (see also Section 4.4). In other neurons, for example in ventral horn cells, Ca^{2+} seems to be admitted with Na^+ into the cell body during impulse generation and to cause the increased g_K responsible for the large after-hyperpolarization mentioned in the previous section. Some investigators suspect that voltage-gated I_{Ca} may hold the key to the understanding of epileptiform seizures (see Section 4.11c).

3.2. The Release of Transmitter from Presynaptic Terminals

Having gained some insight into the biophysics of nerve impulses, we can turn to the mechanism of release of synaptic transmitter substances. Ion currents associated with nerve impulses in presynaptic nerve terminals trigger this release. The sequence of events that liberate transmitter molecules from nerve endings is remarkably uniform at all chemical junctions. This includes not only the neuromuscular and neuron-to-neuron junctions of vertebrates, but also of invertebrates, and both inhibitory and excitatory synapses. The sequence is as follows. Transmitter molecules are stored inside presynaptic nerve terminals in small vesicles that are in some respects analogous to the secretory granules of gland cells (see Fig. 2.15). In some nerve endings there is an additional cytoplasmic pool of transmitter in solution, in others virtually all the transmitter is in the vesicles available for release. Release occurs by exocytosis. That is, the membrane of the vesicle fuses with the surface membrane of the nerve terminal, and the contents are emptied into the cleft between presynaptic and postsynaptic membrane. Transmitter molecules cross the synaptic cleft by diffusion, and then reversibly bind with the receptors in the postsynaptic membranes. Since the distance between the two membranes is very small, the diffusion takes less than 0.5 msec.

In nerve endings at rest, every now and then one of the vesicles pops open. The whiff of transmitter molecules so released causes a small potential deflection of the postsynaptic membrane, called a *miniature endplate potential* (MEPP), or a miniature EPSP (MEPSP), or miniature inhibitory postsynaptic potential (MIPSP), as the case may be. Transmitter is not normally liberated in amounts smaller than what is contained in one vesicle; therefore that amount is called a *quantum*, and release is said to be "quantal" in nature. At the neuromuscular junction of vertebrate skeletal muscles, one quantum consists of 1000–5000 acetylcholine molecules.

When an impulse arrives at the presynaptic nerve terminal, Ca^{2+} ions enter the cytoplasm. Very probably Ca^{2+} is allowed to pass through the membrane by way of voltage-gated channels. At the presynaptic nerve terminal the inward ionic current of the action potential is thus carried in part by Na^+ and in part by Ca^{2+}. Free Ca^{2+} in the cytoplasm of the terminal causes many vesicles to fuse with the surface membrane and to expel their contents (see Fig. 2.15). At the motor endplate of vertebrates hundreds of quanta are released by one nerve impulse. At excitatory synapses of the central nervous system fewer quanta are released per terminal bouton, sometimes less than ten, but then most central neurons are innervated by many boutons and the combined effect of these terminals can be summed. There are exceptions. At some central synapses a single presynaptic terminal can be of (relatively) giant size and it can release large numbers of quanta with each presynaptic impulse.

The mode of action of calcium is not exactly known, but the discovery of small quantities of actin and of myosin in nerve fibers, especially in nerve terminals, provided a hint. These proteins are the moving parts of muscle (Chapter 14) and it is at least thinkable that contractile filaments may pull synaptic vesicles toward the surface membrane. Calcium initiates muscle contraction, and it may play a similar role at the nerve terminal.

Be that as it may, the Ca^{2+} ions needed for synaptic transmission must come from the interstitial fluid around the synapse, for there are no intracellular stores of calcium in nerve fibers. If the interstitial fluid is deficient in Ca^{2+}, neuromuscular and synaptic transmission may be impaired.

Mg^{2+} ions cannot substitute for Ca^{2+} in synaptic transmission. On the contrary, an excess of Mg^{2+} can paralyze nerve-muscle junctions and block transmission at other synapses as well. This very probably is so because excess Mg^{2+} prevents Ca^{2+} ions from entering the Ca^{2+} channels of the membrane. This must be remembered when using salts of Mg^{2+} for therapeutic purpose. Co^{2+} and Mn^{2+} have blocking effects similar to Mg^{2+}, but stronger.

3.2a. AXOPLASMIC TRANSPORT

The enzymes required for the synthesis and metabolism of transmitters can only be manufactured in the perikarya of neurons, for only there is the equipment for making proteins. These enzymes are then moved through the axon to the nerve terminals by a mechanism much like a conveyor belt. Besides transmitters, the materials for forming, repairing and maintaining cell membranes, vesicles and organelles also come from the cell body. For some organelles building materials are moved; others come fully assembled. Time-lapse photography of neurons in cell culture shows whole mitochondria floating down the axon, like barges on a river.

Transmitter substances are synthetized throughout the entire neuron, from cell body to axon terminal, as the enzymes which make the transmitter are moved from cell body to terminal (see Fig. 2.15). The highest enzyme activity and the highest concentration of transmitter are, however, in the terminal boutons. Synaptic vesicles may be transported also; or their component parts may be moved and then assembled and filled at the terminal.

By following the movement of different tracer compounds, three separate and independent axoplasmic transport processes have been identified. The fastest moves at a rate of about 400 mm/day, the slowest barely more than 1 mm/day. The mechanical parts of the system are probably neurofilaments, neurotubules, or both. The fast transport depends on calcium and may utilize a contractile protein related to myosin. Axoplasmic transport requires metabolic energy and can be stopped by certain poisons, such as colchicine.

The mainstream of axoplasmic transport flows from cell body toward the tips of the fiber; in motor nerves it is in the same direction as the impulse traffic, in primary sensory neurons it is opposite in direction to the impulses. Similar perikaryo-fugal transport mechanisms operate in the dendrites of central neurons as well.

Besides the perikaryo-fugal transport there also is transport toward the cell body, called *retrograde axoplasmic flow.* It may return worn or broken-down cell constituents to be recycled but this is not known for sure. Retrograde transport is, however, of undoubted importance for pathophysiology. It seems that this is the vehicle by which neurotropic viruses, such as the agents of herpes zoster, are moved from peripheral tissues into the central nervous system.

3.2b. TERMINATION OF TRANSMITTER ACTION

Synaptic action must be terminated by removing the transmitter molecule. Three methods are available for this, utilized at different junctions to varying degrees: (1) enzymatic breakdown, or inactivation, (2) re-uptake by the presynaptic terminal, supplemented by uptake into peri-junctional Schwann or glial cells; (3) dispersal and dilution into surrounding interstitial fluid.

At most cholinergic junctions acetylcholine is rapidly broken down into choline and acetate by the action of acetylcholinesterase (also referred to as "true" cholinesterase). This enzyme is either built into or attached to the endplate membrane, and thus acts exactly where it is needed (see Fig. 2.15). Lesser amounts of true cholinesterase are found elsewhere, including in all parts of cholinergic neurons and also in such unexpected places as red blood cells. The organism apparently needs safeguards against possible spilling and indiscriminate spread of acetylcholine that could wreak havoc with many tissues.

The principal method of terminating the action of most other transmitters is re-uptake into synaptic terminals. This evidently is also the most economic way, since the material is then available for re-packing into vesicles. The suspected role of glial cells in the turnover of transmitters will briefly be discussed in Chapter 5. For detailed information on the enzymes that make and break transmitter molecules, refer to textbooks on pharmacology.

3.2e. PRESYNAPTIC INHIBITION

IPSPs make neurons less excitable. The effect is indiscriminate since it counteracts all EPSPs, no matter which afferent fibers evoked them (see Fig. 2.14, *B* and *C*). If there was a way to selectively turn off the excitation by a particular presynaptic fiber before it acted on the postsynaptic neuron, then the postsynaptic neuron would remain available for excitation through other inputs. It would seem that such a selective admittance of input signals could serve a useful purpose, for example in shifting attention from one kind of stimulus to another. There is clear evidence that the nervous system of some invertebrate organisms is equipped with such *presynaptic inhibitory junctions*. The evidence is less definitive that such a mechanism operates in the mammalian central nervous system as well. The following account is based in part on fact, in part on hypothesis.

Anatomists have described what appear on electron micrographs as functional junctions between one axon terminal and another (axoaxonic synapses (see Fig. 1.5)). This is the kind of structure that might make presynaptic inhibition possible. In the schematic representation of Figure 3.13, *e* indicates a terminal button that forms an excitatory junction with the postsynaptic neuron. The terminal marked *i* is the supposed presynaptic inhibitory nerve ending. Note that *e* is a "presynaptic" terminal for its target neuron but it is "postsynaptic" in relation to *i*.

To do its presumed job, *i* must limit the amount of transmitter released from *e*. A well known theory suggests that the inhibitory terminal *i* releases a transmitter that depolarizes the excitatory terminal *e*, without affecting the postsynaptic membrane. This polarization persists for some time. Impulses arriving from the excitatory axon in the terminal *e* find the terminal depolarized and therefore its sodium channels partially inactivated. Consequently the amplitude of the spike in terminal *e* will be curtailed (Fig. 3.13a), less Ca^{2+} will enter the cytoplasm, and less transmitter will be released (Fig. 3.13b).

Maybe so, the reader might respond, but does the depolarization of *e* by the action of *i* not trigger impulses in *e*? And if so, does that not cause transmitter release? The truth is that under laboratory conditions, if many dorsal root fibers are stimulated synchronously, antidromically conducted impulses are indeed triggered in other adjacent afferent fibers. This phenomenon, known since the 1930s as the "*dorsal root reflex*," is regarded as a laboratory artefact by most

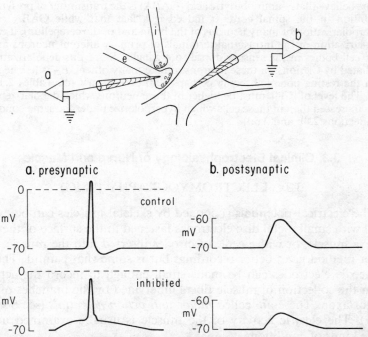

Figure 3.13. A hypothetical experiment investigating the mechanism of presynaptic inhibition. Amplifier *a* is used to record the intracellular potential of excitatory terminal *e*; amplifier *b*, to record the intracellular potential of the postsynaptic cell. The experimenter is equipped to stimulate excitatory fiber *e* as well as presynaptic inhibitory fiber *i*. If an impulse arrives in *i* before an impulse in *e*, then terminal *e* is depolarized, and the amplitude of its own impulse curtailed. Consequently less transmitter is released, and the EPSP generated in *b* is smaller. Unlike IPSPs, presynaptic inhibition does not affect the membrane potential or membrane conductance of the postsynaptic cell. (Note: So far no one has succeeded to record the intracellular potential of presynaptic terminals in the mammalian central nervous system. The theory of presynaptic inhibition is based on recordings made from mammalian afferent fibers at considerable distances from the synaptic terminals and from the presynaptic elements of the giant synapses of squids.)

investigators. If it never happens under physiological conditions, then this may be either (1) because normally the presynaptic depolarization related to presynaptic inhibition is strong enough to trigger impulses; or (2) because the afferent depolarization is too slow, and accommodation prevents excitation of terminal *e*. There are yet other reasons why controversy still surrounds the topic of presynaptic inhibition and this would be a good reason not to say much more about it. There is, however, one more point worth mentioning. Many investigators believe that γ-aminobutyric acid (GABA) is the transmitter of presynaptic inhibition in the spinal cord. It indeed is a fact that while GABA causes hyperpolarization of many neurons of the brain and of the cerebellum, it causes depolarization of the intraspinal terminals of primary afferent neurons and of their cell bodies in the sensory dorsal root ganglia. Since this depolarization is mediated by Cl^- ions, in these neurons, unlike many others, E_{Cl} is less negative than the resting potential, being perhaps -30 or -40 mV (cf. Tables 2.1 and 2.2). The level of $[Cl^-]_i$ must be higher in those neurons which depolarize when g_{Cl} is increased than in those cells which hyperpolarize under the same condition (see Sections 2.4b and 2.5d).

3.3. Clinical Electrophysiology of Nerve and Muscle

3.3a. ELECTROMYOGRAPHY (EMG)

The electrical potentials generated by skeletal muscles can be examined with small metal disc electrodes fastened to the surface of the skin over a muscle, or with needle electrodes inserted into the muscle. The latter method gives better recordings but is somewhat painful. The tip of needle electrodes can be made small enough to record the activity from the collection of muscle fibers innervated by the branches of one motor axon. These are called *motor unit action potentials* (see Section 15.1). The electric activity of the muscle is usually examined under three kinds of conditions.

1. At rest, that is with the subject relaxing the examined muscle, and in the absence of electric stimulation. In normal muscle there is no detectable electrical activity under these conditions, except that produced by the movement of a needle electrode which irritates muscle fibers. Spontaneous activity in a resting muscle can be a sign of abnormality. Impulse discharge by *individual muscle fibers* is called *fibrillation*, and usually indicates that fibers have lost their innervation. If an entire motor unit discharges, the recorded potential is of larger amplitude and more complex in form than fibrillation potentials because the impulses of several muscle fibers are superimposed. The uncalled-for firing of *motor units* is *fasciculation*. If a superficial muscle fasciculates, small twitching movements can often be seen through the skin but fibrillations are too small to be observed without EMG electrodes. Fasciculation frequently occurs in healthy individuals, especially if fatigued, and after excessive caffeine intake, but in combination with other neurological signs it may indicate disease of ventral horn cells or of their axons in peripheral nerves. Myotonia (see Section 3.4d) can often also be recognized from EMG examination of resting muscle.

2. Voluntary contraction is also routinely examined by EMG. The pattern of activation (*recruitment*: see Sections 4.2c and 15.1c) of motor units and the form and amplitude of their action potentials are of diagnostic interest. For example, after partial lesion of the motor nerve, during regeneration, as surviving motor axons reinnervate previously denervated muscle fibers (Section 3.4f), motor unit potentials increase abnormally in amplitude and duration.

3. Compound action potentials of the muscle are usually recorded with electrodes placed on the skin, and are evoked by transcutaneous stimulation of the motor fibers innervating the muscle (Fig. 3.14). One purpose of this technique is to measure motor nerve conduction velocity (see next section and Fig. 1.1).

3.3b. MOTOR NERVE CONDUCTION VELOCITY

If a peripheral nerve is stimulated and the resulting action potential is recorded from a muscle, the time elapsing between stimulus and response (the latent time) is occupied by: (1) conduction of nerve impulses in the motor fibers; (2) transmission across the nerve-muscle junction; and (3) the initiation of muscle impulses by the EPP. In order

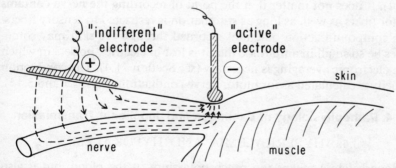

Figure 3.14. Current flow during transcutaneous stimulation. The stimulus is effective where the nerve lies near a cathode placed on the skin, because it is here that the current flows outward through the fibers in the nerve. Since much of the current is shunted through inactive tissues, relatively large voltages and currents must be used. To avoid electrolytic damage to the skin and subcutaneous tissue and to avoid stimulating cutaneous nociceptive fibers (cf. Chapter 6), pulses of the shortest possible duration should be used. The diagram shows monopolar stimulation, but the principle is not different from that using bipolar electrodes, as in Figure 1.1*B* or 3.15.

to measure the conduction time in the motor nerve, the nerve is stimulated at two points. The distance between the two points is the conduction distance and the difference in latent times when stimulating at the two points is the conduction time. Conduction distance divided by conduction time is conduction velocity. This is the principle that Helmholtz used over a century ago to determine nerve conduction velocity; only the equipment has changed (Fig. 1.1).

3.3c. SENSORY NERVE ACTION POTENTIALS AND CONDUCTING VELOCITIES

To examine sensory nerve fibers, a favorable anatomical location must be found. A nerve is chosen which contains mainly sensory and no, or only a few, motor fibers. The digital nerves are frequently chosen. The stimulating electrodes may be in the form of two metal rings which éncircle a digit, or else similar to those shown in Figure 1.1B. The recording electrodes are placed on the skin over the nerve proximally at some distance from the stimulating electrodes. One can either stimulate at one point and record at two different distances from the stimulated point (Fig. 3.15, *left*), or one can stimulate the same nerve fibers at two different points, and make recordings from the same site (Fig. 3.15, *right*). It does not matter if at the point of recording the nerve contains motor fibers as well, as long as stimulation is restricted to sensory fibers. The compound action potential recorded through the skin may sometimes be so small in amplitude that it is lost in electric "noise," in which case electronic averaging is necessary (see Section 21.4). The conduction velocity is calculated as for motor nerve conduction (Figs. 1.1 and 3.15).

3.4. Pathophysiology of Excitation and Junctional Transmission

3.4a. HYPERKALEMIA AND HYPOKALEMIA

Hyperkalemia means too much potassium in the blood, but it also implies excessive levels in other extracellular fluids, with the possible exception of the cerebrospinal, brain interstitial, and intraocular fluids (cf. Chapter 5). Hyperkalemia is common in renal failure and also in disorders of the adrenal cortex. If external K^+ activity is increased near excitable cells without changes in intracellular K^+, the equilibrium potential of K^+ changes (see Section 2.4b). Thus if $[K^+]_o/[K^+]_i$ becomes larger than normal, the result is depolarization. Mild depolarization

Somatosensory Evoked Potentials and Peripheral Nerve Conduction Velocity

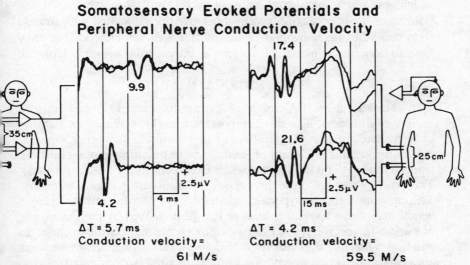

Figure 3.15. Two clinical methods to measure sensory nerve conduction velocity. *Left*, the nerve is stimulated by electrodes on the skin of the wrist; the action potential is recorded through two pairs of electrodes placed over the elbow and shoulder. *Right*, the nerve is stimulated at two points in the arm, and the cortical sensory evoked potential is recorded with EEG electrodes on the scalp. The diagrams show the conduction distances, conduction times and conduction velocites measured in a patient by the two methods. Note different time scales for the two sets of recordings. (Reprinted with permission from Starr et al.: Some applications of evoked potentials. In E. Callaway, P. Tueting and S. H. Koslow (eds.), *Event-Related Brain Potentials*, New York, Academic Press, 1978.)

makes excitable tissue more excitable. Stronger depolarization causes uncalled-for, spontaneous excitation, and severe depolarization blocks impulse generation by inactivating sodium channels.

The tissue that suffers most of hyperkalemia is the heart. At first only the configuration of the electrocardiogram changes without change of rhythm, then ectopic beats and other arrhythmias appear. Severe hyperkalemia can be lethal, causing cardiac arrest.

In potassium depletion (as in hyperaldosteronism) usually both $[K^+]_o$ and $[K^+]_i$ decline. Most of the body's total potassium content is found inside cells. Intracellular potassium therefore serves as a reservoir from which extracellular potassium can be replenished. As long as the ratio $[K^+]_o / [K^+]_i$ remains constant, resting potentials do not change much, even if a significant amount is missing from the total body potassium. Low potassium syndrome is usually associated with muscle weakness, the mechanism of which is not well understood, but may have to do with shrinking cell volume as intracellular solute is depleted.

3.4b. HYPOCALCEMIA

In the laboratory, deficiency of extracellular calcium can cause a variety of disorders. The most important are: (1) increased excitability of nerve and muscle; (2) paralysis of nerve-muscle and other synaptic transmission; and (3) failure of excitation-contraction coupling in some smooth muscles and in cardiac muscle (see Sections 3.1k, 3.2, and 14.3). The first (1 above) of these three groups of disorders is known as *tetany*. The cardinal signs of hypocalcemic tetany are painful muscle cramps which may occur spontaneously, or can be provoked by the examining physician in specific tests. Electrocardiographic signs are common. In children suffering hypocalcemia due to rickets, epileptiform seizures also occur. In other words, the clinical picture is dominated by the instability of nerve and muscle membranes. Hypocalcemic patients rarely if ever suffer muscle paralysis, presumably because the very low level of $[Ca^{2+}]_o$ at which nerve muscle transmission fails is not compatible with survival.

3.4c. HYPOXIA OF NERVE

We all have had an arm or leg "go to sleep" after being held in certain positions for some time. The tingling, numbing and laming of a limb is the result of depolarization in nerves. There are two possible causes: (1) direct pressure on the axons; (2) more frequently, interruption of the blood supply due to pressure on the arteries. Of course both can occur in combination. When the blood supply is interrupted, the main and most immediate cause of impairment is the deprivation of oxygen, but insufficiency of nutrients and the accumulation of waste products make the situation worse.

Withdrawal of oxygen supply stops active transport of ions. Consequently, the cytoplasm of nerve fibers begins to accumulate Na^+ and to lose K^+ ions, and therefore the membrane potential declines. Since the membrane potential is influenced by the ratio of $[K^+]_o/[K^+]_i$ (see Section 2.4b), the depolarization is worse if $[K^+]_o$ increases at the same time as $[K^+]_i$ decreases, than if $[K^+]_i$ alone is changing. The fibers could continue to function for some time if the K^+ ions escaping through the membrane would be cleared away, but since no blood flows, K^+ ions accumulate in the interstitial space. When pressure on the artery is relieved and blood begins to flow again, not only is O_2 readmitted, but excess $[K^+]_o$ is washed away. Consequently recovery occurs in two phases, the first phase being fast as $[K^+]_o$ declines, the second more slow, as Na^+ ions are pumped out and K^+ ions are recaptured.

As long as nerve fibers are only moderately depolarized they are hyperexcitable, since the membrane potential is then closer to threshold. Spontaneous excitation may occur and give rise to the peculiar painful tingling sensation with which we all are familiar. The numbing of fingers and ears in freezing cold weather and the pain associated with re-warming such a numbed body part are also due to hypoxia of nerve fibers. In this case the hypoxia is caused by reflexive constriction of the small arteries.

Large-caliber nerve fibers are more vulnerable to blockade by both pressure and hypoxia than are small fibers. For this reason pain sensation returns into a numbed leg before the appreciation of touch and motor control recover. (cf. Fig. 6.4).

3.4d. MYOTONIA

There is a group of muscle diseases, different in some respects, but having in common a difficulty to relax muscles following a contraction. This clinical sign is called *myotonia*. It occurs in several hereditary conditions, the two most common ones being myotonia congenita and myotonic dystrophy, and it also can be caused by certain toxic agents which affect the muscle membrane.

The diagnostic sign during electromyographic investigation of these patients is a prolonged shower of muscle impulses following contractions, whether voluntary or electrically evoked. If the amplified muscle discharge is made audible with a loudspeaker it gives a characteristic sound due to waxing and waning of the frequency of firing, which EMG specialists call the "dive-bomber discharge."

A similar disease occurs in goats, and their muscles have been examined in great detail. Biopsy samples from human patients have also found their way into the electrophysiological laboratory, and the basic membrane defect causing this condition has been defined rather precisely in at least one form of the disease. The resting membrane conductance is much reduced due to a specific decrease in the chloride conductance, g_{Cl}. In muscle, unlike in nerve membranes, g_{Cl} accounts for most of the "resting" conductance (see Section 2.4b). Pathological decrease of g_{Cl} has two consequences. (1) The depolarizing ("negative") afterpotential is enhanced and prolonged. This afterpotential is caused by the accumulation if K^+ ions outside the membrane during the firing of an action potential (see Section 3.1a), in the case of muscle especially in the T tubules (see Fig. 14.1) from where excess K^+ cannot rapidly diffuse away. With the membrane conductance being too low, the length constant expands (see Section 3.1b), thus depolarization of the T tubule membrane spreads farther into the remainder of the membrane. (2) Less of a Na^+ current is required to start the action potential. The threshold condition in nerve is for I_{Na} to exceed I_K (see Section 3.1a). In normal muscle g_{Cl} is large and I_{Na} has to overcome both $I_K + I_{Cl}$ because both tend to keep membrane potential near the resting level (cf. Section 2.5d). In myotonia g_{Cl} is abnormally low so that one of the two factors opposing excitation is missing. The combined result of these two changes, (1) and (2), is that the myotonic muscle membrane, having fired an action potential, remains depolarized beyond the refractory period due to the prolonged depolarizing afterpotential; this residual depolarization acts on a membrane that is abnormally ready to be excited. The result can be a prolonged burst of repetitive firing.

Whether this description is applicable to all forms of myotonia or only to some is the subject of continuing research.

3.4e. MYASTHENIA GRAVIS

Meaning "grave muscle weakness," this condition was once fatal in the majority of cases within a few years after diagnosis. It is an autoimmune disease in which the immune reaction reduces the concentration of acetylcholine receptor in endplate membranes. An experimental disease resembling human myasthenia has been induced in animals by immunizing them with purified acetylcholine receptor protein. If many of the receptor molecules are missing from the endplate, actylcholine, even though it is normally released, cannot do its job and neuromuscular transmission fails. There is another condition, called *myasthenic syndrome* (of Eaton and Lambert), in which receptors are normal but the amount of acetylcholine released is too small. Although myasthenia gravis and myasthenic syndrome both produce muscle weakness, the pathophysiology is quite different.

Myasthenia gravis can be treated by blocking the enzyme acetylcholinesterase. A variety of drugs, including prostigmine, have this effect. If acetylcholinesterase is inhibited at a normal endplate, then a simple impulse in the motor nerve fiber evokes a brief shower of impulses in the muscle fiber because acetylcholine is not immediately eliminated after it did its job. The extra acetylcholine made available by cholinesterase blockage to a myasthenic nerve-muscle junction enables it to transmit excitation in spite of reduced sensitivity of the endplate membrane. This treatment becomes less effective, however, when the disease has progressed beyond a certain stage. More promising would be correction of the autoimmune condition itself. Operative removal of the thymus gland at an early stage of the disease produces improvement in many patients, perhaps by immunosuppression, although the exact mechanism is unclear. Immunosuppression with corticosteroids and other drugs also causes marked improvement in the majority of patients.

3.4f. DENERVATION OF SKELETAL MUSCLE

Skeletal muscle may lose innervation if motor fibers are torn in an accident or destroyed by disease. After complete and permanent denervation, the muscle atrophies and eventually the muscle fibers are replaced by fibrous connective tissue. If, however, the muscle fibers are reinnervated in time, their function can be saved.

Within a week or two of denervation, skeletal muscle fibers become abnormally sensitive to acetylcholine. This *denervation supersensitivity* is explained in part at least by an expansion of the acetylcholine-sensitive surface. Whereas in normal skeletal muscle fibers acetylcholine receptors are found in the endplate region only, after denervation receptor molecules appear around the endplate and eventually, colonize the entire surface of the fiber. Acetylcholine anywhere in the vicinity of such a fiber causes depolarization. Yet later the supersensitivity disappears, and after some months the fibers no longer respond to acetylcholine at all.

Denervation supersensitivity is not limited to skeletal muscles. For example, Cannon discovered in the 1920s that cutting the sympathetic fibers that innervate the heart causes cardiac muscle to become supersensitive to the adrenergic substances circulating in the bloodsteam. Some investigators consider denervation supersensitivity a universal property of excitable tissues. If so, then some of the disorders caused by lesions of fiber tracts in the central nervous system may be the consequence of such supersensitivity. For example, excessive excitability of spinal neurons after injury of the fiber tracts descending in the white matter of the spinal cord may play a part in causing the spasticity typical of this condition (see Section 15.7).

A few days after denervation of a muscle, fibrillation potentials appear on EMG recordings (see Section 3.3a). Initially, these fibrillations may be caused by small amounts of acetylcholine acting on the supersensitive muscle fibers. Fibrillation persists, however, even after all detectable acetylcholine has disappeared from the muscle. Electrical instability seems to be inherent in the denervated muscle's membrane. Much later, when the muscle has atrophied, it falls electrically silent.

Reinnervation may occur in two ways. In the fortunate case, the severed nerve fibers find their way back into the muscle (*regeneration*) (see next section). If denervation is only partial, then surviving motor axons may also adopt orphaned muscle fibers. To achieve this, the intact axons grow new branches within the muscle (collateral *sprouting*). After reinnervation, the ectopic acetylcholine receptors disappear from the membrane outside the endplate and supersensitivity to acetylcholine subsides.

Whenever reinnervation occurs by the sprouting of new branches of uninjured axons, the end results will be fewer and larger motor units than is normal for that muscle. This condition is recognized by electromyographic examination. In protracted diseases of nerve fibers (neuropathies), signs of denervation and reinnervation may be detected side by side, as some axons degenerate and others sprout new collaterals.

3.4g. THE REGENERATION OF PERIPHERAL NERVE FIBERS

When an axon is cut, its distal half degenerates and dies, but the proximal stump survives. Severed nerve segments wither because they no longer receive sustenance from the cell body. The central stump fares better, because it remains connected to the perikaryon. The deterioration of a disconnected piece of axon is called *Wallerian degeneration.*

In the central nervous system of mammals, severed axons do not regenerate; in peripheral nerves they might. Shortly after its axon has been injured, a cell body reacts in a typical manner that histopathologists call *chromatolysis*. Chromatolysis, once regarded as a sign of retrograde degeneration, is now thought to be a manifestation of increased protein synthesis. Chromatolysis is observed in all injured neurons as these attempt to regenerate the injured axon. In the neurons whose injured axon is in a peripheral nerve, regeneration may succeed; in the central nervous system the attempt always fails. After some weeks or months the unsuccessful central neurons usually die, and *retrograde degeneration* then becomes the correct description of their status.

The exact reason for the failure of regeneration in central axons is not clear. The severed axon does begin to grow, but reaches only a short distance before it stops. A glial scar forms at the site of the trauma, and this has been blamed for stopping the growth process. The proliferation of glial cells may, however, be a reaction to the failure and not its cause.

It has recently been shown that where synaptic sites on central neurons have been vacated by the degenerated terminals of severed axons, newly formed sprouts grow out of surviving healthy fibers and may "colonize" the vacated synaptic sites. Whether these anatomically recognizable newly formed connections actually perform a useful function is not yet known.

The regeneration of severed peripheral axons is guided by Schwann cells. These cells survive after the axon has been cut because, unlike the axon, they retain their own nucleus and other intracellular equipment. Following Wallerian degeneration of an axon, the Schwann cells change shape and line up in cords. These cords guide the growth of regenerating axons. The closer the two cut ends of the nerve remain after an accident, the better the chances for regeneration. Suturing the two ends together as soon as possible helps a great deal.

3.5. Summary of Chapters 2 and 3

1. The membrane potential of excitable cells is determined by (a) the gradient of activities of various ions across the membrane; (b) the relative permeabilities for those ions; and, to a much lesser degree, (c) electrogenic transport of ions.
2. The transmembrane activity gradient of ions is maintained by active transport, fueled by adenosine triphosphate.
3. The great majority of the membrane potential changes that are related to the normal function of nerve and muscle cells are brought about by changes of the permeability to one or more ions (see 1b above). Pathological changes often involve altered ion gradients.
4. Propagated impulses are generated by voltage-dependent permeability changes, effected by the opening and closing of voltage-gated ion channels. The voltage dependence of these ion conductance changes is the key to the positive feedback character of action potentials.
5. The conductance changes that cause generator potentials, receptor potentials, synaptic potentials, and endplate potentials are not voltage-dependent. Their magnitude and time course are governed by agents that are extrinsic to the cell and its membrane, either a sensory stimulus or a chemical transmitter substance.
6. The intensity of the membrane current carried by an ion is determined by the product of its driving potential and the membrane conductance for that

ion. The driving potential is the difference between the equilibrium potential of the ion and the prevailing membrane potential.

7. Generally speaking, the following conductance changes cause depolarization: increased g_{Na} or decreased g_K. The following cause hyperpolarization: decrease of g_{Na} or increase of g_K. An increase of g_{Cl} may cause either depolarization or hyperpolarization, depending on whether E_{Cl} is less negative or more negative than E_m.

8. Action potentials of axons and skeletal muscle fibers are generated by the activation of g_{Na} and then of g_K in rapid sequence. In many smooth muscle cells, in cardiac muscle fibers, and at presynaptic axon terminals g_{Ca} is also increased during the action potential.

9. Endplate potentials (EPPs) are generated by the simultaneous increase of both g_{Na} and g_K, such that the two become very nearly equal. Excitatory postsynaptic potentials (EPSPs) may be generated by an increase of g_{Na} alone, an increase of both g_{Na} and g_K, or a decrease of g_K. Inhibitory postsynaptic potentials (IPSPs) of many central neurons involve an increase of g_{Cl} with a possible lesser contribution by g_K.

10. Excess external potassium activity ($[K^+]_o$) depolarizes membranes, increases excitability and, eventually, blocks impulse generation and conduction. Decreased $[Ca^{2+}]_o$ causes many disturbances, of which the clinically most important is hyperexcitability of nerve and muscle membranes (tetany). Magnesium poisoning causes failure of synaptic transmission, clinically manifested as paralysis of nerve-muscle transmission.

NOTES ON THE RULE OF "ALL OR NONE"

When firing an action potential, an axon membrane is supposed to "give all it has." This is because of the positive feedback represented by activating voltage-gated Na^+ channels (see Fig. 3.1). It is in the nature of positive feedback processes to progress until one or other essential ingredient of the reaction is depleted. Explosions are typical examples, but the "explosion" of g_{Na} during an action potential is limited by inactivation and by the rise of g_K.

The rule of *all or none* does not mean, however, that impulses are of equal amplitude under all conditions. If an impulse is successfully fired in the relative refractory period, it is smaller than usual. If the impulse is fired by a previously depolarized membrane, its amplitude is also reduced (see Section 3.2c). If, due to pathology, $[Na^+]_o$ is deficient, the impulse will be curtailed.

The correct meaning of the all or none rule is that the *magnitude of the response is not determined by the magnitude of the stimulus*. In this respect impulses differ in a very fundamental sense from receptor potentials, generator potentials, EPSPs and IPSPs, the magnitude of all of which depends on the magnitude of an external stimulus or the amount of available transmitter agent. A summary of the differences between all-or-none action potentials and the *graded* potential signals will now follow.

Summary Table of Properties of Conducted and Non-Conducted Nerve Signals

Conducted Signals (Impulses)	Noncanducted Signals: (Receptor Potentials, Generator Potentials, EPPs, EPSPs)
Are conducted without decrement	Spread by electrotonus only
Have threshold	No detectable threshold (theoretically, each molecule of transmitter causes some change of membrane conductance)
Magnitude: all-or-none	Magnitude determined by stimulus, or by amount of transmitter (gradable)
Time course invariant	Time course determined by presence of stimulus and of transmitter, as modified by adaptation (see Section 4.5) and by desensitization (see Section 4.5).
Refractory period	No refractory period
Summation not possible (because of refractory period and all-or-none feature)	Summation possible (see Fig. 4.2).

Summary of Properties Related to Axon Diameter

Large diameter fibers, compared to smaller ones: (1) are more readily excited by shorter and weaker stimulation current pulses (but see recruitment of neurons in a neuron pool in Section 15.1c); (2) have a shorter time constant and a longer space constant; (3) conduct action potentials faster (because of (2) above); (4) are less easily blocked by local anesthetic drugs; (5) are more easily blocked by pressure and hypoxia; (6) recover function more slowly after injury than small fibers.

Further Reading: Chapters 1, 2 and 3

Books and Reviews

Brazier MAB: *The Electrical Activity of the Nervous System.* New York, McMillan, 1963.

Dale HH: Transmission of nervous effects by acetylcholine. *Harvey Lectures* 32:229–245, 1937.

Eccles JC: *The Physiology of Synapses.* New York, Springer, 1964.

Halliday AM, McDonald WI: Pathophysiology of demyelinating disease. *Br Med Bull* 33:21–27, 1977.

Kandel ER: *Cellular Basis of Behavior.* San Francisco, Freeman, 1976.

Katz B: *Nerve, Muscle and Synapse.* New York, McGraw-Hill, 1966.

Krnjevic K: Pre- and postsynaptic inhibition. *Adv Exp Med Biol* 123:271–286, 1979.

Kuffler SW, Nicholls JG: *From Neuron to Brain.* Sunderland Mass., Sinauer, 1976.

Sernka T, Jacobson E: *Gastrointestinal Physiology: The Essentials.* Baltimore, Williams & Wilkins, 1973.

Siegel GJ, Albers RW, Agranoff BW, et al: *Basic Neurochemistry*, ed 3. Boston, Little, Brown, 1981.

Smith JJ, Kampine JP: *Circulatory Physiology: The Essentials.* Baltimore, Williams & Wilkins, 1980.

Articles

Brock LG, Coombs JS Eccles JC: The recording of potentials from motoneurones with intracellular electrodes. *J Physiol (Lond)* 117:431–460, 1952.

Hodgkin AL, Huxley AF: A quantitative description of membrane current and its application to conduction and excitation in nerve. *J Physiol (Lond)* 117:500–544, 1952.

Huxley AF, Stämpfli R: Evidence for saltatory conduction in peripheral myelinated nerve fibers. *J Physiol (Lond)* 108:315–339, 1949.

Llinas R, Sugimori M: Electrophysiological properties of in vitro Purkinje cell dendrites in mammalian cerebellar slices. *J Physiol (Lond)* 305:197–213, 1980.

chapter 4

The Integration of Nerve Signals

How neurons are interconnected and how they interact; how such interactions operate to generate electroencephalographic waves; how their derangement causes seizures.

4.1. Integration in Nervous System

Sherrington's book, *The Integrative Action of the Nervous System*, appeared in 1906. Many reckon the start of the modern experimental study of the physiology of the nervous system from that date. Significant discoveries had, of course, been made before. To name but one, half a century earlier Sechenov inferred the existence of inhibitory processes in the central nervous system from observations he made on headless frogs. But Sherrington introduced the quantitative analytical approach into the study of the central nervous system, and his work stands out because of its lucidity, precision and absence of vague generalizations.

By "integrative action" Sherrington meant the ability of the central nervous system to respond appropriately to the multitude of sensory signals that reach it. Neural integration consists, then, of a weighted summing of the effects of stimuli, some of which may counteract one another, to produce adaptive responses. The environment acts on an organism through the sense organs the signals of which flow in vast streams into the central nervous system. In response the organism acts on the environment with its muscles and, to a lesser degree, its glands. Muscles are stimulated to move by motor neurons and, for this reason, Sherrington called motor cells the *final common path* of nerve signals.

Between primary afferent neurons and motor neurons lie the great majority of the nerve cells that constitute the central nervous system. It was Sherrington who also coined the term *synapse* to describe the functional junctions between neurons. He perceived the pattern of multiple synaptic interconnections to be the anatomical substrate for the integrative action of the nervous system.

The pioneer neuroanatomists of the second half of the 19th century and of the early 20th, foremost among them Golgi and Ramón y Cajal, described the morphology of the cells that make up the central gray matter and began tracing their connections. The great variety of shapes of neurons and of the arborization of their processes became apparent (see Fig 1.4). It was realized that the axon of a neuron may branch to make contact with many, sometimes thousands, of other neurons—the phenomenon of *divergence*. On the other hand any one neuron may receive synaptic terminals from many different cells—*convergence*.

The multiplicity of divergent and convergent synaptic connections makes neural integration possible. At points of confluence nerve signals can intereact. Summation, facilitation, occlusion and inhibition are the elementary interactions between nerve signals. Their mechanism will be the topic of the following sections.

4.2. Reflexes

One of the most used words in the vocabulary of physiology, and one of the least precisely defined, is "reflex." It means, more or less, any *neurally mediated, predictable response to a stimulus,* or to a combination of stimuli. This definition does not specify the level or the component part of the nervous system mediating the response. Many reflexes are spinal, others are integrated in the brain stem, and some are cortical (e.g., see Section 18.4b). Nor is it explicitly stated in this definition whether an action could be called a reflex if it were the result of a conscious decision, of an "act of will." Most writers probably imply when calling a response a reflex that it occurred "automatically" without conscious deliberation on the part of the subject. There is, however, no reliable way to recognize volition in an experimental animal, and for this reason most authors find it expedient to ignore the question when describing animal behavior.

The problem of how to deal with the neural phenomena of conscious processes has vexed generations of neuroscientists. Some seem to wish the problem would just go away. Pavlov, so the story goes, imposed fines on any collaborator who mentioned or implied that a neural process may have anything to do with conscious mind. Numerous other students of human and animal behavior adopted a similarly hostile stance. Unlike theoreticians, medical practitioners could not ignore the conscious feelings of their patients, for such an attitude would invalidate the very foundation of the profession. But, ethics aside, diagnosis would also become unnecessarily difficult if the physician were not allowed to ask his patient how he feels and what it is that hurts him. As a matter of fact, the very first task of the doctor may sometimes be to find out whether the patient is conscious.

Abhorrence of the topic of consciousness is not universal even among experimental biologists, of course, and there have been attempts to discover the neurophysiological basis of conscious experiences. That research in this area is more difficult than in most others should be obvious without elaboration. The little that we do know will not be ignored in this text. But, as far as the concept of a reflex is concerned, we will have to follow the lead of others and simply eliminate the question of volition from consideration, for the reasons already given.

In everyday life, simple reflexes are rare. Most actions of humans and other mammals are not reflexive responses governed by stimuli arising in the immediate environment. Instead, an individual's behavior is shaped by his past, by his individual memory and by the "memory" of his species, laid down in genetic code, and his behavior is directed toward goals he projects into the future. The stimuli that act on his sensory receptors at any one moment serve as navigational aids by which he finds his way towards his goal. The stimuli acting on sense organs therefore neither propel nor fully define an individual's activity, although they do guide it and set its limits.

The simple reflexes that are so often evoked in the diagnostic clinic and in the research laboratory are thus, for the most part, artefacts. As such they are quite useful, of course. Tapping the patellar tendon with a reflex hammer is a useful way to probe the functioning of spinal neural circuits, even if our knees do not usually make similar jerking movements under ordinary circumstances. In research, we consider the study of simple reflexes as a first step toward analyzing more complex neuronal processes.

4.2a. REFLEX ARC

The pathway of a reflex may consist of (1) a sense organ, (2) a set of afferent neurons, (3) interneurons in the central nervous system, (4) a set of efferent neurons, and (5) an effector organ, usually a muscle or a gland. The simplest reflexes are *monosynaptic*. In a monosynaptic arc the afferent neurons excite the efferent neurons directly, and there are no interneurons involved. A monosynaptic reflex is mediated by a *two-neuron arc*. The special case of the *axon reflex* is described in Section 17.3b.

4.2b. UNCONDITIONAL AND CONDITIONAL REFLEXES

The original paradigm* of the Pavlovian or "classical" conditional reflex is well known. A dog was given some meat; he salivated. Then, next time, a bell sounded before the meat was shown. This sequence, bell-before-meat, was repeated several times. Soon the dog salivated at the sound of the bell. We could say that the dog "learned that the bell announced meat," but then we would not be using scientific language. Properly said, the paired presentation of the *conditional stimulus* (the bell) with the *unconditional stimulus* (the meat) is the condition for acquiring a *conditional† reflex.* Thus, unconditional reflexes are *inborn,* conditional reflexes are *acquired.*

While Pavlov made his first observations in Russia, the foundations were laid in America for the behaviorist approach to experimental psychology. Unaware at first of Pavlov's work, behaviorists used terms similar to Pavlov's but meaning something rather different. In the process of *instrumental conditioning* (later, *operant conditioning*) an animal learns to perform certain acts in response to specific sensory cues to achieve certain goals. For example, he operates a lever to obtain food or to avoid an electric shock announced by a flashing light or a sound. Such conditioned behavior differs from classical or Pavlovian conditional reflexes in a very essential respect. In instrumental conditioning the experiment is arranged in such a way that a "correct" response "pays off"; the animal either gets a reward or avoids something unpleasant. In establishing a classical conditional reflex the schedule of stimulations is not influenced by the animal's behavior. The dog does not get more meat if it produces more saliva.

4.2c. FACILITATION, INHIBITION, AND OCCLUSION

Sometimes two different stimuli can evoke the same reflex response. The question then is, if both are presented at the same time, what will the response be? If the response is contraction of a muscle or secretion of a gland, then the answer can be given in quantitative terms. We could, for example, measure the amount of saliva secreted when a dog

---

* Paradigm: Gr. *paradigma,* example or pattern.

† Conditional: In much of the English language literature the spelling is "condition*ed*" instead of "condition*al*" reflex. This, it is said, is due to a mistranslation in an early English edition of Pavlov's work. In other languages the problem does not arise (e.g. *reflexe conditionel; bedinger Reflex; feltételes reflex*).

is given a piece of meat, or when he chews on a bone, and finally when he is given both at the same time.

Such a trial could have one of several theoretically possible results. (1) The magnitude of the response to the combined presentation of two stimuli could be *less* than that produced when one of the stimuli was given alone. In this case one stimulus *inhibited* the effect of the other. (2) The response could be equal to that produced by either stimulus alone, or it could be more than evoked by one, but *less than the sum* of the two responses. This is called *occlusion*. (3) Or, the response to the combined presentation of the two stimuli could be *equal to the sum* of those produced when each stimulus was given separately. In this case the effect of the two stimuli would be simply *summated*. (4) Finally, the response to the combination of the two stimuli could *exceed* the sum of the responses to separate presentations. If so, then there would be *facilitation* between the two stimuli.

The magnitude of a response, be it the secretion of a gland or the contraction of a muscle, is determined by the *number* of efferent *neurons* firing impulses, multiplied by the average *number* of impulses fired by each. If the response takes an appreciable length of time then, instead of total number of impulses, it is more appropriate to speak of the number of impulses per unit time; that is to say the *rate of firing*.

Figure 4.1 illustrates the manner in which convergence of input signals enables the interactions just described. For simplicity, assume that all fibers fire only one impulse, but the number of active input and output fibers varies. Causing more and more neurons to fire is called *recruitment*. Of a *pool* of available neurons, cells are *recruited* into the *discharging fraction* of the pool. A pool could consist of the neurons of a motor nucleus or any other collection of cells which could be activated by convergent afferent nerve fibers.

To explain facilitation, Sherrington postulated that central neurons could be *subliminally* excited. He conceived of subliminal excitation as a state of enhanced readiness to discharge, without actually firing impulses. If two different stimuli would, each by itself, cause a certain group of neurons to be subliminally excited, then the convergent effect of both may recruit them into the discharging fraction (Fig. 4.1*A*). Several decades later Sherrington's former student, J. C. Eccles, demonstrated that neurons in the central nervous system may indeed be depolarized subliminally by impulses fired by afferent fibers, and coined the term excitatory postsynaptic potential (EPSP) to describe it (see Section 2.5b).

A.   Spatial facilitation   B.   Occlusion

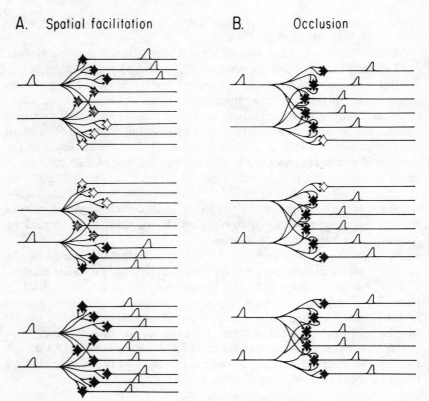

Figure 4.1. The principles of spatial facilitation and occlusion. On each diagram afferent fibers, drawn on the *left* side, make excitatory synaptic contacts with postsynaptic neurons (*center*), whose axons point to the *right*. The conduction of an impulse is indicated by the action potential drawn on the axon. Discharging neurons are *black*, subliminally excited neurons, *shaded*. *A*, facilitation: an impulse arriving in one of the two afferent fibers causes discharge in three and subliminal excitation in three others of the nine available postsynaptic neurons; impulses arriving in both afferent fibers cause the discharge of all 9 postsynaptic neurons. In *B*, occlusion: an impulse arriving in 1 of the 2 afferent fibers is sufficient to cause the discharge of 5 of the 6 available postsynaptic neurons.

Since impulses generated by central neurons are started at the initial segment of the axon (see Section 1.3) but most excitatory synapses are scattered over the surface of the dendrites, the EPSPs generated by these synapses must spread by electrotonus (cf. Section 2.5a) to the initial segment. The more excitatory synapses are active at once, the more the initial segment will be depolarized. The influence that any one of these synapses can have on the membrane potential of the initial segment varies inversely with its distance and directly with the mean cross-sectional area of the dendrites that connect it to the cell body (cf. definition of length constant, Section 3.1b). The effect of different synapses is thus weighted (or biased) according to their "electrotonic distance" from the initial segment.

The mutual reinforcement by synapses scattered over the surface of a neuron is called *spatial summation*. Spatial summation of EPSPs makes *spatial facilitation* of a reflex possible, since it enables the recruitment of otherwise subliminally excited neurons. Besides spatial facilitation, we speak of *temporal facilitation*. This can occur if two volleys of afferent impulses arrive within a short enough time, so that the (subliminal) EPSP evoked by the first has not yet subsided when the second arrives (Figs. 1.6 and 4.2A). Since EPSPs have no refractory period, the second EPSP can be superimposed on the first, and thus it has a better chance to exceed the threshold voltage of the cell.

Facilitation can occur, then, if part of the available neurons are subliminally excited, "on reserve" so to speak, and ready to be recruited into the discharging fraction. Spatial facilitation is possible whenever such subliminally excited neurons are accessible to excitation by two or more sets of convergent afferent fibers. On the other hand occlusion results when a set of neurons is liminally excited by either of two convergent sets of afferent fibers (Fig. 4.1B). Occlusion is similar to getting a "busy signal" when calling a station by telephone. The neurons which have already discharged are not available for further excitation until their refractory period has passed. Inhibition differs from occlusion in that it actually prevents excitation from taking place, or extinguishes it if it already is in progress. The biophysical substrate of inhibition is the inhibitory postsynaptic potential (IPSP), discussed in Section 2.5d, but in some cases may be presynaptic inhibition (see Section 3.2c).

4.3. Potentiation, Rebound and Other Non-Linear Synaptic Processes

In the discussion so far it was assumed that presynaptic nerve impulses always release the same amount of transmitter substance, and that the postsynaptic membrane response is always uniform. Interaction of EPSPs and IPSPs was considered as a linear process, mediated by the passive (electrotonic) processes of the postsynaptic membranes. In real-

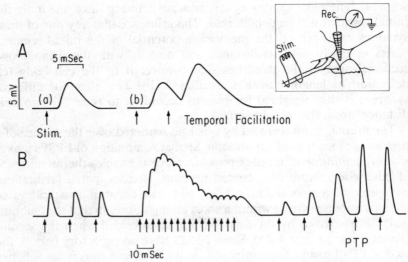

Figure 4.2. Some non-linear processes evoked at synapses by repetitive stimulation. The *inset* shows the recording conditions: an afferent pathway is stimulated electrically, and intracellular recordings are made from one of the postsynaptic neurons. For the sake of illustration all input volleys are assumed to cause only subliminal excitation (EPSPs) in the postsynaptic neuron. A: a, EPSP evoked by a single stimulus; b, by two stimuli in rapid succession. B: to the *left* are the responses to 3 stimuli delivered at low frequency followed by a train of high-frequency stimuli, and then the responses to further 5 stimuli at low frequency. Note that A and B are not drawn to the same time scale, and time relations in B are distorted to fit all responses into the picture. For further explanation see text.

ity synaptic processes are influenced by non-linear processes—some, for example, that depend on the immediate past history of the synapse, in other words whether the synapse has recently transmitted or not.

Figure 4.2B illustrates the result of repeated excitation of a synapse. To simplify this illustration the propensity of the postsynaptic neuron to fire impulses has been neglected and only EPSPs are shown. During high-frequency repetitive stimulation, instead of EPSPs of equal size, one following the other and each added on the top of its predecessor, the amplitudes grow for the first few EPSPs in a "train," but later diminish. Then, after cessation of the repetitive stimulation, individual EPSPs become for a while much larger than in the control state.

The initial growth of EPSPs during high-frequency repetitive stimulation is called *facilitation of the EPSP* (sometimes post-activation potentiation). The difference between facilitation of a reflex and facilitation of the EPSP should be noted. In speaking of facilitation of a reflex, we mean that an increased number of postsynaptic neurons fire an increased number of impulses (see preceding section). By facilitation of the EPSP we mean that the amplitude of individual EPSPs has increased. Facilitation of a reflex could be caused by linear summation of EPSPs. Facilitation of EPSPs may be, but need not be, an additional factor in causing the (temporal) facilitation of a reflex.

The apparent fatigue of the EPSPs seen to follow their facilitation in a prolonged train (Fig. 4.2*B*) may be the combined result of a decrease in the amount of transmitter available for release and of a desensitization of the postsynaptic membrane, about which more will be said presently (Section 4.5).

The great enhancement of individual EPSPs that occurs after a train of high-frequency stimulation has been completed is called *post-tetanic potentiation*. For reasons that cannot be detailed here it seems likely that the mechanisms of post-tetanic potentiation and EPSP facilitation are different. The one factor that the two seem to have in common is the release of a greater than usual amount of transmitter with each presynaptic nerve impulse.

Post-tetanic potentiation is a general property of junctions, including neuromuscular endplates. At the nerve-muscle junction of skeletal muscles it normally plays no role, because each impulse arriving in any motor nerve terminal always releases enough acetylcholine to cause the muscle fiber to discharge an impulse. (Concerning potentiation of contraction, as distinct from transmission, see Section 14.2a.) But in myasthenic muscle (see Section 3.4e) and in muscle paralyzed by curare-like drugs, post-tetanic potentiation is clearly detectable. In these cases some or all of the endplates may fail to transmit when the motor nerve is stimulated by single pulses. Following a brief tetanic stimulation some of the blocked junctions may transmit again.

In the synapses of the spinal monosynaptic segmental reflex (see Section 15.3a) post-tetanic potentiation reaches its maximum about a minute after the repetitive stimulation has ceased and lasts for 4–8 minutes. In some other synapses it may last longer. Warming up for exercise entails the opening of the microcirculation in muscles and getting muscle fibers themselves in an optimal state for doing work. But it is conceivable that post-tetanic potentiation of the central synapses that control the muscles to be exercised is also important for enhancing the speed and vigor of their movements.

A rather different kind of potentiation of excitatory synaptic transmission has recently been discovered in the hippocampal formation. Unlike spinal post-tetanic potentiation, which lasts for a few minutes, the potentiation of hippocampal synapses lasts for hours or days, some say perhaps for the lifetime of the synapse. For reasons that we will discuss in Chapter 20, the hippocampal formation is believed to be a key component of the neuronal circuits involved in memory processes. The *long-term potentiation* of hippocampal synapses may be important in the formation of new memory traces. In simplistic terms these synapses appear to "remember" when they have been excited. There are indications that long-term potentiation is associated with the formation of additional receptor molecules in the postsynaptic membranes, but whether this is the complete explanation of the phenomenon is not yet clear.

Synaptic inhibition is often followed by *rebound excitation*. The phenomenon is reminiscent of post-hyperpolarization (anode-off) excitation (Fig. 3.10), but the mechanism may be more involved in the case of synapses than in nerve fibers subjected to electric current. Post-inhibitory rebound excitation is believed by some to be a key element in generating the rhythmic oscillations of electroencephalograph (EEG) tracings (see Section 4.8)

4.4. Dendritic Spikes

For some years it has been debated whether the dendrites of central neurons generate action potentials. The answer seems to be a qualified yes. Voltage-dependent, self-regenerative, all-or-none responses have been demonstrated in the dendrites of some large neurons, most convincingly the Purkinje cells of the cerebellum (see Section 18.3b). These responses differ in several important respects from impulses conducted in the axons of the same cells. The dendritic responses are longer, sometimes up to 10 msec in duration. Moreover, they seem to depend in part or in whole on an inward current of Ca^{2+} instead of Na^+. It will be remembered that Ca^{2+} inward current also occurs when impulses arrive at the presynaptic terminals of axons, where it triggers transmitter release (see Section 3.2), and during impulse firing of certain cell bodies, where it opens the Ca^{2+}-gated K^+ channels responsible for the after-hyperpolarization (see Section 3.1k).

We do not yet know whether dendritic action potentials, Ca^{2+}-dependent or otherwise, occur in many neurons or only in a selected few. Nor have the theoretical consequences of the dendritic action potentials for the transmission of excitation to cells been thought through. One thing is clear, however: the dendrites of neurons that generate voltage-dependent responses are not passive summators of EPSPs and IPSPs, but highly non-linear reactors.

4.5. Accommodation, Adaptation, Desensitization, and Habituation

Excitation may change as a function of time, even if stimulation remains at a constant level. This happens in various excitable cells, for various reasons, by different mechanisms. Some of these are discussed elsewhere in this text (see Sections 3.1f, 6.1, and 20.3a), but this seems to be a good place for a brief general summary of temporal excitability change to contrast the various forms it can take.

Earlier (Section 3.1f) we became acquainted with *accommodation*, an increase in the threshold depolarization of nerve fibers when stimulated by current of slow rise, instead of sudden onset (Fig. 3.9). A related phenomenon is seen when a nerve cell is stimulated by a prolonged suprathreshold constant current. When so stimulated, neurons usually start firing at a high rate and then slow down (Fig. 4.3). This is sometimes described as *spike frequency adaptation*, sometimes as a special case of accommodation.

We speak of *adaptation of a sense organ* if the organ responds to a

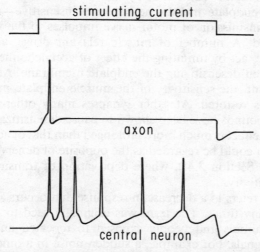

Figure 4.3. Stimulation of a peripheral axon and a central neuron by prolonged suprathreshold current. Note that the spike potential of the axon is followed by a brief and small after-hyperpolarization, and that after the first one no further impulses are fired. Spikes generated in central neurons are followed by large and prolonged after-hyperpolarizations, and impulses are fired as long as the depolarizing current is maintained. Note also spike frequency adaptation of the central neuron.

constant stimulus at first with strong and then with gradually decreasing excitation. Adaptation is a feature of many but not all sense organs. Its significance will be discussed in Section 6.1. At one time it was thought that the adaptation of primary afferent neurons may be related to the accommodation (or spike frequency adaptation) of the nerve fiber. It is now clear, however, that the most important factor causing adaptation of sense organs is usually in the transducing mechanism itself. The crucial difference is this: accommodation involves an increase of the electric threshold, whereas sense organ adaptation is mainly due to a decline of the receptor potential (or generator potential) in the face of constant intensity stimulations.

Some sensory nerve endings do not adapt, but on the contrary they become *sensitized* when exposed to prolonged stimulation. Examples are however fewer than of adaptation (see Section 6.7).

Desensitization means a decreasing effectiveness of a chemical transmitter or other neuroactive compound. An example is the effect of acetylcholine at the neuromuscular junction. Under normal conditions acetylcholine is rapidly eliminated by cholinesterase. If, however, this is prevented the endplate membrane becomes insensitive—so much so that further transmission of motor nerve impulses to the muscle fiber can be blocked. A number of muscle relaxant drugs, among them succinylcholine, act by imitating the effect of acetylcholine, first depolarizing and then desensitizing the endplate membrane. After removal of such an agent, the sensitivity of the muscle endplate membrane to acetylcholine is restored. At other synapses many other neuroactive chemical compounds have been shown to cause desensitization, and in some cases the effect is much more prolonged than that of acetylcholine. Desensitization could be regarded as the opposite of denervation supersensitivity (see Section 3.4f), where deprivation of transmitter causes enhanced sensitivity.

Habituation refers to a decrease in response that occurs as a stimulus is repeated many times. The term was originally used to describe the behavior of animals and people exposed to repeated and otherwise insignificant signals. For example, a sudden noise in a quiet room can at first arouse attention, but if repeated many times it becomes less and less interesting. Habituation is considered to be the simplest form of learning (see Section 20.3a). The term is now used not only to describe the behavior of intact organisms, but also of simple synaptic systems.

Myelinated axons in peripheral nerves usually fire only one or two impulses in response to a constant current, no matter how strong the stimulus (Fig. 4.3). However, pulsatile (as opposed to constant current) stimulation can cause repetitive firing of axons. When the cell body— more precisely the initial segment of the axon—of a neuron, or the sensory terminal of an afferent fiber is depolarized by a supraliminal constant current, it usually continues to fire as long as the depolarization lasts, but the rate usually decreases as a result of adaptation (see above). This is in keeping with the diverse functions of these various parts of neurons, since the myelinated portion of an axon is not normally exposed to constant depolarization, whereas the unmyelinated sensory terminal and the initial segment often are, the former by generator potentials and the latter by EPSPs.

The spike-generating Na^+ channels of myelinated axons are inactivated during long-maintained depolarization and this is the reason that only one impulse is fired. Sensory terminals and central neurons are capable of prolonged repetitive firing because of so called slow voltage- and time-dependent ion conductance changes. Many kinds of excitable membranes seem to be endowed with a number of different "slow" voltage-dependent ion channels and new ones are still being discovered. K^+ ions, for example, can pass through at least six different kinds of channels, but not all six are present in all excitable membranes. For a very simplified scheme of how repetitive firing could be maintained by a constant depolarizing current consider the following sequence: after the first spike has been elicited by the depolarizing stimulus, K^+ conductance increases and remains high for a while (the mechanism of the after-hyperpolarization; see Section 3.1). This K^+ current counteracts the imposed (extrinsic) constant depolarizing current and repolarizes the membrane sufficiently to remove inactivation. Then, as K^+ conductance gradually returns to the resting level, under the continued influence of the depolarizing current the membrane potential slides back into the threshold zone, the next spike is fired, and the cycle repeats itself.

4.6. Spontaneous Excitation

A microelectrode probing the brain of an experimental animal, even if that animal is fully anesthetized, meets countless neurons that fire action potentials without apparent provocation. Some of these cells discharge in a regular rhythm, others at random. Yet others emit little bursts of two or more impulses separated by longer silent intervals. They all seem to be telling the experimenter something, if he but understood their language.

Such unprovoked firing is usually referred to as "spontaneous," and as "background" excitation. The first expression implies that the cells fire on their own without external stimulation, the second that they do so without any specific function. Neither of these two assumptions needs to be true. The discharge may be caused by excitatory synaptic input, without the experimenter being aware of it. And the seemingly aimless firing may in fact have an important function. That periodic excitation can have a function is obvious in the case of those neurons in the brain stem, the discharge of which keeps time with the breathing of the animal. The firing of these cells is related in one way or another to the control of respiration. In other cases, where no such clear link can be detected, the firing may or may not have a definite function.

In the ganglia of some invertebrate animals, researchers have succeeded in tying a fine ligature around the axon of giant neurons, and then cutting the cell loose from its environment. Some of these cells continued to generate oscillatory membrane potentials. In these, the membrane of the neuron was evidently its own pacemaker and required no synaptic input to drive it. Such truly spontaneously firing cells generate slow oscillatory potentials which resemble the pacemaker potentials of vertebrate hearts (see Smith and Kampine, pp. 78–81). The ionic conductance changes of these neuronal pacemaker potentials are not identical with those of the cardiac pacemaker, but the basic principles of operation are similar. Pacemaker potentials belong to so-called relaxation oscillations, where a slow change (the pacemaker potential) leads to an abrupt event (the impulse, or a burst of impulses), after which the initial state is restored, and the cycle starts again. Pacemaker potentials are reminiscent of the oscillations seen during repetitive firing maintained by a constant depolarizing current (see preceding section), except that they are inherent in the membrane and do not require an external current source.

Pacemaker potentials probably drive some of the neurosecretory cells of the hypothalamus. Whether other pacemaker cells exist in the central nervous system (CNS) of mammals is not known at present. It is easy enough to think of synaptic processes instead of pacemaker oscillations which could keep cells firing indefinitely. The simplest possible self-re-exciting, or *reverberating circuit* (or recurrent excitation) is illustrated in Figure 4.4. The assumption is that neuron *A*, which sends its axon to some distant target, also sends a collateral axonal branch to short-axon interneuron *B* which, in turn, sends its axon to neuron *A*. Any time neuron *A* fires, it will excite *B*, which will excite *A* again. Provided that

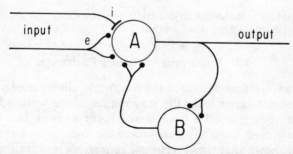

Figure 4.4. Principle of a reverberating (self-re-exciting) neuronal circuit: *e*, excitatory presynaptic terminal; *i*, inhibitory presynaptic terminal. For further description see text.

the synaptic connections are powerful enough to transmit each impulse, and that the conduction time in the loop is long enough so that each new EPSP takes effect at a time when the refractory period of the preceding impulse has passed, this circuit will continue to re-excite itself indefinitely. It may be imagined that the circulation of impulses could be started by a single impulse arriving through excitatory terminal *e*, and it could be turned off again by the convergent inhibitory terminal *i* (Fig. 4.4). While such simple circuits are improbable, more complicated ones that incorporate many more neurons but operate on the same principle may well exist.

Pacemaker potentials and reverberating excitatory systems are not the only two mechanisms that could keep seemingly spontaneous neuronal activity going. For example stable oscillatory discharge bursts could also be generated by multicellular assemblies incorporating recurrent inhibitory loops and featuring rebound inhibition. How this might work will be described in the next two sections of this chapter.

The difficulty of understanding how local circuits actually work lies in unraveling the interactions of the small interneurons which greatly outnumber the larger projection cells but because of their small size are less accessible to study. We do know that in the retina (see Section 9.3a) and in the olfactory bulb (Section 8.3) some of the local circuit cells do not generate impulses, only synaptic potentials, which are conducted by electrotonus from dendritic process to axonal terminal. Whether such impulse-less neurons exist in parts of the CNS other than the retina and olfactory bulb remains to be determined. Some small neurons do not have a proper axon at all; these are called amacrine ("blind") cells (see Fig. 9.8). Among small interneurons we also find dendrodendritic synapses of unknown function. And, to complicate matters further, the ultrastructure of some synapses suggests two-way or reciprocal function: each of the two participating cells seems to function presynaptically at some point and postsynaptically at another nearby point.

4.7. Recurrent Inhibitory Pathways

Ramón y Cajal first described the recurrent collaterals of motor nerve fibers. As motor axons leave the gray matter of the ventral horn of the spinal cord, they give off a branch which curves back into the ventral horn, slightly more medially than where the main axon leaves it. Much later it was shown that these *recurrent collaterals* innervate small interneurons which we now call *Renshaw cells*. The axon of these Renshaw cells inhibits the motor neurons of the same nucleus from which the motor axon originates and some of its synergists as well (see Fig. 15.9). The result is that, whenever motor neurons discharge, they send inhibitory impulses back into their own nucleus. Consequently, the rate at which these cells fire tends to be self-limiting. The story does not end there, however. Renshaw cells are innervated not only by the recurrent collaterals of motor axons, but by excitatory and inhibitory terminals originating in a variety of other structures as well. And they influence the firing of a number of other neurons besides ventral horn cells. Some of the known connections are illustrated schematically in Figure 15.8, and more will be said about them in Chapter 15 (Section 15.3c).

Recurrent inhibitory connections are known to exist in many other parts of the central nervous system besides the spinal ventral horns. Among them are the projection neurons that connect the nuclei of the thalamus to the cerebral cortex. The pyramidal cells of the cerebral cortex, both of the neocortex and the archicortex of the hippocampus, are also equipped with recurrent pathways, but these are not all inhibitory; some seem to be excitatory. Such recurrent excitatory connections could make self-re-excitation of the reverberating variety (Fig. 4.4, possible, but whether this indeed is their function is not clear.

4.8. Recurrent Inhibition and Brain Waves

Electroencephalographic or electrocorticographic tracings often show more or less regular rhythmic voltage oscillations of frequencies between 7 and 13 cps (Fig. 4.5; Table 4.1). In a waking subject these oscillations may continue for many minutes, with their amplitude modulated in a waxing and waning pattern. These are the alpha waves of EEG terminology. During sleep, waves of similar or slightly higher frequency appear and disappear in short bursts called "spindles," interrupted by

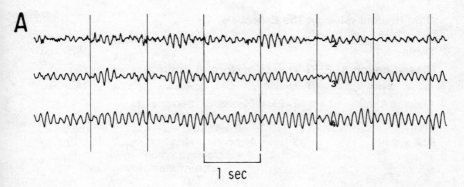

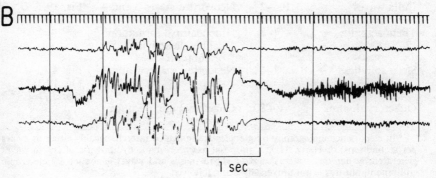

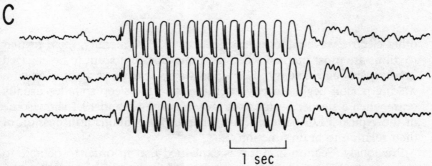

Figure 4.5. Some typical EEG tracings. *A*, normal alpha rhythm; *B*, seizure discharge of a patient precipitated by flashing light stimulation. The marker above the EEG tracings shows the timing of the flashes. (Courtesy of Dr. J. McNamara and Mr. V. Hope, Durham Veterans Administration Epilepsy Center, Durham, N.C.) *C*, spike-and-wave discharge, typical of petit mal (absence) epilepsy. Note remarkable synchrony of spike-and-wave discharges in the three tracings recorded from, respectively, the left frontal, right frontal and left temporal areas. (Reprinted with permission from M. S. Sadove, D. Becka, and F. A. Gibbs: *Electroencephalography for Anesthesiologists and Surgeons*. Philadelphia, J. B. Lippincott, 1967.)

Table 4.1.
Classification of EEG Waves in Normal Brain

Name	Frequency*	Occurrence	Figure No.
Alpha rhythm	7–13	Neocortex; maximal in occipital region; relaxed wakefulness	Fig. 4.5*A*, Fig. 19.1, *A* and *B*
Beta activity	25	Neocortex; alert wakefulness; synonym: desynchronization; low-voltage, fast	Fig. 19.1*A*
Delta waves	0.5–2	Neocortex; stages 3 and 4 sleep	Fig. 19.1, *D* and *E*
Theta activity	4–8	Hippocampal formation; deliberate activity; orientation	
Sleep spindles	8–14	Neocortex; stages 2 and 3 sleep	Fig. 4.7, Fig. 19.1, *C* and *D*
Olfactory rhythm	40–80	Olfactory bulb; pyriform cortex	

* In electroencephalography frequencies are indicated interchangeably either as cycles per second (cps) or Hertz (Hz). A proposal has been made to limit use of cps to waves generated by nervous systems, and of Hz to pulses and waves generated by electronic equipment, but this is not universally being followed.

other electric wave patterns (see Section 19.2). Generally, these regular rhythms are most marked when the brain does not seem to be engaged in any particular activity. The alpha waves tend to disappear when a waking person begins to pay attention, and the sleep spindles usually cease when a sleeper begins to dream. Figures 4.5 and 19.1 show some of the typical EEG patterns, and Chapter 19 contains a discussion of their relation to brain function.

Previously (Section 2.2) it was explained that in order to be able to record potential waves from the surface of the brain or from the scalp, synaptic potentials in a sufficient number of neurons must combine to generate an ordered current field in extracellular space. We now ask: how are the synaptic potentials of cortical pyramidal cells synchronized to make EEG waves? First it had to be decided whether the rhythmic activity is generated within the cortex or imposed on cortical neurons by input originating elsewhere. Cortical tissue contains between 10^4 and 10^5 neurons/mm^3, which in principle is more than enough to produce stable rhythmic patterns. Experiments have shown, however, that if an area of the neocortex is completely deafferented, that is to say deprived of input from all other sources, it usually falls electrically silent for a period. It then resumes "spontaneous" electric activity, but of a distinctly pathological character. Thus, organized spindles and regular alpha wave activity depend on input to the cortex. It has been shown that this input must come, specifically, from thalamic nuclei.

It is also significant that rhythmic activity of thalamic neurons does not disappear when the cortical target area of the thalamic nucleus is removed. In other words, while the cortical rhythm requires input from the thalamus, the thalamic rhythm does not require the input from cortex. The exact mechanism of the rhythm generator in the thalamus is not kown, but a reasonable hypothesis has been proposed. A condensed account of this hypothesis follows (Figs. 4.6 and 4.7).

All regions of the cerebral neocortex receive thalamic input. Specific thalamic nuclei are connected to limited regions of the cortex, and non-specific thalamic nuclei project more widely to larger cortical areas. Thalamocortical projection neurons in all nuclei are equipped with recurrent inhibitory connections. The discharge of an impulse by a projection neuron is followed by an IPSP of 80- to 120-msec duration. This corresponds rather precisely to the cycle length of the thalamically driven cortical rhythms (7–13 cps). Moreover, the IPSPs are regularly followed by a prominent post-inhibitory rebound depolarization (cf. Section 4.3), so much so that many neurons are seen to discharge an impulse in this post-inhibitory phase.

Figs. 4.6 and 4.7 show how these ingredients could generate rhythmic activity. If any one of the projection neurons fires an impulse, it activates an inhibitory neuron in the recurrent pathway. Since the axon of this interneuron is branched, several projection neurons undergo an IPSP, and several of them could then fire an impulse during the post-inhibitory rebound phase. All those that fired on this second round then activate additional inhibitory neurons, which this time would evoke the IPSP-rebound sequence in an even greater number of projection neurons. As a result an ever-widening circle of projection neurons fire bursts of impulses separated by intervals of roughly 100 msec.

This sequence of events explains the waxing of the wave activity, but what about their subsequent waning? Rhythmic activity would be interfered with whenever some of the projection cells in the assembly discharge out of step with the others. Then recurrent inhibition, instead of aiding synchronization, would counteract it. As the zone of rhythmically discharging neurons widens, there is a gradual phase shift at the advancing edge of the discharge zone. The farther the neurons are from the original epicenter of activity, the less well they are synchronized. Finally there will be neurons in the outer reaches of the pool whose IPSP would coincide with the post-inhibitory rebound of the neurons in the center. Once this phase shift occurred in some, it would initiate a reverse wave of cell after cell dropping out of the rhythmical discharge. The gradual recruitment of units would thus be followed by their gradual demobilization,

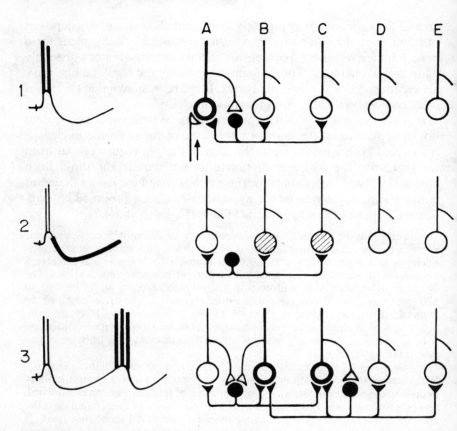

Figure 4.6. A proposed mechanism for the generation of the alpha rhythm and of sleep spindles. *A* to *E*, thalamocortical projection neurons. Those drawn as *heavy circles* are assumed to have just discharged. *Solid circles* represent inhibitory interneurons, excited by recurrent collaterals of the axons of projection cells. In *1*, *A* has just discharged; in *2*, the inhibitory interneuron has discharged and evoked an IPSP in cells *A*, *B* and *C*; in *3* the cells that have been inhibited now discharge in the post-inhibitory rebound phase, and thus excite additional inhibitory interneurons which now evoke an IPSP in *D* and *E* as well, and so the cycle repeats itself. (Reprinted with permission from P. Andersen and S. A. Anderson: *Physiological Basis of the Alpha Rhythm*. New York, Appleton-Century-Crofts, 1968.)

the waxing giving way to waning. The authors of this scheme have programmed a computer and demonstrated that the model they proposed could indeed work.

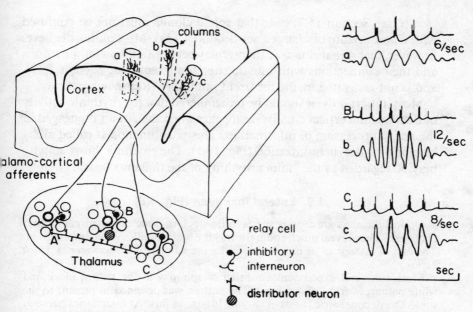

Figure 4.7. Thalamocortical interaction in generating bursts of spindle waves. *Left*, *A*, *B* and *C* represent nests of thalamic neurons generating rhythmic discharge as illustrated in Figure 4.6 and described in text. Discharges in bundles of axons from *A*, *B* and *C* evoke synchronized synaptic potentials in the dendritic trees of the cells in the cortical columns *a*, *b* and *c*. The distributor neuron coordinates the occurrence of spindles in the thalamic nests but does not govern the frequency of discharges within the bursts (which is set by the IPSPs generated by the interneurons; see Fig. 4.6). *Right*, spindle burst discharges: *A*, *B* and *C* from thalamic neurons; *a*, *b* and *c* from the cortical surface. (Reprinted with permission from P. Andersen and S. A. Anderson: *Physiological Basis of the Alpha Rhythm*. New York, Appleton-Century-Crofts, 1968.)

Rhythmic wave activity of one kind or another occurs in other brain structures, for example in the archicortex of the hippocampus (theta waves) (see Section 19.3b) and in the olfactory bulb (Section 8.3). Although recurrent inhibitory connections are a feature of both the hippocampus and the olfactory bulb, the mechanism of wave generation need not necessarily be identical in all cases. Not all recurrent inhibitory pathways develop rhythmic burst firing; the spinal Renshaw connections normally do not. Only under pathological enhancement of excitability do spinal motor neurons develop rhythmic burst discharges, called *clonus* (see Section 15.7; note that spinal clonus must not be confused with clonic seizure discharges: see Section 4.11a). Most authors believe, however, that spinal clonus is an interplay between spinal motor neurons and their connections with muscle stretch afferents (see Section 15.7), and is not generated by the recurrent inhibitory (Renshaw) pathway.

Most importantly, it should be remembered that the rhythmic activity of the thalamocortical circuits disappears when the circuit is engaged in the active processing of information. This phenomenon is called alpha blocking, or desynchronization (Fig. 19.1). The rhythmic burst activity may be regarded as the "idling rhythm" of the thalamocortical circuit.

4.9. Lateral Inhibition (Fig. 4.8)

Optical illusions are among the favorite stock-in-trade of experimental psychologists. They reveal much about the way the brain handles visual information. The one of interest to us now is known by the name of its discoverer as *Mach bands*.

Mach's original experiment consisted of spinning a disc with a black and white pattern in front of a subject. The pattern was designed to present to the subject's eye concentric bands of varying luminous flux. At boundaries between zones of differing luminosity, where the subject should have perceived a uniform light gray zone, he saw a narrow white band embedded in the light gray; and on the darker side, in what should have been perceived as uniformly dark gray, there was seen a narrow black band. Similar illusions can be evoked more simply by staring at patterns consisting of alternating black and white stripes. In each case the subjectively perceived contrast is more abrupt than predicted from the transition in light energy level: the edge of a black band seems blacker than its middle, and the edge of an adjacent white band seems whiter than its central part. To explain the phenomenon, Mach postulated the existence of a mechanism similar to what today we call *lateral inhibition*, much before the electrophysiological demonstration of inhibitory synapses.

Lateral inhibition as a neurophysiological reality was discovered by Hartline in the compound eye of the horseshoe crab. This organ consists of several hundred individual eyelets or ommatidia. Illuminating one of the ommatidia so that no light shines on its neighbors not only excites nerve cells within the illuminated ommatidium, but also inhibits its neighbors. Moreover, if several adjacent ommatidia are illuminated simultaneously, none is excited as intensely as when just one is stimulated, even if the amount of light energy received per ommatidium is equal in both cases. From these and other findings, it appears that each ommatidium is connected to its neighbors by inhibitory synapses. The result of such mutual lateral inhibition is the enhancement of contrast at the borders between illuminated and darkened areas (Fig. 4.8). If a horseshoe crab ever looks at a white and black pattern, he probably perceives Mach bands as we do.

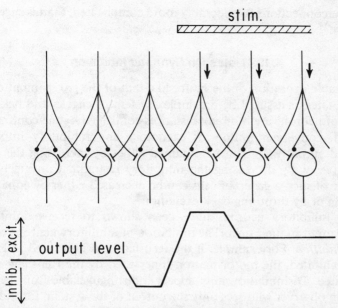

Figure 4.8. The simplest possible form of lateral inhibition. Six afferent fibers and six postsynaptic neurons are shown. Excitatory terminals of branches of the afferent fibers are indicated by *black dots*, inhibitory endings by the *flat terminals*. Three of the six afferent fibers are assumed to have been excited. The distribution of the relative levels of excitation and inhibition of postsynaptic cells is plotted at *bottom*. Lateral inhibition can operate either by afferent collaterals, as shown, or by recurrent collaterals of postsynaptic axons, but in either case the inhibition would usually be mediated by interneurons inserted in the pathway, which have been deleted from this simplified diagram.

After Hartline's work, lateral inhibition of one kind or another has been discovered in the retina and in other parts of the visual pathways of mammals, also in several regions of the central nervous system which receive somatic sensory input. Outside the sensory systems, a form of lateral inhibition seems to operate in the connections between the so-called parallel fibers and the Purkinje cells of the cerebellar cortex (see Section 18.3b and Fig. 18.6.) It seems a general rule that where the excitation of a large number of neuronal elements is arranged in some spatial order and is "mapped" onto another set of neuronal elements, the nervous system often employs some form of lateral inhibition. The number of neurons involved is, of course, always much greater, and their interconnections considerably more complicated, than is suggested by Figure 4.8.

4.10. Notes On Synaptic Inhibition

The stable operation of the brain, like that of the government of the United States, is assured by a complex system of checks and balances. Groups of neurons are in many instances controlled by the continuous, balanced, convergent inflow of excitatory and inhibitory impulses. Increased output may then be obtained either by increasing the excitatory drive or by decreasing the inhibitory restraint. Conversely, the discharge of such a group of cells can be decreased either by enhancing inhibition or by throttling back excitation.

Many inhibitory neurons have been shown to receive inhibitory synaptic input in their turn. The inhibition of inhibitory neurons results in *disinhibition*. For example, if the Renshaw cell illustrated in Figure 15.8 is inhibited, the motor neuron innervated by the Renshaw cell is disinhibited. Disinhibition may appear indistinguishable from facilitation to an observer who sees only the output of the system, for example a reflex movement. Only by analyzing the circuit, for example, by intracellular recording from participating neurons, is it in these cases possible to identify the mechanism.

Nothing demonstrates the importance of inhibitory synapses more dramatically than the effect of poisons that abolish inhibitory effects. If inhibition is taken away, the unbridled excitation may destroy the organism. Strychnine, for example, competes with glycine at glycinergic inhibitory synapses (cf. Sections 2.5e and 4.11b). Consequently, strychnine poisoning blocks synaptic inhibition in the spinal cord, especially in the ventral gray matter, and thereby causes violent muscle spasms. The victim dies of asphyxiation due to cramp of the respiratory muscles. Other poisons, for example picrotoxin, block inhibition mediated by γ-aminobutyric acid (GABA) and so cause convulsions which start in the brain or brain stem.

Less violent, but also severely disabling, are the consequences of lesions that destroy inhibitory neurons in a specific brain area, or the inhibitory connections between areas. Excessive excitation caused by loss of inhibitory restraint is usually referred to as the pathological *release* of a function from control. Many neurological disorders are the mixed result of lost excitatory drive of some neurons combined with the release of others from inhibition. We shall see numerous examples later (e.g. Chapter 18).

4.11. Seizure Disorders

Epilepsy is a condition in which abnormal neuronal excitability results in periodic and unpredictably occurring seizures, but seizures can also be caused by acute brain disturbance due to certain other diseases, for example failure of the liver or of the kidneys. Epilepsy is the most prevalent of all neurological disorders. In fact all mammalian brains are capable of generating seizure discharges if sufficiently provoked. The fundamental and as yet unanswered question in epilepsy research can be formulated in two ways: first, what is it that causes the brain of an epileptic patient to be seized from time to time by paroxysmal discharge? Or, equally importantly, what is it that protects a healthy brain from so being afflicted?

The best known method of inducing an epileptiform seizure in a nonepileptic brain is by electric current. Electroconvulsive therapy is the provocation of a major fit by electric current. As used today in psychiatric practice, overt convulsive movements are prevented by the administration of a muscle relaxant drug, but the electric storm that seizes the brain resembles a major epileptic attack.

4.11a. TYPES OF SEIZURES

Seizures are caused by the excessive and uncontrolled discharge of groups of neurons. This may or may not cause convulsive movements. If it does, then the fit must be differentiated from other types of pathological muscle contractions, for example the involuntary movements characteristic of diseases of the basal ganglia (see Section 18.2). The criteria by which such distinctions are made belong in textbooks of clinical medicine.

Seizure discharges have an eruptive, explosive nature. There are numerous forms, but those suffered by a particular patient tend to remain in character and to be rather stereotyped. They may occur at unpredictable moments, but once started run a predictable course. For these and other reasons it is strongly suspected that there is an element of positive feedback, of pathological self-re-excitation, in the generation of seizure discharges.

A seizure is said to be *partial* if it affects a part of the brain and *generalized* if it affects all or most of it. A seizure may be generalized from the moment it erupts, or it may begin as a partial seizure in a small part of the brain and then become *secondarily generalized.* The distinction is important, for when there is a localized trigger focus, the disorder can be cured by surgery. In these cases, it must be decided what is the greater handicap, the epilepsy or the deficit expected as a result of the surgical lesion. Primary generalized seizures cannot be treated surgically.

A primary generalized seizure strikes without warning. Secondarily generalized seizures may be heralded by an *aura*—a peculiar, distinctly abnormal sensation, sometimes a mood change, usually recognized by the patient from previous episodes. The aura is the consequence of the discharge of neurons in the trigger focus, which may be in a sensory area of the brain. In other patients the seizure may begin as localized twitching of a muscle of one limb which then spreads to other parts of the body. In these cases the initial discharge is in a motor area of the brain. This form is called Jacksonian epilepsy, after Hughlings Jackson (see Section 18.1).

In a typical generalized seizure, or *ictus* (meaning a blow), the patient loses consciousness, falls to the ground with or without uttering a cry, and his muscles tighten in strong maintained contraction. This is the *tonic phase.* It is followed by rhythmic interrupted convulsive movements, the *clonic phase* (not to be confused with clonus or spinal origin). The seizure is terminated by a limp unconscious state, the *postictal depression,* after which the patient ordinarily remains weak and groggy for half an hour or more. Epilepsy characterized by generalized tonic-clonic seizures is often referred to as *grand mal* (literally, "great illness").

Petit mal ("little illness") or absence epilepsy affects children only. It consists of brief spells of unconsciousness or absences, typically of a few seconds, rarely more than a minute in duration. During such an attack the patient retains normal posture and may or may not show minor twitching movements. The EEG tracing shows the so-called "3 per second spike-and-dome" complexes (Fig. 4.5*C*) that are the reliable diagnostic signature of the disease. This EEG pattern appears over both hemispheres at once and is believed to be driven by seizure discharge originating in the diencephalon, probably the non-specific thalamic nuclei. For this reason the condition has also been referred to as *centrencephalic epilepsy.*

One of the ways in which a seizure can be triggered in a brain that is not epileptic is by prolonged excessive hyperventilation. It is worth our while to dwell on this briefly, for it illustrates some important physiological principles. Breathing excessively lowers P_{CO_2} in circulating blood, and as a result, cerebral arterioles constrict. Since CO_2 passes freely through the blood-brain barrier (see Section 5.1), the P_{CO_2} in cerebral tissue is lowered, and the cerebral pH rises. Alkalinization can shift the ratio of bound to ionized calcium in favor of the former. When these three factors—cerebral hypoxia due to vasoconstriction, cerebral alkalosis and lowered cerebral $[Ca^{2+}]_o$—are combined, they can trigger a fit which, once it has erupted, is no longer distinguishable from a seizure. In days when hysteria was common, recognizing such spells was a frequent problem. Today it has been seen in contestants excessively hyperventilating in preparation for an underwater swimming contest.

The diagnosis of epilepsy is usually possible by EEG examination. It is useful but not always necessary to "capture" a seizure on an EEG tracing, especially if video and audio monitoring are also available so the behavior can be correlated with electrophysiology. The EEG of epileptic patients usually has abnormal features also in the seizure-free intervals, known as *inter-ictal* discharges. They take the form of "sharp waves," or "spikes" or isolated "spike-and-dome" complexes.

4.11b. EXPERIMENTALLY INDUCED SEIZURES

In experimental animals acute seizures can be caused by convulsant drugs. One class of convulsant drugs acts by blocking inhibitory synapses. Strychnine induces convulsions of spinal origin by blocking spinal postsynaptic inhibition mediated by glycine. The seizures of strychnine poisoning differ from epileptiform seizures in many respects. Perhaps best known of all convulsant drugs is pentylenetetrazol (metrazol, cardiazol) which, for a few years, had been used in psychiatric practice until it was supplanted by electroconvulsive therapy. The effect of pentylenetetrazol does not depend on the blockade of inhibition.

Penicillin, in toxic amounts, can cause generalized tonic-clonic seizures. Under ordinary conditions penicillin is a safe drug, because little of it passes through the blood-brain barrier. It must be used with caution when there is reason to believe that the blood-brain barrier may have been breached, or if the route of administration is intrathecal: into the subarachnoid space.

Chronic epileptogenic foci can be created in the brains of experimental animals in various ways. One is by the local injection of alumina cream. Another is by the local deposition of cobalt powder. Both procedures cause the formation of a glial scar, and gliotic foci are frequently found also in specimens taken at autopsy or in surgery of human patients suffering from partial or from secondarily generalizing seizures.

When an epileptogenic glial scar has been created in the brain of an animal, it behaves rather like the trigger focus of partial epilepsy in a human brain. That is, it emits interictal discharges, occasionally erupts in a partial seizure, and sometimes triggers secondarily generalized seizures. If the primary focus is in an area of the cerebral cortex that is connected through the corpus callosum with the opposite hemisphere, then seizure discharges in the primary focus evoke similar activity at a symmetrical site of the opposite hemisphere. The discharges in the *mirror focus* are, at first, driven by the activity of the primary focus. However, after some months the mirror focus may start its own autonomous epileptiform activity. If the condition is permitted to exist for a long period, then removing the primary focus no longer cures the epilepsy, for the mirror focus will then itself initiate seizures.

Of the various methods invented to induce experimental epilepsy in animals, perhaps the most interesting is the one to which the picturesque name, *kindling*, is attached. To kindle seizures, a brain area is stimulated by electric current of a moderate intensity that initially causes no epileptiform discharge. If the same mild stimulus is repeated at daily intervals, eventually it becomes epileptogenic. After a few stimulations, *paroxysmal afterdischarges* appear on electric recording from the stimulated area. Later, overt partial seizures and, eventually, secondarily generalized seizures are triggered by the stimulation. If daily stimulations are continued further, true epilepsy develops so that the animal suffers seizures even if no more electric stimulation is administered. The sites commonly used to kindle seizures are the amygdala and the hippocampal formation. These are accessible to stimulation by depth electrodes that are permanently implanted and sealed to the skull (cf. Section 1.2, 1.4b and Fig. 1.3). It probably is no coincidence that homologous regions are the usual primary foci of the discharges causing so-called complex partial seizures—a common form of epilepsy in human patients. The mechanism of kindling is not fully understood, but several investigators have suggested that excessive long-term potentiation (see Section 20.3b) of too many synapses at once plays a part. As we have seen, long-term potentiation is a characteristic of synapses in the hippocampal formation. The evidence linking the two phenomena is suggestive but incomplete at the time of this writing.

The most important lesson learned from the discovery of kindled seizures is that excessive use—abuse if you will—of a certain neuron population, or rather the synapses linking them, can cause lasting and severe cerebral malfunction. Control experiments have established that the mere presence of the implanted electrodes (undoubtedly a foreign body), or any chemical reactions perhaps catalyzed by the electric current, are not the cause of the seizures. To kindle seizures it is both necessary and sufficient to evoke the firing of certain groups of neurons at certain frequencies at certain intervals. The similarity between kindling and the development of an autonomous mirror focus is evident. The consequences of the discovery of kindling for the way we think not only about certain neurological disorders, but perhaps also about psychiatric conditions, are not yet clear but may well be far-reaching.

4.11c. ELECTROPHYSIOLOGY OF EXPERIMENTAL SEIZURES

Artificial seizure foci can be induced not only in the cerebral neocortex and hippocampus, but also in the nuclei of the diencephalon and brain stem, and in the ventral horns of the spinal cord. The patterning and the time course of seizures may differ in certain details, but the eruptive and episodic character of the discharges is similar in all regions of the CNS. Perhaps the only part of the central gray matter that may be immune to seizures is the cerebellar cortex.

What appears on EEG records made with surface electrodes as an interictal discharge, is apparently generated by synchronized waves of intense depolarization of neurons in the epileptogenic focus. These waves are known as paroxysmal depolarization shifts, or PDS. The rising phase of a PDS triggers a burst of high-frequency impulses. During the crest of the PDS, impulse firing is often suppressed, apparently due to inactivation of Na^+ channels caused by the excessive depolarization (see Section 3.1). There is disagreement whether the PDS is a "giant" EPSP caused by excessive release of excitatory transmitter from presynaptic terminals or an abnormal voltage-dependent response of dendritic membranes, perhaps an exaggerated dendritic calcium spike.

A typical experimental seizure focus emits interictal discharges at irregular intervals. From time to time, for unknown reasons, these become more frequent and then coalesce into a seizure. The seizure may be limited to the focus (remain partial), or it may generalize. When seizure activity remains confined, the discharging zone seems to be surrounded by an inhibited zone. Why this protective surrounding is sometimes breached, so that the seizure becomes generalized, is not clear.

During a tonic seizure the neurons participating in the discharge remain depolarized. They may fire impulses at high but irregular frequencies throughout the tonic phase, or impulse firing may become blocked after a while. During the clonic phase, the membrane potential of neurons undergoes rhythmic synchronized waves of depolarization. During postictal depression, the cells that participated in the seizure discharge become hyperpolarized. This is an important distinction between postictal depression and spreading depression (see Section 5.8b), for during spreading depression cells are severely depolarized.

During seizure discharges, especially during the tonic phase, there are important shifts of ion distribution between intracellular and extracellular fluids. Extracellular K^+ activity, $[K^+]_o$, rises from the rest level of 3 mM to about 10 mM, while $[Ca^{2+}]_o$ and $[Na^+]_o$ decrease. It must be assumed that these extracellular changes are accompanied by reciprocal changes of intracellular ion activity, $[K^+]_i$ decreasing and $[Ca^{2+}]_i$ and $[Na^+]_i$ increasing.

4.12. Chapter Summary

1. The concepts of reflexes, conditional and unconditional, and of reflex arcs, is defined.
2. Integration of signals in the CNS depends on convergence and divergence of synaptic connections. Spatial facilitation, occlusion and postsynaptic inhibition are possible where connections converge. Spatial facilitation occurs when the subliminal zones created by two convergent inputs in one neuron pool overlap. Occlusion occurs when the discharge zones of two convergent inputs overlap.
3. Temporal facilitation of synaptic transmission may be caused by two processes. If a presynaptic terminal is fired twice in rapid enough succession for the EPSP caused by the second presynaptic impulse to begin before the first has subsided, the two EPSPs sum linearly. In addition, the second EPSP of a pair may be of larger amplitude than the first (post-activation potentiation, or EPSP facilitation).
4. After a series (train) of input volleys the amount of transmitter released per impulse per presynaptic terminal may at some synapses be enhanced for several minutes (post-tetanic potentiation), and at other synapses for hours or days (long-term potentiation).
5. Accommodation means an increase of threshold due to slowly increasing or continued depolarization. It is caused mainly by inactivation of voltage-gated Na^+ channels and also by activation of K^+ channels. Spike frequency adaptation is due to similar membrane conductance changes. Many central neurons are nevertheless capable of firing repetitively and steadily for indefinite periods in response to a moderately strong constant depolarizing current if their membrane potential is returned to near the resting level by after-hyperpolarization following each spike. Other excitable membranes are not so repolarized after each impulse, and therefore cannot fire repetitively, but become blocked due to inactivation of the Na^+ channels.
6. Desensitization means decreasing responsiveness to a chemical agent caused by exposure to that agent or one of similar action.
7. Habituation is a diminishing response of an organism to oft-repeated stimuli.
8. Neurons in the CNS may be spontaneously active due to (a) the generation of pacemaker potentials; (b) excitation circulating in reverberating (recurrent excitatory) circuits; (c) oscillations generated in recurrent inhibition followed by post-inhibitory rebound excitation.
9. The alpha rhythm and sleep spindles of EEG tracings depend on input from the thalamus to the cortex. These oscillatory potentials may be generated by the mechanism just defined (8c above).
10. Lateral inhibition is a mechanism of contrast enhancement found in spatially patterned neuronal activity.
11. Inhibition of inhibition (disinhibition) can lead to enhanced excitation and spontaneous firing. Prolonged loss of inhibitory restraint causes pathological release of neurological functions.
12. Seizures may also be the result of pharmacological blockade of inhibitory synapses or of irritation by toxic agents and sometimes of unknown causes.

A classification of seizure types is given in the text. Some of the most important experimental methods to induce seizures are also described. The EEG signs of seizures are caused by the paroxysmal depolarization of many neurons occuring simultaneously.

Further Reading

Books and Reviews

Creed RS, Denny-Brown D, Eccles JC, et al: *Reflex Activity of the Spinal Cord.* Oxford, Clarendon Press (reprinted and annotated) 1972.
Sherrington CS: *The Integrative Action of the Nervous System.* New Haven, Yale University Press (paperback edition) 1961.
Smith JJ, Kampine JP: *Circulatory Physiology: The Essentials.* Baltimore, Williams & Wilkins, 1980.
Wheal HV, Schwartzkroin PA (eds): *Electrophysiology of Epilepsy.* London, Academic Press (in press).

Articles

Andersen P, Sundberg SH, Sveen O, et al: Possible mechanisms for long-lasting potentiation of synaptic transmission in hippocampal slices from guinea pigs. *J Physiol* (Lond) 302:463–482, 1980.
Lloyd DPC: Post-tetanic potentiation of response in monosynaptic reflex pathways of the spinal cord. *J Gen Physiol* 33:147–170, 1949.

chapter 5

The Internal Environment of Central Neurons and the Functions of Neuroglia

In what way are the fluids that bathe the cells of the central nervous system different from the extracellular fluids of the rest of the body? How is the composition of fluids of the CNS regulated? How does their composition change in disease, and what are the consequences of such changes? What is the role of glial cells in the regulation of CNS interstitial fluid, and what are the other functions of neuroglia?

5.1. The Blood-Brain Barrier

Around 1910 E. Goldmann, working in the laboratory of Paul Ehrlich, injected live mice with *trypan blue*. At autopsy he noted that all the tissues turned blue except those of the brain, spinal cord, peripheral nerves, eyes and testicles. When the same dye was injected into the cerebrospinal fluid, the brain did take the color, proving that it was not some inherent property of brain that prevented it from being stained. These and other observations led to the conclusion that there must be an impediment to the transfer of certain compounds from blood into these organs, and the term "*Blut-Hirn Schranke*" or "blood-brain barrier" was coined. It would be more accurate but more cumbersome to speak of a "blood-central nervous system barrier," for the spinal cord is similarly insulated. The idea was not universally accepted, and various alternative explanations were sought for these findings. With the advent of radioactively labeled tracers and of electron microscopy the phenomenon could be defined with greater precision, and today there remains no doubt that the interface separating blood plasma from the interstitial fluid of the central nervous system differs from that separating blood from all other tissues of the body.

To understand the transfer of materials into and out of the central nervous system (CNS) we must consider the exchanges at three different interfaces: between blood and cerebrospinal fluid (CSF); between CSF and the interstitial spaces of the brain and the spinal cord; and between blood and CNS interstitial fluid. The last named is the blood-brain barrier proper, but substances can also pass from the bloodstream first into the CSF and then from the CSF into brain, and therefore no bookkeeping of the intake and output of materials by the brain is complete without an accounting of the transfers by way of the CSF. Each of the cell layers forming the interfaces between these three fluids has a different histology, and therefore their permeabilities and transport functions need not be identical either. Before discussing their specific properties, it may be well to briefly review transport processes through cell layers in general.

5.1a. TRANSPORT ACROSS CELL LAYERS

Where two fluids are separated by a layer of cells, materials may be transported by several distinct processes. These are:

1a. *Bulk flow.* If there are gaps between the cells, and there is a hydrostatic pressure difference between the two fluids, then fluid will flow from the compartment under higher pressure toward that under lower pressure. Solutes and solvent are transported by bulk flow together at a rate determined by the pressure gradient and by the resistance to flow.

1b. *Ultrafiltration* is a special case of bulk flow, driven by a hydrostatic pressure gradient, but one in which the passage of large molecules is retarded or prevented altogether.

2. *Free diffusion.* If the membrane has pores for solute and solvent molecules to pass through, then there will be exchange by diffusion even if there is no hydrostatic pressure gradient. As a rule, the rate of diffusion is different for different particles and it is governed by the chemical activity gradient (in the

case of charged particles, the electrochemical gradient: see Section 2.3) and the mobility of the particles.

3. *Carrier-mediated (facilitated) diffusion.* The mobility of a compound through a membrane may be increased by special carrier molecules that are constituents of certain membranes. The substance to be moved is reversibly bound by the membrane carrier. It then is translocated across the membrane, perhaps by a conformational change of the carrier molecule. On the side of the membrane where substrate concentration is high, binding is more probable; where the substrate concentration is low, the bonds are more likely to be broken. Therefore net transport will continue as long as concentrations on the two sides of the membrane are different. The affinity of such a carrier is limited to one chemical compound, or to a class of related compounds. Facilitated diffusion is saturable. Once all carrier sites are occupied, no more substrate can be added. Competition between similar molecules for common sites is another hallmark of carrier-mediated diffusion.

4. *Active transport.* Selected materials may be moved actively, often against a chemical gradient, by the expenditure of metabolic energy.

Bearing these alternatives in mind, we now can proceed to analyze the transfer of materials between CSF and interstitial fluid, and between interstitium and blood. The formation and the absorption of the CSF itself will be the subject of the next section of this chapter (Section 5.2).

5.1b. EXCHANGE OF MATERIALS BETWEEN CSF AND INTERSTITIAL FLUID OF THE CNS

CSF is separated from interstitial fluid in the cerebral ventricles by a single layer of ciliated cells, the ependyma. This layer is quite leaky, except where it covers the choroid plexus (Fig. 5.1*B*). The fenestration between ependymal cells permits the free diffusion of water and of solutes. This is also true of the outer surfaces of the brain and of the spinal cord, which are covered by a dual layer of tissue. The outer layer, the pia mater, is of mesodermal origin. Beneath it a second layer is formed by the end-feet of glial processes, the glia limitans. A basal lamina separates the two cell layers. Like the ventricular ependyma, this fine double sheet of tissue, and the basal lamina in between, are permeable to water and to aqueous solutes. However, since water-soluble material can only pass between the cells and not through them, diffusion is slowed both at the ependymal and at the pia-glial surfaces. This hindrance is not selective, and all water-soluble substances are retarded to the same degree. The important point, however, is this: the slowing of the diffusion does not prevent *near-equilibration of solutes between CSF and interstitial fluid*; not so for the interface between capillary blood and cerebral interstitium, which is our next subject.

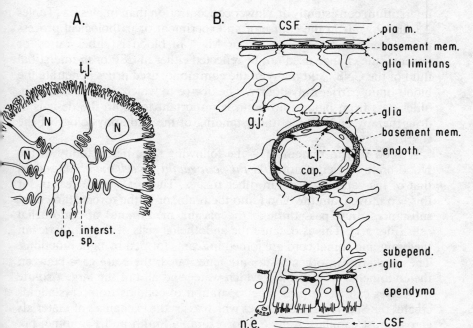

Figure 5.1.   The cell layers separating the fluids of the central nervous system. *A*, the specialized ependyma investing the choroid villi; *B*, the components of the pia-glial membrane of the outer surfaces of brain and spinal cord, of the walls of CNS capillaries, and of the ependymal layers lining the cerebral ventricles. *t. j.*, tight junctions; *N*, nuclei of ependymal cells; *cap.*, capillary; *interst. sp.*, interstitial space; *pia m.*, pia mater; *basement mem.*, basement membrane; *endoth.*, endothelium; *n. e.*, nerve ending in ventricular wall. Note that in the choroid villus the ependymal cells are joined by complete seams of tight junctions, but the capillaries are fenestrated; whereas in the remainder of the CNS tissue capillary endothelial cells are joined by tight junctions and the ependymal and pial cell layers are fenestrated.

5.1c. EXCHANGE OF MATERIALS BETWEEN BLOOD AND CNS INTERSTITIUM

Even though the total surface area of the walls of the capillaries in brain and spinal cord is many times greater than the surface area of the ependyma and of the pia mater combined, many solutes are normally not at equilibrium between circulating plasma and the interstitial fluid of the CNS. For example, potassium and glucose are in CSF and cerebral interstitium consistently at a lower concentration than in plasma (Tables 2.1 and 2.2). If in the course of an experiment or pathological process the concentration of K^+, Ca^{2+} or Mg^{2+} in blood is either raised or lowered, the change need not be reflected either in CSF or in interstitial fluid of the CNS. And many of the commonly used drugs penetrate the blood-brain barrier only poorly. The degree to which drugs and metabolites pass from blood into brain is important for both the designs of drug therapy and for the understanding of the pathophysiology of the CNS.

A good rule to remember is the following. The permeability of the blood-brain barrier is more *like the permeability of cell membranes* than that of the capillary walls in other tissues. There is a good reason for this. To move from the blood into the brain, or in the reverse direction, substances must pass through the plasma membranes of endothelial cells (Fig. 5.1). This is because the endothelial cells of the capillaries in the brain and spinal cord are joined in seams formed by tight junctions. The capillaries in other tissues are fenestrated: there are gaps between the endothelial cells through which water and all but the largest solute molecules can freely pass. The separation of colloids from crystalloids creates the Starling-Landis forces which assist the exchanges of materials across most capillary walls (cf. for example Smith and Kampine, pp. 134–136). Free diffusion and filtration (i.e. bulk flow) are the two means of moving water and aqueous solutes in an out of systemic capillaries. Neither occurs in the CNS capillaries where other mechanisms must prevail.

The capillary endothelium of the central nervous system allows free diffusion only of lipid-soluble substances, for only they can move through the membranes of the endothelial cells. Free passage is thus granted to the respiratory gases O_2 and CO_2 as well as to ethanol, ethyl ether, chloroform and a number of toxic solvents. Water-soluble molecules pass with varying degrees of hindrance, and non-polar, non-ionized molecules move with less hindrance than those electrically charged. Macromolecules are almost totally excluded. Consequently, certain drugs and some of the normal constituents of blood that could permeate the barrier may be prevented from doing so if they are bound to plasma protein. Thyroxine (T_4) is an example. Only 1% of the T_4 present in plasma is free, the remainder being bound to a protein carrier. The free T_4 in plasma is exchangeable with the T_4 in cerebrospinal fluid and so the concentration of T_4 in the fluids of the brain is 1% of its total plasma concentration.

It has recently been reported that even the movement across the blood-brain barrier of radiolabeled water is restricted and variable. The apparent water permeability could, for example, be influenced by catecholamines and by certain peptides. The interpretation of these potentially very important experiments has, however, been criticized, and the controversy has not yet been resolved. It is worth remembering that the collecting ducts of the kidneys and the skin of frogs are also adjustably waterproof and therefore it is at least conceivable that the blood-brain barrier could be also.

So far it may seem that the brain is nearly inaccessible to most solutes carried by the blood. Yet, clearly, there needs to be exchange of certain materials, such as the substrates of cerebral metabolism, of vitamins and of hormones. Waste products of cerebral metabolism must also be eliminated. For these exchanges, the cerebral capillary endothelium appears to possess specialized transport systems. While in other capillary beds diffusion and filtration allow indiscriminate passage of all but the largest molecules, brain capillaries are much more selective.

It is increasingly realized that, in many respects, the blood-brain barrier functions in ways similar to *a secreting epithelium*. The difficulty that had retarded general acceptance of this insight was the fact that histologically, the barrier is an endothelium, not an epithelium. Since numerous studies demonstrated that the endothelial cells of CNS capillaries are unusually richly endowed with mitochondria and enzymes, including Na, K-activated adenosine triphosphatase (see Section 2.4a) required for active transport, the idea has become much more plausible.

As a general rule, non-ionized but water-soluble metabolic substrates move through the cerebral capillary endothelial cells by facilitated diffusion. This process is chemically selective but passive, i.e. it requires no metabolic energy. The specificity of binding by carrier molecules is high, but not absolute. If a drug molecule can be made to "look like" a natural substrate, it could "get a ride" on a carrier. Several distinct carrier systems have been identified at the blood-brain barrier. For example, there is one for the hexoses; one each for neutral, basic and acidic amino acids; one for the carboxylic acid hydrocarbons; and others. Stereospecificity has been demonstrated for some; e.g. D-glucose is accepted, L-glucose is not.

The concentration of glucose in CSF and hence probably in the interstitial fluid of the brain is consistently lower than in blood plasma. The reason is probably that glucose is used in cerebral metabolism at a high rate, and its mobility across the barrier, even with the assistance of a carrier, is restricted. The high rate of glucose consumption lowers its concentration on the brain side, until the gradient across the barrier is large enough so that its rate of supply by diffusion can keep up with its rate of consumption. It is well known from clinical determinations on CSF samples that in pathological conditions where the blood-brain barrier is defective (cf. Section 5.4) the difference in concentration between blood and brain is less than normal.

The activity of potassium is also held at a level lower than its activity in blood plasma (Table 2.1A). But unlike glucose, K^+ evidently is not consumed in cerebral metabolism. The mechanism that keeps K^+ lower in the interstitial fluid of the CNS is *active transport* from brain into blood. It is likely, though not clearly shown in each case, that other ions are also actively transported across the blood-brain barrier. The ion pumps of the endothelial cells are probably similar to those operating in excitable cell membranes (cf. Section 2.4a), and in secreting epithelia. By the activity of these ion pumps the ion activities in the environment of brain cells are regulated more precisely than is possible for the other tissues of the body.

There are, however, two sides to the barrier. Besides protecting against the entry of unwanted material, it may also serve to conserve reusable compounds. Neurons and glial cells have active uptake mechanisms by which they can accumulate certain selected compounds, for example spent transmitter substances (cf. Section 2.5e). A function of the blood-brain barrier may be to prevent the rapid washout of valuable complex molecules by the circulation and thus enable their recycling by brain cells.

While the existence of active transport is well established, the details of the movements of ions are by no means clear. A possible scheme might be that interstitial fluid is formed by the active transport of Na^+ from plasma into CNS interstitium, with Cl^- and water following passively. Cl^- would be obligated to follow Na^+ by electric force, and water would be propelled by osmotic force. It is in keeping with this theory that CSF is always a few millivolts electropositive relative to the blood. This mechanism would in essence be analogous to the formation of saliva and of other saline solutions by secreting tissues, including the small intestine. The handling of other ions, whose activity in the interstitial fluid of the CNS differs from that in plasma, is not immediately obvious, however. They could be transported at rates different from that of Na^+; or there may be a primary secretion similar to plasma which then is modified secondarily by additional transport mechanisms. As we have already mentioned, there is, for example, evidence for the active transport of K^+ from CNS into blood. Current research suggests that the routing of ions between plasma, CSF and cerebral interstitium may rival the complexity of the movements of ions through successive segments of the nephron.

Much speculation concerns the role of the sheath of glial end-feet found around CNS capillaries. For years it has been thought that the glial envelope is the blood-brain barrier, until electron microscopy and other evidence revealed that the glial layer is fenestrated and that it is the endothelial layer which is tight. The pericapillary glial sheath, as does the sub-pial glia limitans, has intercellular gaps large enough to allow the diffusion not only of crystalloid solutes, but also of experimentally introduced macromolecular tracer substances. Nevertheless many investigators feel that there must be a reason for the ubiquity of the pericapillary glial sheaths, and assume that the glial cells assist in the regulation of the composition of interstitial fluid and in the transport of material between it and blood (see also Section 5.9).

Materials may reach central nervous system tissue not only through the endothelium of cerebral capillaries, but they could also be "long-circuited," first secreted into cerebrospinal fluid and thence enter the intercellular spaces. As for the common physiological constituents, such as ions and glucose, the composition of CSF is very similar to, if not identical with, that of the cerebral interstitial fluid. The absence of a significant gradient suggests that transfer of these constituents between the two fluids is limited and the CSF is not an important vehicle for them. There are indications, however, that the CSF serves as a conveyor of special regulatory substances which must reach certain specialized areas or "trigger zones" on the surface of the brain. This will be discussed further (Section 5.3b).

The cerebrospinal fluid may be of greater importance as a vehicle for the removal of waste materials than as a supplier of nutrients. A variety of products of cerebral metabolism find their way into the CSF and from there into the bloodstream. The dumping of wastes into CSF creates an opportunity for investigators to intercept these before they reach the blood. Clinicians and researchers alike tap samples of CSF for diagnosis and for research.

There are altogether three routes for the clearing of wastes from CNS interstitium: (1) by transport through capillary walls into the blood; (2) by washout with the CSF and thus disposal through the arachnoid villi (see Section 5.2c); (3) by way of the nerve roots and the perineural spaces into the lymphatic circulation. The perivascular spaces of brain and spinal cord communicate with the subarachnoid spaces. From the subarachnoid spaces there are two exists: one is through the arachnoid villi and the other through the tissues around the spinal and cranial nerve roots which in turn communicate with the lymphatic spaces outside the skull and the vertebral canal. At least in rabbits this last route has been shown to be a significant fraction of the total waste clearance.

5.2. Cerebrospinal Fluid

5.2a. CIRCULATION OF CSF

The volume of all the CSF of an adult person measures, on the average, 140 ml. About 0.3–0.5 ml of fresh fluid is formed per minute. In other words, the entire CSF is replaced in less than 6 hours. Of the total, about 22 ml is in the ventricles, 45 ml in the cranial subarachnoid spaces, and the balance in the spinal subarachnoid space. Normal CSF pressure in a recumbent subject varies between 5 and 18 cm of saline, measured in the lumbar sac. The main circulation of the CSF is from the lateral ventricles of the cerebral hemispheres through the foramina of Monroe into the 3rd ventricle, and then by way of the aqueduct into the 4th. The 4th ventricle communicates with the cisternae of the subarachnoid space through three openings: the two lateral foramina of Luschka, and the dorsal foramen of Magendie. From the cisternae, which surround the brain stem, most of the fluid streams upward around the cerebral convexities and is then absorbed into the blood of the large venous sinuses in the dura mater. Part of the CSF, however, takes the "southern route" and flows from cisterna magna down into the spinal subarachnoid space, to be absorbed by arachnoid villi into the veins around spinal dorsal roots (Fig. 5.2).

The flow around the spinal cord, however, is not unidirectional. Radiopaque or radioactive material injected into the lumbar subarachnoid space in diagnostic procedures appears within an hour or two in the cranial cavity, demonstrating that spinal fluid flows upward as well as downward. The hydrodynamics of this seeming two-way flow have not yet been determined. The following are possible patterns: (1) alternating flow, now in the caudal, then in the cranial direction; (2) the main current being caudally directed with backflow into the cranial cavity caused by turbulence; (3) actual two-way flow, caudally directed over the dorsal surface and cranially directed under the ventral surface of the spinal cord. The movements of spinal fluid are accelerated by the variable pressure exerted on the spinal canal by contractions of the back muscles, by coughing, and by straining. Even during complete immobility, however, the spinal portion of the CSF is not the "stagnant pool of backwater" it was once supposed to be. If it were, its diagnostic significance would have to be greatly devalued.

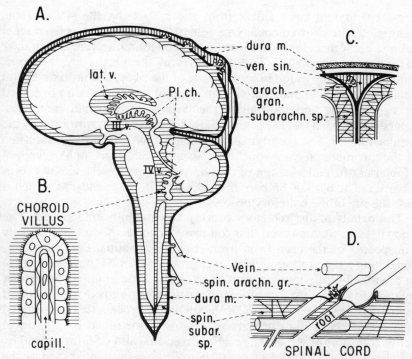

Figure 5.2. Interrelationship of CSF and blood spaces. *A*, the CSF in and around the brain; *B*, choroid villus; *C*, a dural sinus with arachnoid granulations invading its wall; *D*, spinal subarachnoid space. *Pl. ch.*, plexus choroideus; *lat. v.*, lateral ventricle; *III v.*, 3rd cerebral ventricle; *dura m.*, dura mater; *ven. sin.*, venous sinus; *arach. gran.*, arachnoid granulation; *subarachn. sp.*, subarachnoid space; root, spinal dorsal or ventral root. *Horizontal hatching*, CSF; *vertical hatching*, blood. Note that in brain (not shown) as in spinal cord (*D*) the perivascular spaces provide a route for the seepage (bulk flow) of fluid from interstitial space into subarachnoid space and from subarachnoid space into interstitium and lymph vessels outside the skull and spinal canal, as long as CNS interstitial pressure remains higher than interstitial and lymphatic pressures outside the CNS.

5.2b. FORMATION OF CSF

Choroid plexuses are found in all four cerebral ventricles. After several decades of debate, no doubt remains that these structures secrete cerebrospinal fluid. A choroid plexus consists of convolutions of microcirculatory vessels covered by specialized ependyma. The ultrastructure of these ependymal cells differs from those covering the walls of the ventricles. The choroid ependyma resembles the secreting cells of renal tubules and other glandular tissue in both their architecture and in their inventory of organelles. The capillaries of the plexus are, however, similar to the type found in most tissues of the body, and unlike cerebral capillaries. Thus endothelial cells in choroid capillaries are not joined in tight seams, and they allow the passage of all small molecules. Interstitial fluid is formed in the choroid plexus by ultrafiltration of the capillary blood. The ependymal cells then use the interstitial ultrafiltrate as the raw material from which they secrete CSF. Thus, unlike cerebral capillaries, the endothelium of the choroid plexus vessels does not form a barrier. The blood-CSF barrier resides here in the ependyma, which is also the site of the secretory process (Figs. 5.1 and 5.2).

The details of the secretory process are not fully understood. The known facts fit, however, the following scheme. Sodium is actively transported by the ependyma from choroid interstitial fluid into CSF, generating a secretory potential, averaging 5 mV, CSF positive relative to blood. Chloride ions are moved by this electric gradient, and water follows driven by osmotic force. Potassium is pumped from choroid interstitium into ventricular CSF by an active process that is saturated at 3.5 mM. Potassium activity is, however, fine-tuned by additional active transport of K^+ in the reverse direction, from CSF into blood by the choroid ependyma and from CNS interstitial fluid into blood by the cerebral endothelium (see Section 5.1c). The other physiologically important ions, Ca^{2+}, Mg^{2+}, HCO_3^-, have separate transport systems each regulating the activity of its ion independently from the others. The pH in the CSF is determined by the passive movement of CO_2 and by the active transport of HCO_3^-. CO_2 and HCO_3^- are, of course, also generated within CNS tissue by metabolism and by carbonic anhydrase. Whether or not H^+ ions are themselves transported across the blood-CSF and blood-brain barriers is not clear, but any such transport is believed to be less significant than the diffusion of CO_2 and the pumping of HCO_3^-.

The choroid plexuses are not the only sources of CSF. Fluid flows along perivascular spaces and to a lesser degree seeps through the ependymal and pia-glial surfaces of brain and spinal cord, and is then added to the CSF. This extra fluid originates, of course, from capillaries of the CNS, through the blood-brain barrier. It has not been determined what fraction of the total of the CSF originates in this manner. Some investigators estimate nearly half, others believe the amount to be much smaller. Most measurements have been carried out in animals other than man, and differences among species may account for part of the controversy. More to the point, the extrachoroidal contribution to the CSF may change according to circumstances. For example, it is possible that more fluid seeps through the extrachoroidal surfaces when CSF pressure is low.

5.2c. REMOVAL OF CSF

CSF is drained by a process quite different from that which forms it. Arachnoid villi act as one-way valves. Whenever CSF pressure exceeds the pressure of blood in the venous sinus by a critical amount (between 20 and 50 mm H_2O), CSF flows from subarachnoid space into the sinus. But if the pressure gradient is reversed, backflow into the subarachnoid space is prevented. This unidirectional floodgate function has been experimentally demonstrated, but the anatomical structure responsible for it has not definitely been identified. In light- and electron-microscopic examination, the micro-channels of arachnoid tissue forming the villi appear to be blindly ending tubes, with no gaps, flaps, or other visible structures which could act as valves. It is possible, of course, that there are fenestrations which are opened only when CSF pressure rises above the critical level and stretches the arachnoid tubules. If so, then the fenestration would vanish, when low pressure allowed the villi to retract, and this must be the state just before the tissue is fixed for histology. According to an alternative theory, fluid is transported across the cells lining the arachnoid villi in microvesicles formed by pinocytosis. Drainage through lymphatics is an additional route, besides the arachnoid villi, through which part of the CSF is being removed (cf. Section 5.1c).

Through all routes, the clearance rate of all constituents, regardless of molecular size, is the same so that CSF is drained exactly as it exists within the cranial vault. This is a hallmark of bulk flow. Normally only trace amounts of protein are present in CSF. Macromolecules deliberately introduced into the CSF are, however, cleared at the same rate as small molecules, ions at the same rate as uncharged particles.

5.2d. FUNCTIONS OF THE CSF

Some functions of the CSF are fairly obvious. The density of CNS tissue is less than that of the CSF, so that the brain floats, as it were, in a bath. When much of the CSF is removed, as it must be for certain diagnostic procedures such as pneumoencephalography, the patient suffers headache until freshly formed CSF provides flotation again. In the absence of fluid the brain must rest on the hard floor of the cranial cavity, and the meninges are amply supplied with nociceptive nerve endings (see Section 6.7). The headache seems to serve to prevent the patient from suddenly moving his head and thus damaging his brain which does not have its usual fluid protection. Unfortunately, the protection afforded against mechanical trauma by the CSF is not fool-proof. A hard blow to the head will cause unconsciousness, and if there is bleeding or laceration, sometimes lasting brain damage.

There are other functions of the CSF, some of which have already been mentioned. As CSF flows through the ventricles and around the brain and spinal cord, it leaches and so removes metabolic waste products. Bathing the brain in fluid of a composition similar to that of interstitial fluid, CSF assists in maintaining the constancy of the environment of central neurons. And it is suspected that specific chemical messages are carried by the CSF toward receptors located in specialized chemical trigger zones. This will be discussed in the next section.

5.3. Chemoreceptors Within the Central Nervous System

The central nervous system contains specialized regions sensitive to chemical stimulation. Some sample blood, others the CSF.

5.3a. BRAIN REGIONS WITHOUT A BARRIER AND A CHEMICAL TRIGGER ZONE RESPONSIVE TO BLOOD-BORNE STIMULI

There are parts of the brain where blood is not separated from interstitial fluid by the usual barrier. These regions are said to lie outside the barrier. There seem to be two different purposes for such breaches of the perimeter: to permit either access of substances produced in the brain to the bloodstream, or of blood-borne substances to the brain. For example, where hormones are made by neurosecretory cells, these must be secreted into the circulation. Thus in the neural lobe of the neuro-hypophysis, in the pineal gland, and in the tuber cinereum-median eminence regions, endothelial cells offer no hindrance to the permeation of neurohumors into blood.

Chemical agents are allowed to pass in the reverse direction, from blood into brain, at a specific site, the *area postrema*. This is a narrow strip of tissue astride the midline beneath the floor of the caudal end of the 4th cerebral ventricle. Dyes administered intravenously that are kept out of the CNS elsewhere stain this tissue. Capillaries in this region are not "tight," but are fenestrated, much like those of somatic tissues. On the other hand, the ependyma lining the 4th ventricle over the area postrema is much less permeable than the ependyma elsewhere. This prevents substances that leak through the capillary walls into the area postrema from seeping into the CSF. Nothing hinders diffusion from the area postrema into adjacent parts of the medulla oblongata, but the exchange of material by this route is considered to be insignificant.

The principal response to chemical stimulation of the area postrema is vomiting. Apomorphine, a non-narcotic derivative of morphine, appears to exert its strong emetic action here. Certain other drugs, cardiac glycosides among them, which do not penetrate the blood-brain barrier elsewhere, have access to the area postrema and thus trigger vomiting. It is a reasonable guess that blood-borne toxic products of bacteria, or of diseased tissues, may also cause vomiting by their effect here.

Vomiting is a complex response involving activation of numerous neuronal circuits, the various components of which are coordinated in the medulla oblongata. The area postrema acts as a trigger zone, but not all the programming of the response occurs in this small volume of tissue. Other neural inputs can also evoke vomiting, including excessive stimulation of the labyrinths (motion sickness) (Section 13.3b) and certain stimuli acting in the stomach or on the pharyngeal mucosa.

5.3b. CHEMICAL SENSOR ZONES FOR CSF

Certain areas on the surface of the brain are sensitive to specific chemical stimuli. On the ventral aspect of the brain stem there are several small zones with such specialized sensitivities. Appropriate chemical stimulation of these zones elicits coordinated responses, mainly involving visceral functions. Respiratory responses can be evoked by stimulating one zone, vascular responses by stimulating another, the release of vasopressin into the bloodstream by yet another.

Acetylcholine and other cholinergic drugs, monoamines, and some neuropeptides have been shown to elicit these responses, each having a specific effect limited to one or other of the chemoreceptive zones.

The sensitive elements are believed to be neuronal and lie 100–300 μm beneath the pia-glial surface. The natural stimuli which normally act on the chemosensitive areas may be neuroactive substances, including peptides and monoamines, which have been found in the CSF. As already mentioned, products of cerebral metabolism find their way into CSF. Whether intact neurohumor molecules simply spill into the CSF or are secreted into it has not been determined. The axon terminals of some neurosecretory cells do, however, reach the ependyma, and some actually protrude into the lumen of the ventricle (Fig. 5.1B). Such terminals could well be the source of neuroactive substances carried by the CSF from the ventricles to the chemosensitive target areas of the cerebral surface. This method of chemical information transfer would be intermediate between endocrine and neuronal modes of signaling.

A special case is the sensitivity of the ventral surface of the medulla to acid. Acidification of the environment of cells in the brain stem, caused by the penetration of CO_2 through the blood-brain barrier, has been recognized as the centrally acting chemical stimulus for the control of respiration (see West, p. 117). It is because CO_2 penetrates the barrier easily, whereas H^+ ions do not, that respiratory acidosis stimulates both peripheral and central chemoreceptors, whereas metabolic acidosis has an effect only on the former.

At first it was thought that neurons of the respiratory centers are themselves stimulated by the lowered pH caused by excess CO_2, but subsequent tests indicated that these neurons are not sensitive to acid. When it was discovered that H^+ ions in contact with the ventral surface of the medulla do stimulate respiration, the mystery of the central chemoreceptors appeared close to being solved. Unfortunately not all questions have been answered, and for several reasons which cannot be detailed here, the central chemoreceptors sensing pH changes cannot yet be regarded as definitely identified.

5.4. The Breaching of the Blood-Brain Barrier

There are circumstances under which the blood-brain barrier can become abnormally permeable for a shorter or longer period of time. In experimental animals the barrier can, for example, be opened by suddenly raising the arterial pressure. The pressure must approach or exceed the limit below which autoregulation can keep cerebral blood flow relatively constant (see Smith and Kampine, pp. 159–160, 187–188). Another method to open the barrier is to cause maximal cerebral vasodilatation by hypercapnia. Yet another is to rapidly infuse a small volume of highly hypertonic solution into the internal carotid artery.

In all these cases the opening of the barrier outlasts the provoking stimulus. Generally, however, in such experiments, the impermeability of the capillaries is restored in a relatively short period, for example 15 minutes. The mechanism of the temporary increase of the permeability of the blood-brain barrier under such experimental conditions is a subject of controversy. One theory holds that clefts open between endothelial cells. According to another view, material is transferred in pinocytotic vesicles and in submicroscopic channels through the endothelial cells, not between them. Both mechanisms may operate to various degrees under different conditions.

The clinician must count on a partial or complete opening of the barrier in certain pathological conditions, such as meningitis. In a way this can be helpful, because it enables delivery of certain antibiotics to the central nervous system. Yet it also contains a danger. Penicillin, which usually is an innocuous drug, becomes a powerful convulsant if too much of it is taken up by the brain or spinal cord.

X-rays and other ionizing radiation can cause damage to the blood-brain barrier. Surprisingly, hypoxia leaves the blood-brain barrier intact for a considerable period of time. Neurons die of oxygen starvation before the barrier opens. Eventually it does, however.

Virus particles can reach the central nervous system, though not through the barrier. They enter either peripheral nerves or dorsal root ganglia and move by axoplasmic transport into the CNS. The access to the CNS of the antibodies of autoimmune diseases has not yet been discovered.

5.5. Other Endothelial Barrier Systems

The brain is not unique in being relatively insulated from blood by a selective access system. The barrier of the retina is entirely similar. After all, retina is brain tissue of a sort. But other compartments of the eye are also invested with a barrier and so is the inner ear.

When one of the dyes customarily used to test blood barriers has been administered, the perineurium of peripheral nerves is stained, but endoneurium and nerve fibers are not. The barrier of peripheral nerves and the composition of their interstitial fluid are not yet understood in detail. The exposed terminals of peripheral sensory nerve fibers, the dorsal root ganglia, and the ganglia of the autonomic nervous system stain in the same way as non-nervous tissues.

Some parts of the testicles have a barrier which in some respects is similar to the one between blood and brain. That organ is, however, outside the scope of this text.

5.6. Cerebral Edema

The interstitial space of the brain has in years past been estimated by some investigators to occupy as much as 30% and by others as little as 4% of the total volume of the tissue. The most recent and best estimates were obtained by adding inulin to both CSF and blood of experimental animals until identical steady concentrations were reached in both fluids, and then measuring the inulin content of the brain. With this method central interstitial space (not including vascular and CSF spaces) was found to occupy an average of 15% of the total tissue volume. This volume can change somewhat even under normal conditions. During neuronal activity, there is a net gain of intracellular salt and water causing extracellular space to shrink by 1 or 2%. During seizures, spreading depression (see Section 5.8b) and hypoxia, changes of interstitial fluid volume can be much more drastic.

If cells swell at the expense of interstitial space, the volume of the organ as a whole does not change. If, however, extra water is transferred from blood into brain, its volume actually increases. This condition is *cerebral edema.*

Cerebral edema can have several causes. Lowering of the osmotic pressure of the blood is one of them. It can be either the consequence of hemodilution, as in water intoxication or during inappropriate secretion of antidiuretic hormone; or it can be caused by the loss of NaCl, as in Addison's disease. When extracellular osmotic pressure is lowered in peripheral tissues, it is mainly the cells that swell. In systemic tissues the capillary walls are permeable, and the cell membranes are semipermeable. Therefore osmotic gradients develop across cell membranes, not the capillary wall. The CNS reacts differently, because the blood-brain barrier is itself a semipermeable structure. Thus while peripheral cells act as osmometers, the brain as a whole acts as an osmometer. Therefore, the water content of the whole organ can be modified by changes of osmotic pressure in the blood. This peculiarity makes emergency treatment of brain edema possible. For if low osmotic pressure of the blood causes the organ to swell, high osmotic pressure has the opposite effect. Neurologists and neurosurgeons indeed administer hypertonic solutions for the immediate relief of cerebral edema. But the hypertonia induced as a therapy must not be so high that it opens the blood-brain barrier. The administration of a hypertonic solution is a first aid, and must be followed by correction of the disturbance that originally gave rise to the edema.

This first aid can, however, be life-saving. If the volume of the brain increases, then an equal volume of either CSF or of blood or both are squeezed out of the cranial cavity. Compression of blood vessels raises their resistance to flow. Moreover the swelling of the brain stem can compress the aqueduct of Sylvius, which is the outflow path of CSF from the cerebral ventricles. The consequent rise of ventricular CSF pressure is then added to the already raised intracranial pressure and, in the worst cases, a vicious circle is set up, threatening the life of the patient.

Besides hypotonicity of the blood, cerebral edema can also be a consequence of cerebral trauma, of capillary bleeding in the tissue, of inflammation and of careless manipulation in surgery. The mechanism of the edema in these cases in not always clear. Opinions differ whether tissue hypoxia, uncomplicated by other factors, can also cause edema or merely movement of water from interstitial space into cells. Edema has also been attributed to disturbances of the blood-brain barrier. In so called vasogenic edema the barrier is opened so much that plasma protein passes from blood into cerebral interstitium. Consequently there is net filtration of fluid from vessels into interstitial spaces, propelled by the hydrostatic pressure gradient.

5.7. Hydrocephalus

The clinical term for too much CSF is hydrocephalus, literally "water on the brain." Quite generally, it occurs when CSF is produced faster than it is removed. It can be accompanied by raised intracranial pressure, but in a chronic process this is not always the case. If there is an obstruction in one of the apertures connecting the ventricles or between the ventricular system and the subarachnoid space, it is termed non-communicating hydrocephalus; if the flow of CSF through the cerebral cavities is unimpeded, we speak of communicating hydrocephalus. In the latter case the trouble can be obstructed outflow through the arachnoid granulations or overproduction at the sources of CSF. Chronic hydrocephalus is frequently associated with enlargement of the ventricular system and decrease in the mass (atrophy) of cerebral tissue.

5.8. Perturbations of Interstitial Ion Activities

Since neurons exchange ions when they generate synaptic and action potentials, and since such exchanges take place within a milieu of limited volume, the composition of the interstitial fluid may change transiently during neuronal activation. The transport processes of the blood-brain barrier regulate the average overall composition of the interstitial fluid. The question is whether ion activity levels may be perturbed transiently and locally, by neuronal activity, and if they do, how they are restored to the normal, "resting" level. Recently, it has become possible to measure the extracellular activities of some ions with probes whose tips measure only a few microns in diameter. These instruments revealed that the activities of certain ions do indeed change as neurons get excited and inhibited, and more so by pathological events.

5.8a. TRANSIENT CHANGES OF INTERSTITIAL ION ACTIVITIES DURING NORMAL NEURONAL ACTIVITY

When an experimental animal is kept in a dimly lit environment and then shown a bright visual stimulus of strong contrast, extracellular potassium activity $[K^+]_o$ increases in those parts of the central nervous system to which the visual pathways project. Similarly, when a cat's fur is stroked, or its tail is squeezed, $[K^+]_o$ rises in the dorsal gray matter of the excited spinal segments. Such stimulation causes $[K^+]_o$ to rise from its resting level of 3.0 mM to, perhaps 3.5, rarely above 4.0 mM. Glial cells probably limit changes of $[K^+]_o$ as explained in Section 5.9b.

Since with each nerve impulse K^+ is exchanged for Na^+, $[Na^+]_o$ should decrease as $[K^+]_o$ increases. A change of 0.5 or 1.0 mM of $[Na^+]_o$ against a resting background of 140 mM is, however, not detectable with present techniques. A decrease of $[Ca^{2+}]_o$ by 20 μM or so from its resting level of 1.0 to 1.1 mM is sometimes demonstrable. It will be recalled that Ca^{2+} enters presynaptic terminals as a prelude to synaptic transmission and also postsynaptic target neurons with impulse discharge (see Sections 3.1k and 3.2). There are also small local changes of pH, $[Cl^-]_o$, and a shift of water from interstitial to intracellular space.

The changes of extracellular ion activities that accompany the normal workings of a healthy brain are probably small enough not to disturb neuronal function. This is not the case with the much larger perturbations seen during pathological conditions, to be discussed next.

5.8b. INTERSTITIAL ION ACTIVITIES DURING PATHOLOGICAL PROCESSES

Strong electric stimulation, which activates many neurons of unrelated function, causes ion levels to depart from their resting condition much more than natural (adequate) stimuli ever can. More importantly, during seizure discharge, $[K^+]_o$ can rise to a level between 8.0 and 12.0 mM, and $[Ca^{2+}]_o$ can sink to between 0.4 and 0.6 mM. These ion activities are grossly abnormal. The acidification of the interstitial fluid, the changes of $[Na^+]_o$ and $[Cl^-]_o$, and the associated osmotic entry of water from intercellular into intracellular space are all more noticeable during seizures than during excitation of healthy CNS tissue. Whatever the primary cause of the seizure (see Section 4.11), the greatly altered ionic milieu cannot fail to influence the course of the seizure discharge. High $[K^+]_o$ acts as a stimulus in itself, and may be one of the factors of positive feedback (Section 3.4a) that maintain a tonic paroxysm. Lowering of $[Ca^{2+}]_o$ also enhances the excitability of neurons, but then as it is more and more lowered it also causes synaptic transmission to fail and so it may actually assist in finally quenching paroxysmal discharge.

The worst ionic disturbances in live CNS tissue occur in the condition known as *spreading cortical depression of Leão*. Intense stimulation of the cerebral cortex at one point may, after an initial burst of seizure discharge, be followed by the suppression of electroencephalographic (EEG) waves. This silencing of the normal electrical activity then spreads over the cortical surface at the very slow pace of roughly 3 mm/min. Recovery of activity at any one point may take 1–10 minutes.

Intense local electric stimulation, a small weight falling on the cortical surface, a small crystal of KCl, and several other stimuli can provoke spreading depression. Other than in the neocortex, the phenomenon can be produced in most parts of the central nervous system, for example, in the cerebellar cortex, in subcortical brain nuclei, and in the retina, but *not* the spinal cord. Dehydration and hypoxia favor its development; immature brains are, however, relatively resistant to it.

During spreading depression the extracellular electric potential of the affected region shifts in the negative direction by 10–35 mV, because for a few minutes all cells, neurons and glia alike, are severely depolarized. At the same time $[K^+]_o$ rises, $[Ca^{2+}]_o$, $[Na^+]_o$, and $[Cl^-]_o$ fall, reaching levels never otherwise measured in live brain. The exact mechanism of the depressive process is not understood, but the changes of ion levels are bound to be links in the causal chain of events. $[K]_o$ rises high enough to account for the depolarization of neurons and glial cells, and hence also for the consequent silencing of EEG activity. The low $[Ca^{2+}]_o$ would, however, by itself be sufficient to interrupt all synaptic transmission.

Spreading depression is accompanied by vasodilatation and shrinkage of interstitial space (cell swelling). Oxidative metabolism in the electrically depressed tissue is greatly augmented during and after a depressive episode, and the extra energy developed is probably utilized to transport ions in order to restore the normal condition. The recovery of normal ion distribution takes only 1 or 2 minutes, but spontaneous electric activity is not resumed for several additional minutes.

Spreading depression in human pathology. There is no definite proof that spreading depression occurs in human brains, but there are at least three common neurological conditions which it might explain. The first is the immediate effect of sudden hypoxia. In experimental animals either the sudden interruption of blood flow or sudden deprivation of oxygen causes cerebral tissue to enter a state resembling spreading depression in almost every respect. The difference is that hypoxia affects the whole brain at once, so that the depression is not "spreading" but the whole brain goes through the cycle of depression and recovery at the same time. If the supply of oxygen is interrupted for a short time only, recovery is possible. Permanent damage results if a part, or the whole of the brain is deprived of oxygen for more than a few minutes. The transition from reversible depression to irreversible damage is not understood.

Another condition possibly related to spreading depression is the coma caused by a severe blow to the head. This concerns those cases where there is no inwardly displaced fracture of the skull, or bleeding inside the cranial cavity. It is known that mechanical stimulation of the cortical surface can initiate spreading depression. If the intact skull is hit to cause sufficient acceleration, the brain may bounce in its case, and the depressive process could be triggered simultaneously at several points. If the depressed state generalizes to the entire cortex and perhaps to the subcortical nuclei, this could cause unconsciousness for several minutes, and then a period of being dazed which may last much longer.

A third process, attributed by some investigators to spreading depression, is the scotoma of migraine. Many, though not all, patients suffering with migraine experience a blind spot that moves slowly across their visual field during an attack. The distinguished investigator K. Lashley, himself a victim of this condition, timed the apparent movement of his own scotoma. Making the assumption that the march of his blind spot was related to a disturbance moving across his cerebral cortex, he calculated its rate of progression based on the known dimensions of the visual projection in the human brain. The calculated rate with which the supression of visual function seemed to move across the cortex corresponded to the known velocity of spreading cortical depression. While this coincidence may be fortuitous, it does suggest that the two processes could be related. Needless to say, this theory does not explain the whole migraine syndrome, only one of its manifestations.

5.9. Neuroglia

Toward the middle of the last century, Virchow reasoned that the brain, like all other organs, must contain connective tissue. Examining brain tissue by gross dissection and under the microscope, he thought he recognized such a tissue component, but he also felt that in some ways this was different from connective tissue found elsewhere. He, therefore, coined a special name, *neuroglia*, literally "nerve glue," or "nerve putty." It took many decades of patient work and the better staining methods used by the leading histologists of the latter half of the 19th century for it to become clear which cells of the central nervous system are neurons and which are something else. By the turn of the century it also became clear that, unlike connective tissue, glia is not of mesodermal origin but is derived from the same embryonal ependyma from which nerve cells also arise and, therefore, is of epithelial type. In the adult organism glial cells nevertheless behave in ways quite different from their cousins, the neurons.

Glia is by no means a minor component of the CNS. Glial cells outnumber neurons in most parts of the gray matter but, on the average, they are smaller than nerve cells. They occupy between 20 and 45% of the brain volume, varying according to region and cytoarchitecture. Generally speaking, there is more glia in neuropil than in nuclear layers.

Four types of cells are classified as neuroglial. *Astrocytes, oligodendrocytes* (oligocytes), *ependymal cells* and *microcytes* (or microglia). Of these four, astrocytes and oligocytes are the most numerous, and they constitute the true glia. The number of microcytes in healthy CNS tissue is very small. Many more are found at sites of injury and of inflammation. The few microcytes that are there under normal conditions may perhaps be regular residents of the CNS, but the vast number appearing in lesioned tissue are considered invaders, or wandering histiocytes, which arrive with the bloodstream and whose function is to remove the debris left by injury. Oligocytes and perhaps even astrocytes are said to be capable of phagocytic activity when properly provoked, but they are amateurs besides the professional phagocytes, the microcytes.

The principal known function of oligocytes is to invest axons in the CNS with myelin, to maintain this sheath, and repair it if necessary (Fig. 5.3). They are the functional central counterparts of the Schwann cells of peripheral nerves. Whether or not oligocytes have other functions, sharing some of those attributed to astrocytes, is not clear at present.

About the adult ependyma much has already been said, and there is little to add. During embryonic development the ependyma is the germinal layer from which all cells of the central nervous system migrate toward the site they will occupy in adult life. During this migration a special kind of embryonic glia leads the way. Fibrous processes of this *radial glia* provide the scaffolding along which primitive nerve cells move toward their destination. Once cell populations have organized into the layers and nuclei of the adult CNS, the long guide ropes of the radial glia vanish, and the embryonic glial cells are transformed into the adult form. In the retina and in the cerebellar cortex adult glial cells retain a radial orientation, and are known as the Müller and Bergman cells, respectively.

5.9a. THE FUNCTIONS OF ASTROCYTES

It seems unlikely that glial cell which make from a quarter to a half of the bulk of the CNS are simply, as Virchow thought, the putty (*Nervenkitt*) that holds the neurons together. Astrocytes especially have fascinated researchers for decades. Much has been learned about their staining properties, their biochemistry, their electrophysiology, but still firm conclusions concerning their true functions have eluded us. Here follows a brief summary of the most important suggested functions of astrocytes, some better founded on facts than others. It is also possible that some of these functions are shared with oligocytes.

The repair of CNS tissue. Two types of astrocytes are distinguished

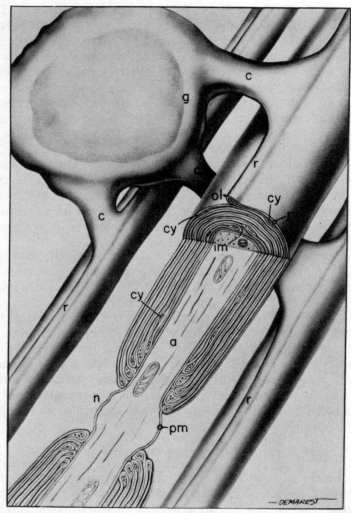

Figure 5.3.   An oligodendrocyte (*g*) wrapping myelin around several axons (*a*) in the central nervous system. *pm*, plasma membrane; *n*, node of Ranvier; *cy*, remnant of cytoplasm of oligocyte between myelin layers; *r*, ridge formed by free edge of myelin, which on transverse section appears as a loop (*ol*) of oligocyte plasma membrane; *c*, process connecting oligocyte cell body with myelin sheath. (Reprinted with permission from M. B. Bunge, R. P. Bunge and H. Ris: *Journal of Biophysical and Biochemical Cytology,* 10:67–94, 1961.)

by microscopic examination. *Protoplasmic astrocytes* are typical of healthy CNS. *Fibrous astrocytes* abound at the sites of injury. Whether the latter are a transformation of the former, or whether fibrous astrocytes are an altogether different species of cell which proliferates after injury, is not known. After microcytes have cleaned up the debris of injury, the remaining cavity is filled by astrocytic tissue. Pathologists call this process *repair* to distinguish it from *regeneration*. Adult mammals cannot replace lost neurons (but see Section 20.5). Thus, injured CNS tissue is, after a while, replaced by a *glial scar* which in the long run tends to shrink. Such glial scars frequently become *epileptic foci* (cf. Section 4.11). The epileptic activity originates from neurons in the transitional border region of the scar, and not from the glial cells within it.

Astrocytes and transmitter substances. Early histological investigations of the CNS revealed that wherever one neuron touches another, extensions of glial cells surround the junctions. For example, where the surface of a dendrite is studded with the terminal buttons of many different nerve fibers, the endings usually are segregated by glial elements. Further, where dendritic and axonal tips of several neurons enter into complex relationships known as synaptic glomeruli, as in the cerebellum and the thalamus, the complex is invested by an astrocytic capsule.

Several interpretations have been offered for this prevalence of glial dividers between synaptic junctions. They may serve as dams limiting diffusion of transmitter substances. This could aid the buildup of an adequate concentration of transmitter within the synaptic cleft, and at the same time insure that transmitter released at one synapse should not act on its neighbor.

Astrocytes have also been shown to be capable of actively accumulating certain transmitter molecules, for example, γ-aminobutyric acid (GABA) and some of the monoamines. The uptake may have a role in *terminating synaptic action* (cf. Section 3.2b). The captured transmitter molecules may be chemically inactivated or, alternatively, recycled to nerve terminals.

Besides inactivating or recycling transmitters, glial cells may have a role in their synthesis *de novo*. Indeed, glial cells possess the enzymes required to synthesize some transmitter substances or their precursors. According to one recently proposed scheme, glial cells produce glutamine from glucose. Glutamine is then transferred to presynaptic nerve terminals where it is made into glutamic acid, an excitatory transmitter (see Section 2.5e).

A hard-to-explain fact is that glial cells contain transmitters, specifically GABA, in parts of the nervous system where there are no known GABA-ergic synapses (*i.e.* synapses utilizing GABA as transmitter) or for that matter any synapses, as in dorsal root ganglia. To some investigators this means that glial cells may have unsuspected functions in regulating overall excitability of neural tissue or in transmitting actual signals. So far these theories have not been proven, and it may be that GABA in these cells is a metabolic intermediate, with no direct involvement in nervous function.

Membrane properties of astrocytes. Glial cells have a resting membrane potential as high as, or slightly higher than, that of neurons. If K^+ activity changes in the environment of a glial cell, the cell's membrane potential behaves as the Nernst equation for potassium (Equations 2.5 and 2.6) predicts (assuming a constant internal $[K^+]$), except at external $[K^+]$ lower than any that prevails in living tissues. Glial membranes follow the Nernst equation more closely than neuronal membranes because the glial membrane is even less permeable to Na^+ than the resting neuronal membrane (cf Section 2.4b).

The membrane of glial cells is not electrically excitable: it is incapable of generating action potentials and so far there has been no convincing demonstration that it responds to chemical stimulation. The exception is potassium, which does cause the glial membrane potential to change, but it too leaves the membrane conductance unaffected.

Astrocytes, and perhaps also oligocytes, are joined one to another by so-called *gap junctions*. These junctions have a low resistance to electric current. It is believed that the narrow gaps separating the adjacent membranes at these junctions are actually bridged by ion channels, and these channels allow the passage of ions from the cytoplasms of one cell directly into that of its neighbor (see also Section 2.5c). Being randomly connected through gap junctions, astrocytes form an electrotonic network, which sometimes is referred to as a "functional syncytium." Since there is no continuity of proptoplasm, this is not a true syncytium.

5.9b. THE SPATIAL BUFFERING OF $[K^+]_o$ BY ASTROCYTES

Earlier we have seen (Section 5.8) that $[K^+]_o$ can rise in the vicinity of active neurons. The glial cells exposed to the excess $[K^+]_o$ will be depolarized. But if some glial cells are depolarized and others are not, a voltage gradient is created and current flows through the gap junctions. Potassium being the predominant intracellular cation, and being more mobile than the intracellular anions, the current will be carried mainly by K^+. As K^+ ions move away from the depolarized (i.e. less negative) toward the resting (more negative) cells, they must be replaced. Since the glial membrane admits K^+ in preference to all other cations, K^+ will enter the depolarized cells, and an equivalent amount of K^+ will leave the resting cells. In this manner some of the excess K^+ that caused the depolarization in the first place is carried away and deposited in the resting region. The intracellular current must be matched by an extracellular return current, equal in magnitude but opposite in direction.

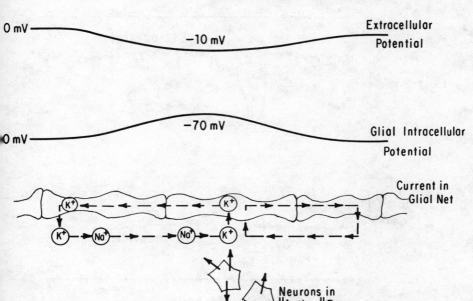

Figure 5.4. Diagrammatic representation of the current generated by an electrotonic net of glial cells, and the potential gradients associated with it. Near the center of the hypothetical row of glial cells activated neurons have released an excess of K^+ ions into the interstitial fluid, depolarizing the glial cells from their resting potential of -90 mV to -70 mV. This causes current to flow from the cytoplasm of the depolarized into that of the resting glial cells, and extracellular current in the reverse direction. For further description see text. (Reprinted with permission from G. Somjen: Physiology of glial cells. In *Physiology of Non-Excitable Cells*, edited by J. Salánki. Budapest, Académiai Kiadó, 1981, pp. 23–43.)

Since Na^+ is the predominant extracellular cation, it will carry most of the return current.

This circulation is illustrated in Figure 5.4 and recordings of glial depolarization are shown in Figure 5.5. The net result of these ion currents is that K^+ is carried away from the region where it had been in excess, and it is replaced by Na^+. This function of the network of glial cells has been described as *spatial buffering*. This redistribution of K^+ can occur over sizable distances very rapidly, because ion currents flow with the speed approaching that of light (remember the analogy of the closely packed billiard balls: (see Section 2.1b)).

If in the course of normal impulse discharge K^+ would accumulate in

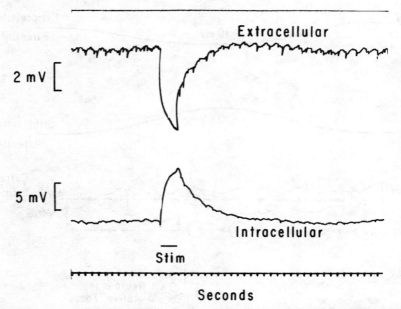

Figure 5.5. Recordings in and outside a spinal cord glial cell. During the time marked by the *horizontal bar* an afferent nerve was stimulated, which caused excitation of the neuron population in the vicinity of the recording electrodes. The depolarization (positive shift of intracellular potential) of the glial cell was the consequence of increasing K^+ caused by the release of K^+ ions by the excited neurons, as suggested in the drawing of Figure 5.4. The spatial profiles of extracellular and intracellular potential illustrated in Figure 5.4 are reconstructions based on numerous recordings similar to those illustrated in this figure. (Reprinted with permission from G. Somjen: *Progress in Neurobiology* 1:199–237, 1973.)

a large excess, this would cause depolarization of neurons, which would change their excitability, and also alter the functioning of synaptic nerve endings. The spatial buffering by glial cells limits the local accumulation of K^+, and hence protects the stability of CNS function. During seizures, and in spreading depression, the limits of the buffering capacity are apparently exceeded (see Section 5.8b).

Glial cells in the regulation of interstitial fluid composition. As was mentioned in Section 5.1c, and illustrated in Figure 5.1, glial processes line blood vessels of the microcirculation in the CNS, and the pia glial membrane. If ependyma is a variety of glia, then glia is in intimate relationship with all the interfaces of the CNS with the "outside," be that blood or CSF. This suggests that one function of glia may be the regulation of the internal environment of the CNS, setting ion levels, removing toxic wastes and perhaps adding nutrients. This theory is strengthened by the knowledge that the glial cell membrane is capable of transporting ions. The demonstration that a variety of organic products, including some transmitters, are transported by glial cell membranes further reinforce the idea. It then takes but a small leap of the imagination to assume that glia may indeed regulate the interstitial fluid of the CNS. The spatial buffering of K^+, explained in the preceding section, would then be just one specialized aspect of this more general function. Unfortunately, this theory remains as yet unproven.

Other suggested functions. From time to time other roles have been suggested for glial tissues. These included endocrine secretion; overall regulation of neuronal excitability; the storage of memory traces (Chapter 20); and yet more. Until founded on more solid experimental evidence, we must forego discussion of these admittedly fascinating ideas.

5.10. Chapter Summary

1. The interstitial fluid of brain and spinal cord is separated from blood by a barrier that is relatively impermeable, not only to large molecules, but also to all water-soluble substances and especially electrically charged ones.
2. The CNS is supplied with essential nutrients by carrier-mediated diffusion.
3. Ion activities in the interstitial fluid of the brain are regulated by active transport.
4. The tissue that forms the barrier and pumps ions between blood and CNS is the capillary endothelium which differs from endothelium in other parts of the body in several respects. In addition, glial cells may have a role in regulating the composition of cerebral interstitial fluid.
5. Metabolites and drugs are cleared from CNS tissue by three routes: (a) by transport through capillary walls; (b) by way of cerebrospinal fluid and the arachnoid villi; (c) by bulk flow along nerve roots into lymphatic vessels.
6. Cerebrospinal fluid (CSF) is formed by secretion by the ependymal lining of the choroid plexuses of the cerebral ventricles. Fluid is also moved from blood into CNS interstitial spaces by the capillary endothelial cells, and this fluid seeps through the ventricular ependymal lining and the pia-glial membrane and is then added to the CSF.
7. CSF is drained by the arachnoid villi in the arachnoid granulations and Pacchioni bodies by unidirectional bulk flow, ensured by the one-way valve action of the villi.
8. CSF protects the brain mechanically, aids in maintaining a stable internal environment, provides an additional channel for the removal of waste, and probably also acts as a vehicle for neuromodulator substances involved in regulating vital functions. For the action of these regulator substances there are chemosensitive trigger zones on the surface of the brain stem.
9. Under certain abnormal conditions the blood-brain barrier becomes more than normally permeable to certain substances. Such failure of the blood-brain barrier is one of several possible causes of cerebral edema.
10. During intense neuronal activity excess K^+ accumulates locally in interstitial

fluid. $[Ca^{2+}]_o$, $[Na^+]_o$, $[Cl^-]_o$ and pH may locally be also perturbed to lesser degrees. During seizures the increase of $[K^+]_o$, the decrease of $[Ca^{2+}]_o$, lowering of pH, and the swelling of cells at the expense of interstitial space are larger than during normal function, and these changes of the internal environment then affect neuronal function.

11. Spreading cortical depression is an example of transient but extreme perturbation of ion distribution in CNS tissue. It may occur in cerebral hypoxia, after traumatic injury of the brain, and perhaps in migraine.

12. The chief known function of oligodendrocytes is the formation of myelin.

13. Microcytes are believed to be wandering histiocytes that invade the CNS from the bloodstream at sites of injury or inflammation.

14. Fibrous astrocytes form glial scars.

15. For protoplasmic astrocytes numerous functions have been suggested, none proven. These include: regulation of the concentration of solutes in interstitial fluid by (a) passive spatial buffering and (b) active transport; uptake and elimination of transmitter substances; synthesis and release of transmitters and other neuroactive substances. More speculative theories include the proposal that glial cells store memory traces.

Further Reading

Books and Reviews

Bradbury M: *The Concept of the Blood-Brain Barrier.* Chichester, John Wiley, 1979.

Davson H: *Physiology of the Cerebrospinal Fluid.* Boston, Little Brown, 1967.

Smith JJ, Kampine JP: *Circulatory Physiology: The Essentials.* Baltimore, Williams & Wilkins, 1980.

Varon SS, Somjen G: Neuron-glia interaction. *Neurosci Res Program Bull* 17:1–239, 1979.

West JB: *Respiratory Physiology: The Essentials,* ed 2. Baltimore, Williams & Wilkins, 1979.

chapter 6

Sensory Receptors and the Somatic Senses

The first part of this chapter deals with the general questions of how receptors transduce stimuli and how sensory information is coded in primary afferent neurons. The second half examines the properties of the sense organs of skin, joints and muscles.

6.1. Introduction to the Physiology of Sense Organs

Sensory receptors gather information by converting small energy changes into electric nerve signals. They are thus *transducers* of one form of energy into another. The transducer element of some sense organs is a specialized receptor cell (see Fig. 8.1), in others it is the membrane of the peripheral terminal of a sensory nerve fiber (Fig. 6.1). The signal generated by a receptor cell is a receptor potential, that of a sensory nerve terminal a generator potential (cf. Section 2.5). The nerve cell whose fiber connects a sensory receptor to the central nervous system (CNS) is called a *primary* (or first order) *afferent neuron*; the central neurons which connect lower to higher sensory nuclei are 2nd, 3rd or *n*th order afferents. A primary afferent neuron with the sensory receptors of all its branches form a *sensory unit*.

Each sensory receptor is especially sensitive to one particular kind of stimulation, its *adequate stimulus*. In this context the word "adequate"

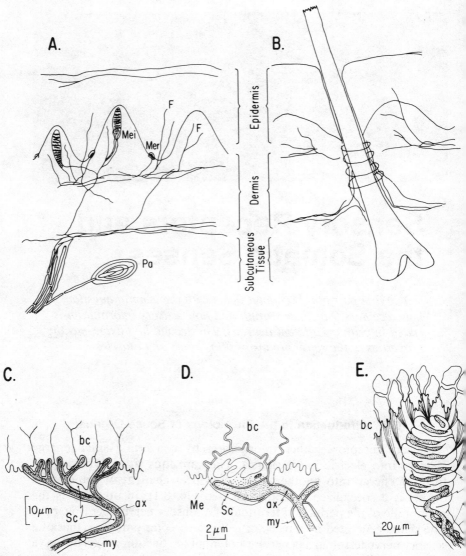

Figure 6.1. Types of sensory nerve endings in skin. *A* and *B*, schematic representation of nerve endings as they appear under the light microscope, *A* in glabrous skin, *B* in hairy skin. *Mei*, Meissner's corpuscle; *Mer*, Merkel's disk; *F*, free nerve endings; *Pa*, Pacinian corpuscle. *C, D* and *E* are simplified diagrams based on electron microscopy. *C*, cold-sensitive nerve terminals; *D*, Merkel disk; *E*, Meissner's corpuscle. *bc*, basal cell of epidermis; *Sc*, Schwann cell; *my*, myelin sheath; *ax*, axon; *Me*, Merkel cell; *pr*, perineural sheath. (*A* and *B* reprinted with permission from G. Somjen: *Sensory Coding*, New York, Plenum, 1975; *C*, *D* and *E* modified and redrawn after H. Hensel: Cutaneous thermoreceptors. In *Somatosensory System*: *Handbook of Sensory Physiology*, vol. 2, edited by A. Iggo, Berlin, Springer, 1973, pp. 79–110; A. Iggo and A. R. Muir: *Journal of Physiology* 200:763–796, 1969; and K. H. Andres and M. von Düring: Morphology of Sensory receptors. In *Somatosensory System*: *Handbook of Sensory Physiology*, vol. 2, edited by A. Iggo, 1973, pp. 3–28.)

means "of the right kind" and not "of a sufficient amount." Sensory receptors are classified according to their adequate stimuli as follows: (1) *mechanoreceptors*; (2) *thermoreceptors*; (3) *chemoreceptors*; (4) *photoreceptors*. Some fish have also electroreceptors, but we terrestrial creatures have none, and could not use one if we did. Within each class there are several subclasses. Among photoreceptors, the rods and the three types of cones are sensitive to different parts of the visible spectrum (Chapter 9, Figs. 9.6 and 9.7). Auditory receptors are a special kind of mechanoreceptor. And shortly we shall get acquainted with the numerous subclasses of mechanoreceptors and thermoreceptors found in the skin and in the connective tissues.

The specialization of sensory receptor is not absolute. Some of the mechanoreceptors are also excited by strong, sudden cooling of the sensory nerve terminal although their adequate stimulus is a small indentation of the skin. And a blow to the eye (a mechanical stimulus) can excite the photoreceptors of the retina, even though their adequate stimulus is light. Such inadequate stimulation evokes an improper sensation, in this example the proverbial stars and flashes perceived when a blow lands in the eye. What distinguishes one kind of receptor from another is that its sensitivity is greatest to its own adequate stimulus.

The central nervous system recognizes stimuli for what they are, because (1) the different sense organs are specialized to transduce different kinds of stimuli; and (2) the central connections of different kinds of afferent neurons vary according to their specialization. If the skin is cooled without being touched, a particular class of afferent neurons (thermoreceptors) is excited, and this excitation is transmitted to a special population of central neurons. If the skin is touched without change of temperature, it is another set of fibers, the mechanoreceptors, which convey excitation to another set of central neurons.

As a general statement it is true that excitation of different kinds of sensory receptors evokes different kinds of subjective sensations. We speak of different *modalities* of sensation. There is, however, not always a simple one-to-one correspondence between type of receptor and the quality of sensation. In some cases the relationship is simple. Excitation of Pacinian corpuscles evokes the sensation of vibration (see Section 6.4). In others, for example color vision, the relationship between receptor activity and subjective experience is quite complex (cf. Sections 9.2d and 9.2g); in fact the closer one examines the issue, the more complex it becomes. Much is controversial in this area. We have neither the need nor the opportunity to examine these problems in any detail here, but the interested reader should consult the specialized monographs cited at the end of the chapter.

We are not aware of all afferent neural input. The excitation of some receptors, e.g. of those of the carotid bodies, is subjectively never experienced. Excitation of other sense organs may or may not enter conscious awareness. In part this is a matter of intensity: the louder a noise, the more likely it is to intrude. In part it is a matter of *attention*. Other circumstances, for example, the presence of competing stimuli (masking) may also influence subjective perception. Under optimal conditions a single impulse in a single cutaneous mechanoreceptor can be noticed by the subject. The minimum intensity of a stimulus that is subjectively perceived is its *psychophysical threshold*. This is not a fixed quantity, but can vary according to the state of the CNS and the conditions of the experiment.

The *physiological threshold* of a primary afferent neuron (as distinct from the psychophysical threshold) is the stimulus intensity just sufficient to evoke an impulse in the afferent fiber. Lesser stimuli are subliminal, even if they do evoke a generator potential (or receptor potential) (cf. Fig. 1.6).

The stronger the stimulus, the greater the amplitude of the receptor (of the generator) potential, up to a maximum or ceiling level. The ceiling is reached when all the available ion channels have been activated (see Section 2.5). Once threshold has been reached, the stronger the stimulus, the higher the frequency of firing of impulses by the afferent axon. In most sense organs the rate of firing is a non-linear function of the intensity of stimulation. The function linking firing rate to stimulus intensity has a decreasing slope (Fig. 6.2); equal increments of stimulus intensity cause greater increments of firing rate when the stimulus is weak than when the sitmulus is already strong to begin with. Consequently we can discriminate the magnitudes of two weak stimuli more precisely than of two strong stimuli.

The rate of firing of many primary afferent neurons can approximately be described by an empirically fitted power function with an exponent less than unity, of the general form:

$$F = a \cdot S^n \qquad (6.1)$$

where F is the rate of firing; a is the proportionality constant; S is the stimulus intensity; and $n < 1.0$.

This equation is but one of several suggested to describe the dependence of excitation on stimulation. Each fits the behavior of some sense organs better

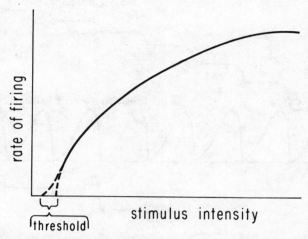

Figure 6.2. Generalized stimulus-response function of primary afferent nerve fibers, showing the dependence of firing frequency on stimulus intensity. Note that near threshold the magnitude of the response is uncertain; note also that the curve has a decreasing slope and it has a maximum (or ceiling) level.

than others. Equation 6.1 is similar in form to the psychophysical magnitude estimate function of S. S. Stevens. The reader interested in quantitative analysis of the relationship of sense organ function and subjective experience should consult, for example, the paper by Mountcastle (1966) cited at the end of this chapter.

Equation 6.1 does not describe the response of afferent fibers to very strong stimuli, for whereas a mathematical power function increases monotonically to infinity, the firing rate of nerve fibers has a definite maximum or ceiling. No fiber can fire faster than about 1500 impulses/sec, and few can sustain firing rates higher than 400/sec for extended periods of time.

Since afferent fibers of otherwise similar function have different thresholds, the stronger the stimulus, the more afferent fibers will begin firing. An increase in the number of activated neurons is called *recruitment*. Assuming that excitation from several afferent fibers converges on secondary afferent neurons in the CNS, the input to the CNS is the product of the number of afferent fibers recruited and the mean firing rate of each.

Many sense organs adapt to stimulation (cf. Section 4.5). If adaptation is complete, then excitation fades after a few impulses have been fired, even if a stimulus continues to act on the receptor (Figs. 6.3 and 6.4A). Such completely and rapidly adapting sense organs respond equally

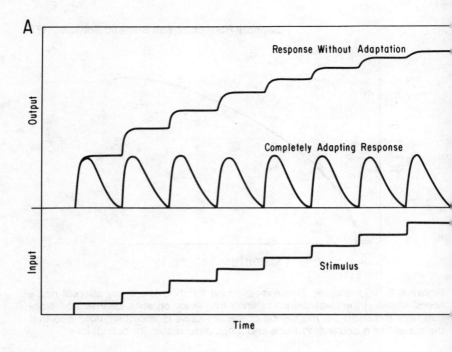

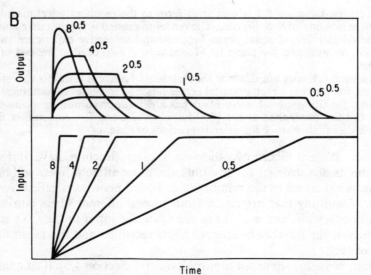

Figure 6.3. The significance of receptor accommodation. *A*, the graphs labeled *output* show the responses of two hypothetical sense organs, one that adapts rapidly and completely and another that does not adapt at all to step-wise increases of stimulation (*input*). *B*, the responses of a rapidly adapting sense organ to stimulations increasing at different rates. The relative velocities of stimulus increase (*dS/dt* of the inputs) are 0.5, 1, 2, 4 and 8, respectively. The responses reach relative maximal amplitudes calculated from Equation 6.2, assuming $n = 0.5$. (Reprinted with permission from G. Somjen: *Sensory Coding in the Mammalian Nervous System*. New York, Plenum Press, 1975.)

each time a stimulus is step-wise increased. Sense organs that do not adapt but obey Stevens' law (Equation 6.1) show less and less increase of firing with each step-wise increment of stimulation (Figs. 6.2 and 6.3A). To be fully informed, the nervous system needs both rapidly and slowly adapting sense organs.

If a stimulus acting on a completely adapting sense organ is gradually rising in intensity, the afferent fiber will fire as long as the stimulus is increasing and cease firing when stimulation becomes steady (Fig. 6.3B).

The rate of firing is a function of the rate or velocity of increase of the stimulus. The relationship is usually non-linear, and can be described by the empirical equation:

$$F = a\left(\frac{dS}{dt}\right)^n \tag{6.2}$$

This is a modified Stevens' function, where the magnitude of the stimulus, S, is replaced by its first derivative with respect to time, dS/dt (Fig. 6.3B).

Most texts classify sensory units as either *rapidly adapting* or *slowly adapting*. The former are the ones that have been described as completely adapting. The latter group includes those sensory units that adapt so slowly that for all practical purposes they can be regarded as non-adapting. It seems useful to define a third class. These units adapt rapidly at first, and slowly or not at all later. For the sake of simplicity call them incompletely adapting, although this name does not describe their behavior entirely accurately. Incompletely adapting afferent units fire at a fast rate while a stimulus is increasing, and then continue to fire at a lower or at a slowly decelerating rate when the stimulus settles to a steady level (e.g. see Figs. 6.6B and C, 6.9A and 15.5). While the stimulus is changing, the excitation of these afferents is influenced both by its actual magnitude and by its rate of change. While the stimulus is steady, these neurons respond to the actual stimulus magnitude. While the stimulus is decreasing, (dS/dt negative), the firing rate of such units decreases below that expected from the momentary stimulus intensity. The response to changing stimulus levels is called the *dynamic response*, to steady stimuli, the *static response*.

There are also afferents which respond only transiently even to stimuli that are on the increase. The excitation of these has been related to the second derivative of the stimulus level, in other words to acceleration. These units have been called transient detectors, sometimes jerk-sensors.

As a rule, the peripheral end of a primary afferent neuron is branched.

For example, a cutaneous afferent nerve fiber can be stimulated either from a number of points scattered over a limited surface area of skin, (punctate excitability), or from a contiguous zone of the skin. Similarly, a retinal ganglion cell can usually be excited not by a single photorecep- tor, but by many photoreceptors occupying a certain limited area of the retina. The zone from which an afferent unit can be excited is its *receptive field* (e.g. see Fig. 6.5). We can also speak of the receptive fields of a central, i.e. second and higher order, afferent neuron. In the case of central afferent neurons, the effect of stimulation of some portion of the receptive surface may be one of inhibition. We then speak of *inhibitory* and *excitatory zones* of the receptive field (see Figs. 7.2, 9.9 and 10.1).

6.2. Somatic Sensory Receptors

The sense organs of the skin have been classified as *exteroceptors*, those of the muscles and connective tissues as *proprioceptors*. The former term is somewhat obsolete, the latter still widely used. It is clinically useful to classify somatic sensibility as *superficial* or *deep*, corresponding, respectively, to excitation of cutaneous sense organs and proprioceptors. Information flowing from both classes of receptors serves to recognize an object we cannot see as we explore it with our moving fingers. Recognition is much more difficult if the object is placed into a passive hand so that only the skin is stimulated. During active exploration, exteroceptive and proprioceptive information and feedback from the motor apparatus blend to facilitate recognition.

Signals from cutaneous and proprioceptive sense organs are also required to guide movements. To a large degree, the control of move- ments proceeds without our conscious attention. Information from somatic sense organs flows in several channels in the spinal cord and brain stem. Some channels serve the cognitive brain processes; others provide for the feedback required in the guidance of motor output (Chapter 16). Somatic afferent nerve fibers are also the first link in spinal reflex arcs. Thus, for example, signals from a single stretch receptor in a skeletal muscle can be transmitted to spinal centers, the cerebellum and the cerebral cortex through three different systems of interneurons (Chapter 7).

In most if not all somatic sensory receptors, the sensing element, or transducer, is the membrane of the afferent nerve terminal. Some are equipped with a capsule or other accessory apparatus of more or less complex structure. Nevertheless energy of the stimulus is transduced into nerve signals by the nerve ending itself, not by the accessory structure. In an almost literal sense we feel the world with the tips of our nerves. A possible exception is Merkel's disk, where the epithelial Merkel cell is perhaps the transducer.

There are three functional classes of cutaneous receptors: (1) *mechanoreceptors*, whose adequate stimulus is deformation of the nerve ending under the impact of physical force; (2) *thermoreceptors*, responding either to warming or to cooling; and (3) *nociceptors*, which respond to stimuli that threaten to damage tissues. The relationship of the excitation of nociceptors to the feeling of pain will be discussed in Section 7.9. Each of these major classes can further be subdivided into subclasses, as we will presently see.

Most afferent nerve fibers branch near their peripheral receptors. How generator potentials of the several sensory terminals of a single parent axon interact is a poorly explored question. In some cases action potentials may be triggered in any one peripheral branch; in others, it may be necessary for generator potentials of several branches to sum in order to trigger impulses at their point of confluence.

The cell bodies of somatic primary afferent neurons reside either in the dorsal root ganglia or, in the case of the Vth cranial nerve, in the semilunar ganglion of Gasser. Somatic primary afferents are pseudo-unipolar, that is the seemingly single axonal process divides in the shape of a "T" (Fig. 1.4*A*). Afferent impulses arriving from the periphery may invade the cell body as well as the central branch of the "T." In other cases, impulses continue towards the spinal cord but do not activate the cell body.

6.3. The Skin as Sense Organ

Toward the end of the 19th century, Goldscheider and Blix, independently of one another, made the same discovery. They both tested the sensibility of their own skin and that of their friends with fine-tipped probes. They found that sensitivity was not uniform but *punctate*: maximal sensitivity was limited to small spots. More remarkably, those spots maximally sensitive to touch were insensitive to the pain of a pinprick, and *vice versa*. Further, spots sensitive to warming were not sensitive to cooling, or to touch or pinpricks. Later, von Frey continued this work and elaborated the theory. These and similar observations have led to the definitions of the *modalities* of skin sensation, touch-pressure, warm, cold and pain. An inference from these psychophysical observations was that each modality of sensation has its single specific sense organ.

For decades the doctrine of the specificity of cutaneous sense organs was the subject of heated debate, in part scientific and in part philosophical. Theoretical debate has stimulated work in the laboratory. Evidence now available supports the contention that individual sensory fibers are specialized and excited by a limited spectrum of stimuli. By combining the methods of morphology, electrophysiology and psychophysics, it has been possible in several instances to establish the structural characteristics of a sense organ, define its responses and describe the elementary sensations to which its excitation gives rise.

Some of the mechanoreceptive nerve endings have accessory structures which are readily recognized on stained sections with the aid of a light microscope. For a long time it seemed that endings without accessory structures had no distinguishable features. The rule was this: endings with complex accessory structures were mechanoreceptive; endings without such structures could be mechanoreceptive, thermoreceptive or nociceptive. More recently it was discovered that some of the seemingly featureless free endings in fact have recognizable ultrastructure, and are associated with a particular function. The cold-sensitive ending illustrated in Figure 6.1C is an example. We still do not know, however, what biophysical or chemical peculiarity accounts for the specialized sensitivity of receptor membranes. The list of receptor types in Table 6.1 is far from complete. The many different morphological structures of somatic nerve endings have been variously grouped into larger, more inclusive classes. For example, encapsulated endings include Ruffini's and Golgi's organs, among others. Lamellated endings include Pacini's and Meissner's corpuscles, and several more that exist only in animals other than man.

The endings which have complex accessory structures have myelinated nerve fibers of larger caliber, which fall in the beta range according to Gasser's classification (see Fig. 3.12). Free endings have either small-caliber (delta) myelinated or unmyelinated (C) fibers (Fig. 6.4).

It is fair to say that the principles of the encoding of information by peripheral afferent fibers are today understood, even if all the factual details have not yet been discovered. How the elementary messages of primary afferent neurons combine in the brain to enable, for example, the recognition of an ice-covered brick wall, or an experience such as, "I have found my housekey in my pocket," is still uncertain. Neurons in certain sensory nuclei, including most of those in the dorsal column nuclei, the ventroposterolateral and ventroposteromedial (VPL and VPM) nuclei of the thalamus, and in the primary sensory area of the cerebral cortex, receive excitatory input from but one class of primary afferent

Table 6.1.

Form and Function of Some Mechanoreceptors

Morphology	Location	Response Characteristics and Adequate Stimulus
Ruffini's corpuscles: encapsulated, branched, with collagen fiber anchorings	Dermis; joint capsule	Slowly adapting (type II) Stretching of skin or of connective tissue
Golgi's endings: similar to Ruffini's	Ligaments, tendons	Slowly adapting, stretch
Merkel's disks (Fig. 6.1)	Dermal ridges; hairy and glabrous skin	Partially adapting (type I); indentation of surface; very low threshold
Hair endings (several morphological types)	Around hair bulbs (very numerous)	Different types: respond to velocity and acceleration of bending of hairs
Meissner's corpuscles (Fig. 6.1)	Mostly glabrous skin; some in hairy skin	Completely adapting; velocity of skin indentation; low-frequency vibration
Krause's end bulbs	Glabrous skin	Similar to Meissner's
Pacinian corpuscles (Figs. 6.1 and 6.7)	Subcutaneous tissue; connective tissue membranes; joints; mesentery	Very rapidly adapting; brief mechanical transients; high-frequency vibration
C fiber mechanoreceptors; unencapsulated endings	All skin areas	Respond to slow rates of deformation; stimuli moving slowly over skin surface: "crawl detectors"

neuron, thus preserving the specificity of the message. Elsewhere in the CNS, including the dorsal horns of the spinal cord and many parts of the brain, some neurons can be either excited or inhibited by several different kinds of sensory signals. Somewhere, somehow, elementary messages must be woven into meaningful patterns, which then can be recognized by comparing current input with information stored in memory.

6.4. Mechanoreceptors

The elementary sensations evoked by the excitation of mechanoreceptors are traditionally described as touch, pressure and vibration. Distinguishing between touch and pressure may be vague, but the feeling of vibration is quite distinct.

Mechanoreceptors have in common that they respond to a deformation of the sensitive nerve ending, in other words to a displacement of

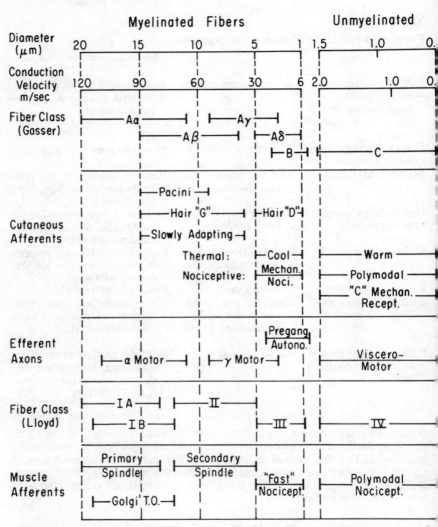

Figure 6.4. Fiber diameters and conduction velocities of different types of axons in peripheral nerves. The axons of olfactory neuroepithelial cells (Fig. 8.1A), which are 0.2–0.3 μm in diameter, fall outside this chart.

the receptor membrane. Changes in hydrostatic pressure are not effective unless the pressure is distributed unevenly so that it actually moves the ending. Mechanoreceptors differ in (1) the degree of *adaptation*; (2) the

A   B

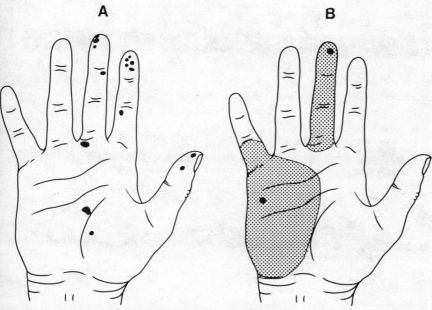

Figure 6.5.   Receptive fields of sensory fibers in the ulnar nerve of a human subject. Micro-wire electrodes were inserted through the skin and into the nerve, until the impulses of a single fiber were recorded (Fig. 6.6). The receptive field was then mapped with the aid of an electrically controlled mechanical stimulator. *A*, the *blackened areas* show the receptive fields of 15 rapidly adapting sensory units, probably Meissner's corpuscles. *B*, the *blackened areas* show where two other fibers, probably of Pacinian corpuscles, could be stimulated by near-threshold stimuli; the same fibers could also be excited by stronger stimuli (about 5× threshold) applied to the *shaded areas*. (Reprinted with permission from A. B. Vallbo and R. S. Johansson: Tactile sensory innervation of the glabrous skin of the human hand. In *Active Touch: The Mechanism of Recognition of Objects by Manipulation*, edited by G. Gordon. Oxford, Pergamon Press, 1978.)

extent of the *branching* of their terminals and the location of their endings in the tissue; (3) the properties of the *accessory equipment* associated with the endings.

The adaptive properties of an ending determine whether it responds to the *position* of the stimulus (the amplitude of the displacement of the membrane); to the *velocity* of the stimulus (rate of displacement); or to *transients*, such as shocks, taps, jolts and vibration (acceleration of displacement) (Fig. 6.6). Some mechanoreceptors combine dynamic

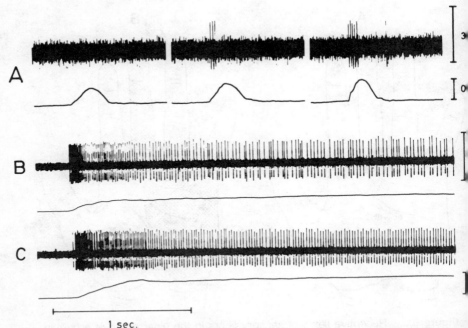

Figure 6.6. Recordings of the impulses of human cutaneous primary afferent fibers, made as described in legend of Figure 6.5. *A*, a rapidly and completely adapting unit; *B* and *C*, a partially adapting unit. The *upper tracings* are the recordings of diphasic action potentials; the *lower tracings* the force exerted by the mechanical probe used to stimulate the skin, calibrated in newtons. (Reprinted with permission from M. Knibestöl and A. B. Vallbo: *Acta Physiologica Scandinavica* 80:178–195, 1970.)

and static responses, and thus signal both position and velocity (partially adapting).

The distribution of the terminal branches is one of the main factors in determining the shape and size of the receptive field. The manner in which the endings are anchored in the tissue is another. The spindle-shaped capsule of Ruffini's and Golgi's end organs has collagen fibers attached. If the skin is stretched, the nerve endings are pulled by the collagen fibers and the receptor is stimulated. Thus if the tip of a pencil indents the skin, it stimulates the displacement sensors (e.g., Merkel disks, see Fig. 6.1 and Table 6.1) under the tip, but also the encapsulated stretch-sensitive endings in a much wider area around the tip. In the human hand the sizes of cutaneous receptive fields vary widely from about 0.5 mm to 20 mm in diameter (Fig. 6.5). Some are round, others oval, some irregular in shape. Those of adjacent units overlap widely. The sensitivity of some mechanoreceptive units is punctate: within their receptive field there are highly sensitive points surrounded by less sensitive zones. For others, sensitivity is more evenly distributed within the receptive field. The average size of the receptive fields is smallest at the fingertips and largest in the skin of the back, but there is considerable variation in all areas. The shape and the size range of receptive fields is characteristic for each type of mechanoreceptor.

The mechanical properties of the accessory tissue associated with some mechanoreceptors can decisively influence its adaptive properties. In the next section we will see how this works in Pacinian corpuscles. In some cases the accessory structure favors the action of stimuli acting in a particular direction. Stretch-sensitive endings are maximally excited when the surrounding tissue in pulled in the direction of the anchoring fibers. Some of the nerve endings around hair bulbs respond best when the hair is bent one way, not when it is moved in other directions.

A peculiarity of the mechanoreceptor C fibers is that they are best stimulated by small objects moving slowly over the skin. It has been suggested that they are specialized to detect crawling insects, and perhaps contribute to the sensation sense of itch and/or tickle.

To illustrate some of these general principles, I will now describe the corpuscles of Pacini, which are one of the most studied of the somatic sense organs.

6.4a. CORPUSCLES OF PACINI

These small beads, shaped like grains of rice about 0.2–1.5 mm in length, are just visible to the unaided eye. They are located in subdermal connective tissue, in the ligaments and capsule of joints, the interosseal membrane of lower arm and leg, and in the mesentery; therefore, they are not cutaneous sense organs in the strict sense of the word. Vibration applied to the skin does stimulate them, however, and they are often described with skin receptors.

Pacinian corpuscles consist of a capsule formed of lamellae of connective tissue reminiscent of the layers of an onion. At the core is the terminal of a single myelinated nerve fiber. Unlike most somatic afferent fibers, those of Pacinian corpuscles are rarely, if ever, branched. The terminal of the fiber is not myelinated; but the first segment of the myelin sheath and the first node of Ranvier are enclosed within the capsule (Fig. 6.7*F*).

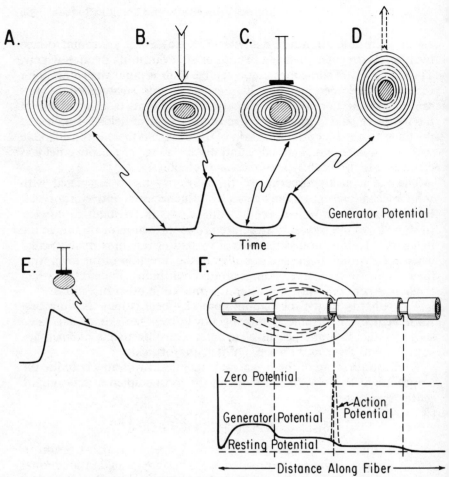

Figure 6.7. The working of Pacinian corpuscles. *A* to *D* illustrate the mechanics of the capsule. *A*, at rest. The *hatched circle* in the center represents a cross-section of the axon, surrounded by the concentric layers of connective tissue of the capsule. *B*, sudden indentation of the capsule causes deformation of the axon and evokes a generator potential. *C*, during sustained deformation of the capsule the inner layers of elastic connective tissue regain their circular cross-section, thus relieving the axon so that excitation ceases. *D*, the compressing force is lifted, the elastic force stored in the outer layers is released, and causes renewed deformation of the axon and thus renewed stimulation. *E*, the sensitive axon terminal stripped of its connective tissue capsule still produces a generator potential when it is deformed; such a denuded terminal adapts more slowly than the intact corpuscle. *F*, the generator potential of the unmyelinated terminal portion of the axon draws current from the first node of Ranvier, where the impulses are triggered. (Reprinted with permission from G. Somjen: *Sensory Coding in the Mammalian Nervous System*. New York, Plenum Press, 1975.)

When a Pacinian corpuscle is lightly depressed by a fine probe, its nerve fiber fires an action potential; another is triggered when the probe is removed, but the fiber remains silent while the corpuscle is steadily compressed. Because of its great sensitivity and its very fast adaptation, this organ is exquisitely sensitive to jolts and to vibration (Fig. 6.8).

The capsule can be peeled away by microdissection except the inner-

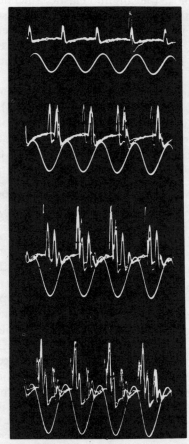

Figure 6.8. Impulses recorded from fibers of several Pacinian corpuscles, stimulated by mechanical vibration acting on the corpuscles. From the *top* of the figure *down*, the amplitude of vibration was increased so that more and more units were recruited. (Reprinted with permission from C. C. Hunt: *Journal of Physiology*. 155:175–186, 1961.)

most layer. The stripped nerve terminal still produces a generator potential when deformed ever so slightly. The naked terminal adapts, however, much slower than the complete organ (Fig. 6.7E). This experiment proved two important points: (1) that the true sensing element is the nerve terminal and not the capsule; (2) that the capsule is a high-pass mechanical filter, which is to say that it allows high-frequency vibrations to act on the terminal and prevents low frequencies from doing so. This is because the stiff and elastic lamellae of the capsule can slide upon one another. When the outer layer is suddenly deformed, force is transmitted to the nerve terminal, but when the outer shell is steadily compressed, the spring-like inner layers have a chance to regain their original shape and so remove the pressure on the nerve ending (Fig. 6.7).

Pacinian corpuscles are most sensitive to mechanical vibrations in the range of 200–300 Hz (Hz = cycles per second). At this frequency the human sense of vibration has the lowest threshold. This, with other arguments which cannot be detailed here, suggest that Pacinian corpuscles mediate the sense of vibration, as it is clinically tested with a tuning fork (see Section 7.10).

6.5. The Mechanoreceptors of Proprioception

6.5a. STRETCH RECEPTORS IN SKELETAL MUSCLE

Skeletal muscles are equipped with a specialized mechanosensor apparatus. These will be discussed at some length in the chapters concerned with motor control (Chapters 15 and 16). They are mentioned here only for the sake of completeness.

The two types of specialized sense organs in mammalian skeletal muscle are *muscle spindles* and *Golgi tendon organs*. Active contraction of the muscle excites Golgi tendon organs, but silences the spindles. Passive stretching excites the spindles, but it leaves Golgi tendon organs relatively unaffected. This contrasting behavior occurs because Golgi tendon organs are mechanically *in series* with the muscle fibers, whereas spindles lie *in parallel* with them. Muscle spindles are in addition excited by the contraction of their own internal contractile fibers known as intrafusal muscle (see Section 15.2a and Figs. 15.3–15.5).

6.5b. MECHANORECEPTORS OF JOINTS AND OTHER CONNECTIVE TISSUES

Mechanically sensitive nerve endings are present in perhaps all connective tissue, especially in the capsules and the ligaments of joints.

Other unusually richly innervated deep tissues include the periodon-
tium, which is quite sensitive to tapping and pressure; the eyelids and
the sclera; and the genitals. Mechanoreceptors of the circulation, the
airways, and the other viscera will briefly be described later (see Section
17.2).

According to structure, many sensory endings in the capsule and
ligaments of joints are of the branched and encapsulated variety, either
Ruffini's or Golgi's end organs. The adequate stimulus for these is very
probably the stretching of the connective tissue within which they are
embedded. Pacinian corpuscles are also found here and, as elsewhere,
are stimulated by transient or vibrating stimuli. Besides the encapsulated
ones, there also are free nerve endings.

Most of the specialized receptors in joints respond to rotation of the
joint. In the case of hinge joints such as the knee, some of the receptors
are excited by flexion, others by extension, but some respond indiscrim-
inately to movement in both directions. In joints which have more
freedom of movement there may be several categories, corresponding
to movements in different directions, but this has not yet been shown
experimentally. The majority of the sense organs of joint rotation are
completely adapting mechanoreceptors: their excitation is a function of
the velocity of movement and drops to zero when the joint is stationary.

A minority of the afferent fibers innervating joints are incompletely
adapting, firing rapidly during movement and at a slower rate when the
limb is held motionless. Some of these are maximally excited when the
joint is fully extended, others when the joint is fully flexed. Few, if any,
respond when the joint is stationary at an angle halfway between the
extremes.

6.5c. THE UNSOLVED RIDDLE OF THE SENSES OF JOINT POSITION AND OF KINESTHESIA

One of the routines of neurological examinations of patients is a test of their
ability to detect, without looking, the position of or the direction of the
movement of their joints (see Section 7.10). *Kinesthesia* is precisely defined as
the sense of passive movement of body parts but is often used to mean both the
sensing of position as well as of movement. Our sense of movement is, however,
keener than our sense of position, possibly because the dynamic responses of
mechanoreceptors are more accurate than static responses. To some extent we
actually may depend on sensing velocity to determine position. Mathematical
integration of velocity with respect to time yields position. Said in another way,
we can know where we are if we can remember where we were and how we
have last moved. This cannot fully explain joint position sense, but the memory
of movement very probably does play a part.

Otherwise, the topic is controversial. One view holds that kinesthesia depends on receptors in joints. The rival view is that joint angle and joint movement are determined by the brain with the aid of stretch receptors in muscle. There are certain difficulties with both opinions.

The controversy was brought closer to solution by observations of patients whose hip has been replaced by a prosthesis. These patients lose all the nerve endings of the hip joint, but nevertheless do not lose the ability to tell the position of their thigh relative to the pelvic girdle. This has proved that receptors of the hip joint cannot be the sole organs of kinesthesia for the upper leg.

The excitation of spindles in the muscles that span a joint could in principle supply all the information required to determine the angle of that joint. Flexing a joint stretches the extensor muscles, and therefore excites the spindles in the extensors; extending the joint does the same for the spindles of the flexors. Supporting the idea were experiments in which vibration was applied to muscles of human subjects in such a way as to preferentially excite primary spindle endings. This stimulation evoked the illusion of limb movement. The difficulty is that as soon as a muscle contracts, the excitation of stretch receptors within it is altered. Thus while muscle stretch receptors seem suitable to gauge joint angle as long as muscles are relaxed, their signal becomes ambiguous when muscles contract. To still compute the movement or the position of a limb from the firing of spindle afferents the brain would have to make appropriate corrections, taking into account the active contraction of the muscles. While this is by no means impossible, it seems a rather roundabout way of achieving a simple goal.

Without further elaboration of data and arguments, the best evidence available today can be summarized in the following points:

1. Awareness of movement and position of joints is normally not mediated by a single class of sense organs. Rather, it depends on a computation in which the brain takes account not only of the input from several categories of sense organs, but also of its own motor output.

2. For kinesthesia of the large joints of the limbs, the most important data are supplied by muscle stretch receptors, with joint receptors and mechanoreceptors in skin and fascia playing less significant roles. In the kinesthesia of the hands, receptors of the interphalangeal joints and perhaps of the skin may be important.

3. When one input channel is destroyed, or temporarily suppressed in an experiment, the CNS can use data supplied by the others to compute joint position and movement with only little loss of precision.

6.6. Thermoreceptors

Temperature affects all biophysical processes and biochemical reactions, and the excitation of nerve and muscle is no exception. Consequently, the sensitivity of all sensory units is, to some degree, influenced by the prevailing temperature. There are, however, nerve endings that respond to temperature changes with a sensitivity that greatly exceeds the temperature dependence of other cellular processes. Excitation of these specialized receptors mediates the feelings of cold and warmth, and the same receptors supply input for certain spinal reflexes and also for the hypothalamic temperature regulator (see Section 17.5a).

A human observer can detect differences of temperature or changes of temperature more accurately than he can estimate a prevailing steady temperature. The minimal temperature difference (or minimal change of temperature) that is just detected is about 0.1–0.2°C when the prevailing temperature is near the subjectively neutral range. The error made in guessing ambient constant temperature may amount to several degrees. Yet the core of the body is kept at its prescribed temperature within a margin of less than ± 0.2°C. Clearly, the central regulator of body temperature must be supplied with information of which we are not conscious. Special sensors are believed to be cells within the hypothalamic region of the CNS, but which cells they are has not been established (see Chapter 17).

Thermoreceptive nerve endings are numerous in the skin and in the mucous membranes of mouth and pharynx. They also exist in the lining of esophagus and stomach. Cold-sensitive endings are branched, slightly expanded terminals of small (delta) myelinated parent fibers (Fig. 6.1C). The fibers of warm-sensitive thermoreceptors of most skin regions of most species are unmyelinated.

Thermoreceptors are partially adapting, which means that their excitation is determined by the rate of change of the temperature, plus by the actual level of the temperature. As shown in Figure 6.9A, a cold-sensitive thermoreceptor will give a dynamic response during the cooling of its receptive field that is determined mainly by the rate of cooling. When the skin temperature settles to a steady level, so does the firing of the cold-sensitive fiber. The adapted or static rate is lower than that obtained while the temperature is falling. When the skin is being warmed, cold-sensitive fibers tend to fall silent. Warm-sensitive fibers are, by definition, those that are excited while the temperature is rising.

A unique feature of temperature receptors is the bell-shaped curve of static firing rate as a function of temperature (Fig. 6.9B). In other sense organs excitation increases until a maximal rate is reached, but the excitation of temperature receptors actually decreases when temperature is moved beyond the point of maximal stimulation. The bell-shaped functions of Figure 6.9B describes only the adapted levels excitation; the "dynamic response" is a positive function of the rate of cooling, even in the range of the descending limb (the left-side half) of the bell-shaped curve. Moreover, in the low range of temperatures (20–25°C

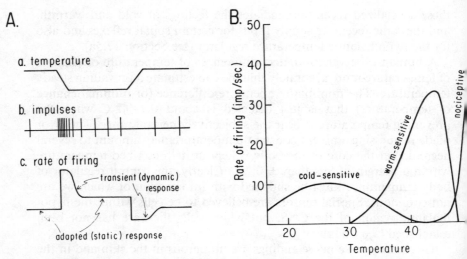

Figure 6.9. Responses of thermoreceptive primary afferent fibers. *A*, the responses of a cold-sensitive fiber first to cooling and then to re-warming of the skin. *a*, intradermal temperature; *b*, diagrammatic representation of impulses of the fiber; *c*, the response represented as rate of firing. (Modified and redrawn after H. Hensel: *Allgemeine Sinnesphysiologie*. Berlin, Springer, 1966.) *B*, the adapted (static) firing rate of different classes of thermally sensitive primary afferent units: cold-sensitive, warm-sensitive and polymodal nociceptive. The *abscissa* is the intradermal temperature (not air temperature). (Based on data from H. Hensel and D. R. Kenshalo: *Journal of Physiology* 204:99–112, 1969; and data from P. Besson and E. Perl: *Journal of Neurophysiology* 32:1025–1043, 1969.)

intracutaneous) the firing pattern of cold receptors changes from an even rhythm to a bursting pattern, in which groups of high-frequency discharges are separated by short pauses. These bursts may be powerfully exciting at central synapses and cause the feeling of cold discomfort at low temperatures.

The relationship of the excitation of thermoreceptors to the subjective awareness of temperature has not completely been clarified. As everyone knows, when we dive into cool water, we feel chilled; but after a few minutes the water may feel quite pleasant even though its temperature has not changed (cf. Fig. 6.10*A*). Such alterations of the appreciation of temperature are in part explained by alterations of cutaneous blood flow, which can influence the skin temperature and counteract the effect of the ambient air temperature. They may also have to do with the

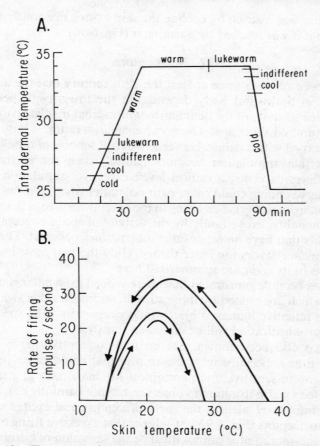

Figure 6.10. The sense of temperature is relative. *A*, the temperature sensations reported by a human subject while the skin was first warmed and then cooled. The graph shows the intradermal temperature; the subject's reports are marked on the graph. (Modified and redrawn after H. Hensel: *Ergebnisse der Physiologie* 47:166–368, 1952.) *B*, the adapted firing rates of a cold-sensitive primary afferent fiber. The skin was first cooled in steps, and then warmed in steps. Note that the fiber fired at a higher rate when any given temperature was reached from a higher level than when the starting temperature was lower (compare with Fig. 6.9*B*). (Modified and redrawn after H. Hensel, A. Iggo and I. Witt: *Journal of Physiology* 153:113–126, 1960.)

adaptation of thermoreceptors and a phenomenon termed *hysteresis*. At any given temperature, a cold receptor will fire more intensely if that temperature was reached by cooling the skin from a previously warmer level than if it was reached by warming it (Fig. 6.10).

6.7. Nociceptors

It has been obvious since at least the 18th century that the ability to feel pain in limbs and body depends on the integrity of peripheral nerves. Serious study of the neural mechanisms that mediate pain began about a hundred years ago. The accumulated literature is large, much of it concerned with a debate between two rival schools of thought. One view was that stimulation becomes painful when the excitation of afferent fibers exceeded a critical level; excessive stimulation of any sensory nerve ending could cause pain no matter what kind the sensory unit is (*intensity theory*). According to the other theory, pain is a separate sensory modality, evoked only by the activity of specific receptors and nerve fibers that have no other function (*specificity theory*). The weight of the evidence favors the latter theory. Only the two most important arguments in its favor are summarized here.

1. It has been demonstrated that there indeed exist cutaneous nerve endings which are excited by those stimuli, and none other, which in a conscious attentive human subject would cause pain. (The special case of receptor sensitization will be discussed shortly.)

2. It has also been shown that no non-nociceptive nerve endings respond in any special way to the stimuli that could cause pain. For example, warm-sensitive thermoreceptors fire maximally at a temperature that feels warm to a human observer, but not painfully hot. Heating to the painful level silences the thermoreceptors and excites a special class of nociceptors (Fig. 6.9*B*). It follows that excessive firing of warm-sensitive thermoreceptor cannot mediate the sensation of burning. Similarly, the firing of mechanoreceptors becomes maximal or near-maximal before the stimulus reaches a potentially painful intensity, at which point nociceptors commence firing.

Before the advent of single-fiber electrophysiology, psychophysicists had defined two kinds of pain. One was termed "fast" or "sharp," the other "slow" or "diffuse." The skin was credited with being able to feel both kinds of pain; viscera with only the slow, diffuse variety. Muscle and joints have both, although their sharp pain is different from that of skin.

Electrophysiological investigations of cutaneous nerve fibers have subsequently revealed the existence of two main classes of nociceptors. One type is supplied by small-diameter (delta) myelinated fibers, the other by unmyelinated (C) fibers. The peripheral endings of both types appear as "free" nerve terminals under light microscopy, but specialized features have been revealed on electron micrographs.

Most nociceptive endings with Aδ fibers respond only to mechanical stimuli, such as pressure of painful intensity, or the pinching, pricking or cutting of the skin, and are quite insensitive to burning heat and to irritant chemicals. There are a few, however, which respond not only to noxious mechanical stimulation, but also to very cold temperatures.

Nociceptive unmyelinated (C) fibers respond to damaging mechanical stimuli, as well as burning heat, and a variety of chemicals. They respond weakly or not at all to extreme cold. These afferents are called *polymodal* nociceptors to distinguish them from the *unimodal* mechanoreceptive nociceptors.

Nociceptors are not excited by chemical agents applied to the skin surface as long as the skin is intact. The mucous membranes of the mouth and nose are less resistant. However, once the skin is cut or abraded, many chemicals act as cutaneous irritants, as we all know well enough. The chemical sensitivity of damaged skin is not specific, and even innocuous materials, such as salt and sugar, can cause pain if they come in contact with a wound in hypertonic solution. There are, however, other compounds whose irritant potency is exceptional. Capsaicin, found in a family of hot peppers, is one of them. Much of the flavor of certain exotic dishes comes from the effect of capsaicin on polymodal nociceptors in the trigeminal innervation field in the mucous membrane of the tongue.

Certain compounds produced in animal tissue cells can also stimulate polymodal nociceptors. These include acetylcholine and histamine, but perhaps the most powerful among them is the polypeptide bradykinin. Intradermal injection of these substances is painful. It has been suggested that the true adequate stimulus of the apparently polymodal nociceptors is bradykinin and that all other stimuli act indirectly by causing the release of this agent from tissue cells. The best evidene favoring this theory concerns nociceptive nerve endings in abdominal viscera, but even here the case is not yet completely settled. It has also been suggested, but not proved, that the analgesic action of acetylsalicylate (aspirin) can be explained in part or in whole as a blockade of the excitatory effects of bradykinin. Bradykinin does not stimulate mechanoreceptive (unimodal) nociceptors.

The skin is said to be "burned" not only when it literally is charred and consumed by flames, but also when it is more moderately damaged.

The conspicuous surface manifestations of such a burn are erythema (reddening) and blisters. The degree of damage depends not only on the temperature but also the duration of the exposure. Heating the skin to about 48 or 50°C, if maintained long enough, can cause damage; heating it between 45 and 48°C may already be painful. The pain thus serves as an advance warning signal to remove the exposed part from harm's way before it is too late. Since the pain of burning has a threshold similar to that of the polymodal nociceptors, the sensation is probably evoked by these receptors. Prolonged exposure to heat renders these polymodal nociceptors supersensitive to mechanical stimulation. Ordinarily, they cannot be excited by mild mechanical stimulation, but after having been excited by heat for a period of time, gentle touching of the skin can set them off. The *sensitization* of nociceptors is very probably the physiological explanation of the tenderness of burnt skin.

Fair skin can also be "burned" by ultraviolet radiation without being heated and, therefore, without the warning signal of pain. The pain of sunburn comes after the damage has already been done. Skin that has no pigment to protect it against sunburn is a biological anomaly, made possible (or even necessary) by breeding for many generations under a Northern European sky.

Nociceptors exist in most tissues of the body, including skeletal and cardiac muscle, joints and other connective tissue, peritoneum, specific parts of the hollow viscera, and the meningeal lining of the brain. Stimulation of CNS tissue itself does not usually cause pain, except at special points, where presumably neurons are processing nociceptive signals. The perivascular tissue in the meninges is on the other hand well endowed with nociceptive endings. Changes in the caliber of meningeal vessels are the probable cause of at least some types of headaches.

A powerful stimulant of nociceptors in both skeletal and cardiac muscle is a failure of the local blood supply, or ischemia. Whether nociceptors are stimulated in this case by hypoxia, by an acid shift of pH, by the release of K^+ ions or of some other intervening secondary agent such as bradykinin, remains to be seen. In any event, ischemia is the cause of the pain of *angina pectoris* (chest pain due to coronary artery narrowing) and of *claudicatio intermittens* (leg pain during walking), to name but two common clinical conditions.

The pain of frostbite may, in large part, also be caused by ischemia due to local vasoconstriction. In a severely cooled limb, nerve fibers and their endings cease to function, and the limb is numbed. Pain occurs only as the temperature drops and again during rewarming, when nerves are able to function even though they are partially depolarized, the depolarization causing excessive and continuous firing. If sensory units of different function, mechanoreceptors, thermoreceptors and nociceptors are all excited, a mixture of feelings is experienced that can be highly arousing and quite unpleasant. This happens in several situations and evokes a similar sensation: a frostbitten limb (the sensation sometimes actually resembles that of burning); as a leg that has "gone to sleep" recovers (also usually caused by interruption of blood flow to a nerve by pressure, less frequently by direct pressure on a nerve); and by strong repetitive electrical stimulation of nerves of mixed function.

It has been thought that the sensation of itching is caused by low-grade stimulation of polymodal nociceptors. It is possible that itching is a separate sense modality served by specialized sensory terminals. The feeling of itch may, however, also be the result of the combined excitation of several kinds of afferent units, for example the C fiber mechanoreceptors together with polymodal nociceptors. Histamine in low concentration causes strong itching, but it causes pain in higher concentrations. Certain other chemicals as well as some mechanical stimuli can evoke an itch.

6.8. Reinnervation After Injury to Sensory Nerves

If a peripheral nerve is cut, the fibers in the distal stump degenerate (Wallerian degeneration: see Section 3.4g). The area of skin supplied by the sensory fibers in the nerve then loses all feeling. If all goes well, sensibility can return to the denervated area by two processes. The first and more important one is regeneration of the cut nerve. A less important contribution may be made by the sprouting of new branches from neighboring intact fibers in the perimeter of the denervated region. The first to reappear are unmyelinated fibers, followed by finely myelinated ones, while the large-caliber myelinated fibers recover last. It is not clear, many decades after this question was first asked, whether small fibers regenerate faster, or whether all axons grow back at the same rate, but it takes extra time to recover new myelin sheaths. In either case, the regenerating small-caliber fibers begin to function first, as judged by the return of pain sensibility before other sensory modalities and the recovery of sweating before the control of voluntary muscles.

As sensory fibers degenerate, the accessory structures associated with specialized mechanoreceptors disappear from the denervated skin. If and when reinnervation by large myelinated fibers succeeds, these end organs reappear. The process of Wallerian degeneration begins in a day or two and is completed in 2–4 weeks. Reinnervation may take many weeks or months, depending on the size of the denervated region, and the distance over which regenerating fibers must grow.

During the second decade of this century, the British neurologist Henry Head had a surgeon friend first cut and then resuture one of his own cutaneous nerves. His purpose was to experience at first hand how it felt when an area of skin first lost and then regained sensibility. His example was followed by others in what seemed to become a tradition among neurologists and experimental psychologists. From their description, and from interview and examination of patients, we know that incompletely reinnervated skin feels peculiar. In the center of such a region sensation may be dull and threshold elevated. This *hypesthestic* center may be surrounded by a zone of *hyperesthesia*, where sensation is abnormally strong and unusual as well as unpleasant in quality (*dysesthesia*). There may also be areas where the threshold is high, but when the threshold is exceeded the sensation evoked is painful even to stimuli that are usually not painful (*hyperpathia*).

Head has built around this and other observations a dual theory of cutaneous innervation. In his view one kind of sensory units serve a crude, emotionally laden kind of sensation which he called *protopathic*; another set of sensory units, the finely discriminating and emotionally neutral *epicritic* senses. The two sets were mutual antagonists and, in normal skin, kept each other in balance. If the balance was altered, for example after nerve injury, pathological sensations arose. While much of Head's theory proved incorrect, his observations were, in part at least, accurate and the terms protopathic and epicritic are sometimes still used to describe qualities of sensations. In the next chapter (Section 7.9b) we will learn that, under certain conditions, input from mechanoreceptors can inhibit transmission of input from nociceptors. Some neurologists feel that this insight is a modern version of some of Head's ideas.

6.9. Chapter Summary

1. Sensory receptors are specialized to transduce specific kinds of stimuli, each its adequate stimulus. The transducing element of somatic sense organs is the membrane of the nerve terminal, which has properties different from the membrane of the main conducting portion of the fiber. In the organs of special senses the transducers are specialized epithelial receptor cells.
2. The amplitude of the generator (receptor) potential of most sense organs is a non-linear function with decreasing slope of the stimulus intensity; consequently, the firing rate of the primary afferent fibers is also a function of the stimulus, with decreasing slope.
3. Stimuli of increasing intensity recruit increasing numbers of primary afferent sensory units.
4. Afferent units that adapt rapidly and completely signal either the rate of change (velocity) of the stimulus or its acceleration. The excitation of

afferent units that adapt partially is expressed in two components, the dynamic response and the static response.

5. Somatic sensory receptors of different kinds have afferent fibers of certain ranges of caliber and hence of conduction velocity. The fast-conducting coarse myelinated fibers all belong to low-threshold mechanoreceptors. Small myelinated (delta) fibers belong to thermoreceptors, high-threshold mechanoreceptors and mechanoreceptive nociceptors. Unmyelinated (C) fibers serve thermoreceptors, polymodal nociceptors and certain types of low-threshold mechanoreceptors.

6. The peripheral terminals of afferent fibers usually branch, sometimes profusely, but all branches serve receptors of similar function.

7. Corpuscles of Pacini are receptors of mechanical vibration and of small jolts. They are exquisitely sensitive, especially in the range of frequencies between 100 and 800 Hz.

8. Other low-threshold mechanoreceptors respond to the bending of hairs; the indentation or the stretching of the skin, and the stretching of skeletal muscles and of the fibers in ligaments of joints, in tendons, and in other connective tissues. The common denominator is deformation of the membrane of the mechanoreceptive nerve terminal.

9. The senses of limb position and of limb movement (kinesthesia) are probably served by stretch receptors of skeletal muscles as well as mechanoreceptors of the ligaments and capsules of joints. The relative importance of the contribution of different sense organs to kinesthesia is controversial.

10. There are two kinds of thermoreceptors, one type sensing cooling, the other sensing warming. Thermoreceptors show both dynamic and static responses, and their static responses are subject to hysteresis.

11. Nociceptors are of two main classes, the mechanoreceptive nociceptors and the polymodal nociceptors (see 5 above). The polymodal nociceptors are sensitive to certain chemicals such as bradykinin, to noxious mechanical stimuli and to noxious heat. They can be sensitized to gentle mechanical stimuli, for example by previous exposure to burning heat.

12. Hypoxia of muscle tissue is a powerful stimulant of nociceptors, causing clinically important ischemic pain.

13. If injury severs sensory nerve fibers, the peripheral stump degenerates. Reinnervation is possible by the growth of new branches of intact fibers in adjacent undamaged areas and also by regeneration of the severed fibers.

Further Reading

See at end of Chapter 7.

chapter 7

Somatic Sensory Pathways and Centers

How the signals sent by somatic primary afferent units to the CNS are processed. The consequences of injury to somatic pathways and centers. The clinical testing of the somatic senses.

7.1. The "Classical" Spinal Pathways

Until recently sensory information was thought to travel over three main avenues toward the "higher" centers of the central nervous system (CNS): (1) the dorsal (white) columns (funiculi); (2) the anterolateral spinothalamic pathway; and (3) the spinocerebellar tracts. The dorsal columns were regarded as the conduits of signals serving the senses of fine touch, vibration and kinesthesia. The spinothalamic tracts were believed to be reserved for the sensory modalities of pain, temperature, pressure and crude touch. The spinocerebellar paths were thought to mediate those proprioceptive signals, needed for the control of movement, of which the subject need not be consciously aware.

This relatively simple scheme turned out to be incomplete and in some respects erroneous. The first observations clearly incompatible with the traditional scheme were reported as early as 1948. In that year the spinal dorsal columns of a small group of patients were cut in a surgical operation. The purpose was to relieve so-called "phantom" pain of an amputated limb (see Section 7.9e), but this was not achieved. In subsequent neurological examination these patients did not show the signs traditionally attributed to damage of the dorsal columns, in spite of the surgically controlled interruption of that pathway.

Research conducted in the intervening years defined more accurately the processing and forwarding of afferent signals in the spinal gray and white substance. Much of this newer information is of importance for the diagnosis of spinal injury and disease. Many questions are still unanswered. This chapter is an attempt to integrate the old and new observations into a coherent picture.

7.2. The Uncrossed Pathways

7.2a. THE DORSAL COLUMNS

The anatomical dorsal columns contain more than the functional dorsal column pathway, by which term most physiologists and clinical neurologists mean only those primary afferent axons that course uninterrupted from periphery to the dorsal column nuclei (See Figs. 7.1*A* and 7.3). Those nuclei are located at the dorsal aspect of the junction of the spinal cord with the medulla oblongata. Such primary afferent fibers make up only about 25% of the dorsal white matter. The remainder consists of fibers connecting one spinal segment with another and also some second-order afferents that originate in the dorsal horn and whose destination is in the dorsal column nuclei.

Among the primary afferent neurons forming the functional dorsal column pathway are found nerve fibers that extend from the tip of the toe to the base of the skull; in a giraffe this is no mean distance. These fibers behave in exactly the same manner as peripheral primary afferent fibers, since they, in fact, are the central extensions of peripheral neurons.

The funiculus gracilis, which contains the fibers from the lower half of the body, lies medially to the funiculus cuneatus, which contains fibers from the upper body. Within each tract, the fibers are arranged in an orderly sequence, those coming from the most caudal segments always lying more medially than those of more rostral origin. This ordering comes about because from segment to segment, from tail to neck, new fibers are always added to the dorsal columns laterally to those already there (see Carpenter, Fig. 4.1).

All the axons of the dorsal column pathway are myelinated and of medium to large caliber. Most of the fibers in the funiculus gracilis are the axons of rapidly adapting cutaneous mechanoreceptors, while in the cuneate tract a number of proprioceptive afferents from the upper limbs mingle with the cutaneous units.

7.2b. SPINOCERVICAL TRACT

In the dorsolateral white matter, medial to the dorsal spinocerebellar tract, lie axons whose cells of origin are in the dorsal horns of segments below. The axons of these cells remain on the same side of the midline as the cell bodies: the spinocervical tract is an uncrossed pathway (Figs. 7.1*A* and 7.3).

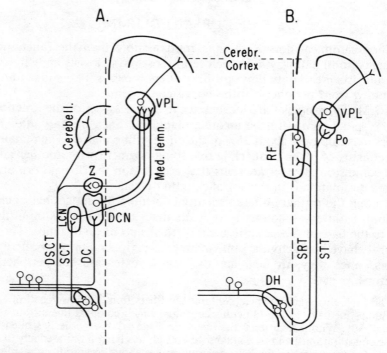

Figure 7.1. Schema of the principal ascending pathways of the spinal cord. *A*, uncrossed pathways: *DSCT*, dorsal spinocerebellar tract; *SCT*, spinocervical tract; *DC*, dorsal column pathway; *LCN*, lateral cervical nucleus; *DCN*, dorsal column nuclei; *Z*, Z nucleus; *Med. lemn.*, medial lemniscus; *VPL*, ventroposterolateral nucleus of the thalamus. *B*, crossed pathways: DH, dorsal horn; *RF*, reticular formation of the brain stem; *SRT*, spinoreticular tract; *STT*, spinothalamic tract; *Po*, posterior nuclear group of the thalamus.

Originally discovered in the cat, this tract was first thought to be peculiar to carnivores. Its existence in primates has, however, been firmly established, and the recent clinical literature tends to confirm its importance in man.

Unlike those forming the functional dorsal column pathway, the neurons of the spinocervical tracts are second-order afferents. The interposition of synapses gives an opportunity for the message to be transformed, for the code to be rewritten.

The main input to the neurons of the spinocervical tract comes from peripheral mechanoreceptors. However, inputs from other sense organs have a detectable influence on some spinocervical tract neurons. For example, nociceptive input can facilitate or inhibit the excitation of some of these units but cannot by itself cause their discharge. It seems that the spinocervical tract, like the dorsal column pathway, conducts information relating to mechanical stimulation.

The target of the spinocervical tract is a group of neurons lying in the upper end of the cervical spinal cord at about the same level as the dorsal column nuclei. In some species these neurons form a circum-scribed mass of gray matter, the lateral cervical nucleus. In man there is no such distinct structure, and it was in part for this reason that the existence of the tract had been in doubt. Neuroanatomists assume today that the cells which form the lateral cervical nucleus in certain species are more diffusely scattered in man.

7.2c. SPINOCEREBELLAR TRACTS

The nature of the input to the cerebellum is described later (Section 18.3a). Here we will describe only the relationship of the spinocerebellar tracts to the other ascending pathways of the spinal cord.

In segments T1 to L3 of the spinal cord we find a column of cells known as the dorsal nucleus, or Clarke's column. The axons of these cells form the dorsal spinocerebellar tract. Many Clarke's column cells receive input from stretch receptors of muscles, others from other proprioceptive afferents, and some from cutaneous mechanoreceptors. Near the junction of spinal cord and brain stem the pathway divides. The main tract continues toward the inferior peduncle (restiform body) of the cerebellum, but branches also enter the so-called Z nucleus. This nucleus lies rostral of the nuclei of the dorsal columns and serves a similar purpose. Third-order afferent fibers emerging from the Z nucleus join those from the dorsal column nuclei to form the medial lemniscus.

The dorsal spinocerebellar tract is thus recognized today to conduct signals not only to the cerebellum but also toward the forebrain.

The ventral spinocerebellar tracts contain fibers of varied function. They have no known relationship to the afferent paths addressed to the forebrain.

7.2d. THE SENSORY NUCLEAR COMPLEX OF THE SPINOMEDULLARY JUNCTION

Gracile and cuneate nuclei, the lateral cervical nucleus and the Z nucleus, all have a similar function. They transmit information from spinal segments to the forebrain, principally to the contralateral ventro-posterolateral (VPL) nucleus of the thalamus. Their output pathway is the band of white matter known as the medial lemniscus (ribbon) which crosses the midline in the medulla oblongata.

The majority of the neurons in the nuclei of the dorsal columns receive input from one functional class of primary afferents. Thus, if one of these cells is excited by mechanoreceptors innervating hair bulbs, that cell will not be excited by other types of afferents such as those of Pacinian corpuscles or Ruffini's organs.

Besides limitation of the type of stimulus, there also is a limitation of the geometric extension of the input. As in the case of primary afferents, one can speak of the *receptive field* of neurons in the dorsal column nuclei. Each one of these cells can be excited by stimulation of mecha-noreceptors lying within a limited area of the skin; or in the case of proprioceptive input, from a single joint or muscle.

The neurons within the two nuclei are ordered so that the most medial cells receive input from the most caudal parts of the body; cells lying more laterally, from the more rostral parts of the body. In this way the topographic order of the fibers of the dorsal white matter (see above) is preserved in their projection. Superimposed on this topographic order is a systematic division of stimulus modalities. The most rostral parts of the dorsal column nuclei receive proprioceptive input; the more caudal parts, the cutaneous mechanoreceptive input. Within each of these two broad categories, further subdivisions according to type of receptor input can be found.

Two more remarks should serve to illustrate the interrelatedness of the three principal uncrossed ascending pathways. (1) All large-caliber myelinated primary afferents run for some length in the (anatomical) dorsal column. Many depart, however, from it after a few segments, to synapse with second-order afferent neurons either in the dorsal horn or in Clarke's nucleus. (2) Not all the input of the dorsal column nuclei arrives there by way of the (functional) dorsal column pathway. Some of the input fibers are second-order, not first-order afferent neurons. The dorsal column nuclei sort information according to receptor type, not according to input pathway.

7.2e. A NOTE ON "RELAY" NUCLEI

The word "relay" conjures up the picture of something carried forward or handed over in unchanged form. The concept of the "relay nucleus" got accepted into neurology under the assumption that, in certain parts of the gray matter, messages from peripheral sense organs are transmitted more or less as they are received to the higher centers of the brain. The nuclei of the dorsal columns were thought to be examples of such relays interposed between the first-order neurons of the dorsal column pathway and the second-order neurons of the medial lemniscus.

In a certain sense the dorsal column nuclei live up to this reputation of message-forwarders. As we have seen, neurons in these nuclei receive, as a rule, input from but one type of sense organ, from a limited receptive field. Thus the signals they send on to the forebrain resemble those they receive: the transmitted message retains specificity with respect to both modality and to body topography. It is also true, however, that the dorsal column nuclei contain, besides *projection cells* with long axons addressed to the thalamus, *short-axon interneurons*. The latter form synaptic circuits, the existence of which suggests that some manner of signal processing occurs here. An example of signal processing is lateral inhibition (Section 4.9). Cells receiving impulses originating with hair bulb mechanoreceptors have a small excitatory receptive field. Either flanking from one side, or completely surrounding the excitatory zone, there is in most cases an inhibitory area. The inhibition is probably mediated by intrinsic interneurons of the nucleus.

Lateral inhibition operates in several parts of the CNS concerned with the processing of sensory information (Fig. 7.2; see also Fig. 4.8), not only in the somatic system but also in the visual (see Figs. 9.9 and 10.1) and auditory systems (Fig. 12.2). What is its significance? We have seen that the receptive fields of adjacent primary afferent units overlap (see Sections 6.1 and 6.4). The same is true of central neurons in the sensory pathway. Consequently, whenever a sharply bounded stimulus acts on a receptive surface, for example, when a coin in placed on the skin, at the edge of the stimulus the distribution of excitation is blurred. This is because the receptive field of some sensory units is entirely, and that of

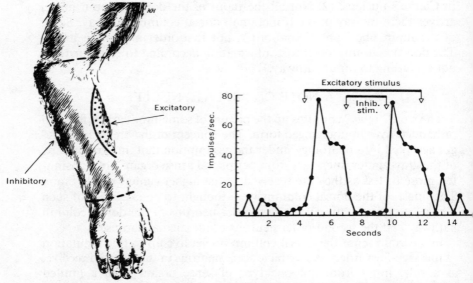

Figure 7.2. Lateral inhibition in a somatic sensory system. The impulses fired by a neuron in the primary somatic receiving area (SI) of the cerebral cortex was recorded. Mechanical stimulation within the excitatory zone of the receptive field evoked firing, stimulation of the surrounding inhibitory zone suppressed this firing. (Reprinted with permission from T. P. S. Powell and V. B. Mountcastle: *Bulletin of the Johns Hopkins Hospital* 105:133–162, 1959.)

others partly, under the edge of the stimulus (the coin in the example). Lateral inhibition sharpens and accentuates the transition between excited and unexcited zones (Fig. 4.8).

The reader may well ask why the nervous system could not be designed without such a problem, for example by making receptive fields smaller, and arranging them to adjoin without overlap, as in a mosaic. The overlap of fields has, however, three advantages: (1) It provides a safety factor in reception; if one unit drops out, the other still functions. (2) Having several receptors innervate the same patch of skin allows grading of signals by recruitment of units (see Section 6.1). (3) Units of different modality innervating the same point allow discrimination of the quality of the stimulus. Arranging receptive fields to overlap, and then superimposing lateral inhibition gives all these advantages, and still allows detection of sharp boundaries.

Besides intrinsic interneurons, sensory nuclei also contain terminals of fibers of *descending tracts* which may interact with the transmission of signals arriving from the spinal pathways. Many of the descending fibers inhibit, and others facilitate, transmission through the "relay" synapses of the dorsal column nuclei. Some arrive here by way of the corticospinal (pyramidal) tract (cf. Section 18.1a). It is as though the forebrain could censor news it receives, favoring some, suppressing others. Such *efferent control* of afferent relays may, in part at least, explain our ability to focus *selective attention* on some stimuli while ignoring others.

7.3. Dorsal Horns and Crossed Ascending Tracts

The dorsal horns are the largest of all sensory nuclei. A more correct but rarely used term is dorsal gray columns, for they resemble "horns" only in cross-section, and then not very closely.

The gray matter of the spinal cord has been divided by Rexed into 10 cytoarchitectonic zones or layers (Fig. 7.3; see also Carpenter, Figs. 3.15 and 3.16). The first 6 of these form the dorsal horns. Lamina I, lying most dorsally, is also known as *Waldeyer's marginal (or posteromarginal) zone.* Lamina II is synonymous with the *substantia gelatinosa Rolandi* of classical neuroanatomy; laminae IV, V and VI form the *nucleus proprius* of the dorsal horn, so named by Ramón y Cajal. Lamina III was originally considered part of the substantia gelatinosa, but is now thought to be a transitional zone between it and the nucleus proprius.

Layer I is the principal target of small-caliber (delta) myelinated afferent fibers, the substantia gelatinosa of the C fibers. Fine-caliber fibers arrive at the spinal cord in the lateral parts of the dorsal roots, whereas the coarser myelinated fibers run in the more medial parts of the dorsal roots (see Carpenter, Fig. 3.19). The largest myelinated fibers enter from the dorsal root directly into the dorsal white columns where, as we have just discussed, they may either run all the way to the dorsal column nuclei or, after a few segments, leave the dorsal column to enter the nucleus proprius or Clarke's nucleus of the dorsal horn. Some large and intermediate size myelinated afferent fibers follow, however in an arch the medial border of the dorsal horn to enter directly into the deeper layers of the dorsal gray matter without a sojourn in the dorsal white column.

Thus the most dorsal layers of the dorsal horns are the target of small-caliber afferent fibers, the deeper layers of large fibers. Signals from small primary afferent fibers reach the deeper layers also, however, albeit indirectly, forwarded by short-axon interneurons of layers II and III to the cells of layers IV and V. The great majority of the substantia gelatinosa cells are small interneurons, but projection cells with long axons have also been found. Short-axon interneurons are present in all

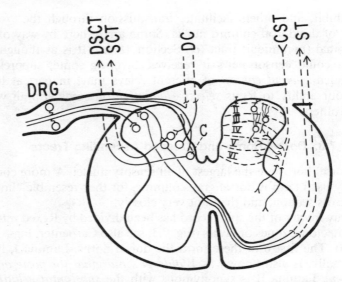

Figure 7.3. Location of some of the neurons of sensory function within a spinal segment. The *left side* shows examples of primary afferent terminals and of cell bodies of projection neurons; the *right side* the boundaries of cytoarchitectonic laminae and examples of short-axon interneurons. *DRG*, dorsal root ganglion; *DSCT*, dorsal spinocerebellar tract; *SCT*, spinocervical tract; *DC*, dorsal columns; *C*, Clarke's nucleus; *I–VI*: Rexed's cytoarchitectonic laminae; *CST*, corticospinal tract showing some of its fibers terminating in dorsal horn layers; *ST*, spinothalamic tract. Remember that coarse (Aα and Aβ) afferent fibers are concentrated in the medial part of the dorsal root, and either continue into the dorsal columns or send their terminals (mainly) to layers III–V; the fine (Aδ and C) fibers in the lateral part of the dorsal root send terminals mainly to layers I and II. Note that *DC* contains both primary afferent and (second-order) projection fibers.

the layers of the dorsal horn, which suggests that the information received from primary afferents is processed in each in some way before being transmitted to the sensory nuclei of the brain.

The cell bodies of the neurons the axons of which form the crossed ascending tracts are found in all layers of the dorsal horns, but there are more of them in layers I, IV, V and VI than in the substantia gelatinosa. The projection cells of lamina I are excited either by the mechanonociceptive or by the thermoreceptive (cold-sensitive) delta myelinated fibers, rarely by both, and never by low-threshold mechanoreceptors.

Among the projection cells of the nucleus proprius there are some that are excited by low-threshold mechanoreceptors. Many of these belong to the uncrossed ascending tracts, sending their axons either into the dorsolateral (spinocervical) or dorsal white columns. The axons of some, however, do cross the midline and join the spinothalamic tracts. For this reason it is no longer valid to consider the spinothalamic tract as serving exclusively the "crude" sensations of pain and temperature.

Nor, so it seems, is it entirely true that the dorsal columns conduct only the signals from low-threshold mechanoreceptors. A few investigators have insisted for decades that there are nociceptive afferents in the dorsal columns. Their view was recently supported in an experiment in which the dorsal columns of monkeys were transected on one side. These animals appeared to have a raised threshold for pain on the side of the lesion, compared to the intact side. Cutting one of the dorsolateral tracts caused the opposite, namely *hyperesthesia* (increased sensitivity) to noxious stimuli. Loss of pain perception is, however, *not* a sign of dorsal column lesion in man; if it occurs, it is too subtle to be detected by clinical tests.

While some of the neurons in the nucleus proprius of the dorsal horns are unimodal, receiving input from one type of primary afferent only, others are influenced by several types of input. Some receive antagonistic messages. For example, neurons have been found which were excited by nociceptors and inhibited by mechanoreceptors, or the reverse. Their role in the flow of information has not been determined, although there has been much speculation in this respect. Since cells of origin of both the crossed and the uncrossed ascending pathways reside, not very far from each other, in the nucleus proprius, there is opportunity for interaction between them. Experimental observations confirm that the crossed and uncrossed systems influence one another. The meaning of these interactions is not yet clear, however.

Like the nuclei of the dorsal columns, the dorsal horns receive input from the forebrain by way of descending fibers. Some of these fibers originate from the cerebral cortex and run in the corticospinal (pyramidal) tract, yet have no motor functions. They inhibit transmission of impulses from peripheral afferents to spinothalamic projection cells. This particular group of corticospinal tract fibers originate in the postcentral (sensory receiving) area of the cortex (see Section 18.1a). Inhibition can also be exerted from the raphe magnus nuclei of the brain stem through fibers of the raphe spinal pathway. The synaptic transmitter of the raphe spinal fibers is serotonin (5-hydroxytryptamine, 5-HT) (see Section 2.5e and Fig. 2.16).

There is a segmental ordering of spinothalamic fibers in the anterolateral white matter. Those originating in the most caudal segments are most lateral, those from more rostral segments lie in successively more medial layers. This is the reverse of the order in the dorsal columns, where caudal segments are represented medially (see Section 7.2a). This difference reflects the way in which fibers enter the two tracts. In the dorsal columns, fibers from each successively more rostral segment join those already in the tract from the lateral side; spinothalamic fibers join the tract after having crossed the midline and therefore always from the medial aspect (see Carpenter, Fig. 4.3).

7.4. Clinical Signs of the Lesions of Ascending Spinal Tracts

If the spinal cord is torn or crushed, the body parts innervated by segments below the injury lose all feeling and are no longer controlled by deliberate acts of the patient. We speak either of *paraplegia* or *quadriplegia* (tetraplegia) depending on whether only the lower body and two legs or all four limbs is involved.

If the continuity of spinal cord is not completely interrupted, then *paresis* (weakening of voluntary movements) and sensory loss need not be total. A peculiar condition, first accurately described by the neurologist Brown-Sequard, can result if one lateral half of the cord is transected. The patient loses much or all voluntary control of the muscles innervated by the segments below the lesion, on the side of the lesion, but retains essentially intact motor power on the contralateral side. He also loses fine touch on the side of the injury below the level of the lesion and is not able to feel the position of his joints or recognize mechanical vibration as such. On the contralateral half of his body, below the level of the lesion, he feels neither temperature nor pain. Such selective loss of sensory faculties is known as *dissociated sensory loss.*

The boundaries of the sensory loss caused by spinal lesions are determined by the dermatomal distribution of afferent fibers. Charts of dermatomes and the relationship of the spinal cord segments to the vertebral segments may be found in textbooks of anatomy and of clinical neurology.

7.4a. DISSOCIATED SENSORY LOSS

Sensory dissociations in cases of partial spinal injury have led to the discovery that signals from most low-threshold mechanoreceptors travel in the uncrossed spinal tracts, while those from nociceptive and temperature-sensing afferents only in the crossed tracts. Both the observation and the inference were in the main correct, except for one significant error. This was the belief that the finely discriminating, low-threshold mechanoreceptive afferents were represented in the dorsal columns and nowhere else.

As we have mentioned in Section 7.1, transection of the dorsal columns alone, whether in man or in experimental animals, is not followed by those sensory losses customarily described as "dorsal column signs." The most important of these signs are: loss of vibration sense; diminished two-point discrimination; loss of kinesthesia on the side of the lesion below the segmental level of the lesion; and preserved pain and temperature sense. It is now clear that to suffer this complex of disabilities, injury must extend to both the dorsal and dorsolateral sectors of the white matter (Fig. 7.4).

The clinical usefulness of dissociated sensory loss as a localizing sign has not diminished. It was, and is, a reliable sign by which damage to the dorsolateral spinal quadrant can be distinguished from ventrolateral lesions. The newer information refines clinical diagnosis. There is one sensory deficiency that, in experiments on monkeys, has reliably been linked to lesion of the dorsal funiculi. It is a loss of the ability to recognize the direction in which a cutaneous mechanical stimulus is moving. Normal monkeys can easily decide whether their fur is brushed with or against the grain, whereas monkeys whose dorsal columns have been cut cannot. Isolated lesion of the dorsal columns is rare in humans,

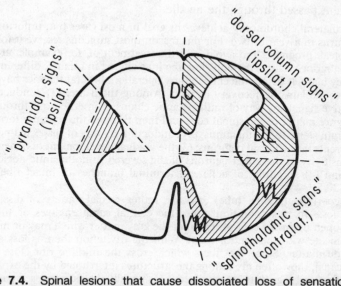

Figure 7.4. Spinal lesions that cause dissociated loss of sensation. The *shaded areas* show the parts of the white matter that must be destroyed to cause sensory loss as indicated. *DC,* dorsal column; *DL,* dorsolateral column; *VL,* ventrolateral column; *VM,* ventromedial column.

but it does occur. The one faculty these patients all lack is the ability to "read" numbers "written" on their skin with a blunt instrument (without looking, of course). One might expect this from the experiments on monkeys, because the tracing of numbers on the skin is a moving stimulus.

Injury to anterolateral white matter on one side causes loss of contralateral pain and temperature sense below the segmental level of the lesion. The most common cause of such a lesion has become a surgical intervention termed *anterolateral chordotomy*, a last resort in incurably painful conditions when analgesic medications no longer offer relief. For pain arising in abdominal and pelvic viscera, the transection must be bilateral. The operation can be performed under local anesthesia, with the aid of a needle introduced into the cervical spinal cord, guided by x-ray. As the needle approaches the tract, an electric stimulus is applied. If it evokes pain radiating into the painful body parts of the opposite side, the needle is correctly aimed. If, instead, the stimulus evokes an "electric" or vibrating sensation, or a contraction of muscles, then the needle is either on the wrong track, or not advanced far enough. When the target is reached the white matter is cut by electric coagulation by current passed through the needle.

Anterolateral chordotomy achieves its goal in most cases but, unfortunately, pain returns in a year or two. For this reason most surgeons reserve it for cases with a bleak prognosis and avoid it in the treatment of, for example, arthritis. When pain does return, patients describe it as altered in quality, different from what they had felt before the chordotomy operation. Several theories have been offered to explain the recovery of pain. Among them are: (1) conduction of nociceptive signals by way of multisynaptic chains of interneurons through the central gray matter of the spinal cord and then through the reticular formation of the brain stem, to the thalamus; (2) conduction by way of suspected nociceptive afferents in the dorsal columns; (3) the gradual development of denervation supersensitivity of the target neurons of the severed spinothalamic nociceptive fibers; and (4) sprouting of collateral terminal branches of intact fibers (see Section 20.5).

Syringomyelia (*syrinx*, tube) causes a rather special variety of dissociated sensory loss. In this condition either the central canal enlarges or tube-like cavities open up in the central region of the gray matter which may or may not communicate with the central canal. With the cavitation there is loss of gray and white matter. Since the fibers which cross the midline run close to the central canal, they often are among the structures interrupted by the expanding cavity. If several segments are involved, as is usually the case, crossed pathways are destroyed in a wide band. The patient then suffers loss of pain and temperature sense in an area that girdles his body or extends into his limbs along dermatomal boundaries. Light touch and other mechanical sensibilities are not diminished in these cases.

7.5. The Trigeminal System

For primary afferents of the face, the trigeminal ganglion of Gasser takes the place of the dorsal root ganglia. In this large ganglion the cell bodies of most of the first-order primary afferent neurons of the skin of the face and of the connective tissues of the head are gathered. The cell bodies of the primary afferents innervating the stretch receptors of the jaw-closing muscles and the periodontal mechanoreceptors are, however, in the mesencephalic sensory nucleus of the trigeminal nerve (see Carpenter, Fig. 6.19). This is the one and only case where the cell bodies of peripheral sensory fibers are within the central nervous system, not in a ganglion.

Besides the mesencephalic nucleus, the trigeminal system contains an elaborate complex of sensory nuclei that extends the length of the brain stem and dips into the spinal cord. Anatomists divide this complex into (1) the principal sensory nucleus and (2) the partes oralis, interpolaris and caudalis of the nucleus of the spinal tract of the Vth nerve (Carpenter, Fig. 6.19). The pars caudalis is, more or less, continuous with the laminae I, II and III of the cervical spinal cord and has been considered by some to be their rostral extension. Other investigators emphasized the differences between the functions of the pars caudalis of the nucleus of the Vth nerve and the substantia gelatinosa. Anatomically, the caudal end of the nucleus of the Vth nerve lies close to the cuneate nucleus.

In a general sense, the components of the trigeminal nuclear complex are indeed similar in function to the various parts of the spinal dorsal horn. Clinical experience suggests that the caudal portion of the trigeminal nuclear complex serves mainly nociceptive and thermoreceptive functions, since lesions here interfere with pain and temperature sensations of the face, but not with mechanical sensibility. The rostral components of the nucleus of the spinal tract and the principal sensory nucleus are thought to serve mainly, if not exclusively, the finely discriminating senses. Physiological experimentation has revealed neurons in the trigeminal nuclear complex with properties resembling those found in the nuclei of the spinal pathways. A detailed listing of their similarities and differences has no place in this text.

7.6. Somatosensory Nuclei in the Thalamus

The ventroposterolateral (VPL) nucleus of the thalamus is the common target of the medial lemniscus and much of the spinothalamic projection. The adjacent ventroposteromedial (VPM) nucleus, with which the VPL nucleus is practically continuous, receives somatosensory input from the trigeminal system. The two together are sometimes referred to as the ventrobasal (VB) complex.

As are the nuclei of the dorsal columns, the somatosensory nuclei of the thalamus are ordered according to both body topography and type (modality) of input. The topographic layout is the reverse of that in the dorsal columns: the snout is represented most medially and the tail most laterally. This is easy to remember if the association of VPM nucleus with the face and of VPL nucleus with the innervation of the body is kept in mind.

As a rule, any one cell in the VPL or VPM nucleus responds to but one type of sensory input. Moreover, cells of like modality are collected in continuous layers of tissue. There are discrepancies in the charting of the representation of various sensory modalities in the thalamus, which have been published by different investigators. In part this is due to the real differences in the organization of the thalamus of different species. The important point to remember is this: the cells in VPL and VPM nuclei are ordered according to both body topography and type of adequate stimulus. The two sequences, one of body parts and the other of adequate stimulus, intersect in such a way that any small cluster of neurons within the thalamus will respond to stimulation of one particular kind coming from one particular part of the body.

It will be recalled that all input to the VPL nucleus crosses the midline, though not all at the same level. Fibers of the spinothalamic pathways cross in the spinal cord, whereas fibers collected in the medial lemniscus cross in the brain stem. The final result is that the right VPL nucleus is connected to the left side of the body, and *vice versa.*

Part of the spinothalamic pathway terminates not in the VPL nucleus, but in the posterior group of nuclei (Po) of the thalamus. At one time this part was believed to be the main target of signals of nociceptive and temperature receptors. Some investigators identified the function of the Po group with the protopathic sensations and the VPL-VPM nuclei with the epicritic sensations as defined by Head (see Section 6.8). Subsequently however, nociceptive input was found to reach the outer zone of VPL and VPM nuclei. Moreover, in human patients operated under local anesthesia, stimulation by stereotactically introduced needle electrodes (see Section 1.2) caused pain in certain limited zones of the ventroposterior thalamus. It seems that much work remains to be done before the representation of nociceptive and temperature input and the relationship of thalamic function to conscious sensation can be analyzed.

The large, long-axon neurons of VPL and VPM nuclei project to the somatosensory receiving areas of the cerebral cortex. There also are short-axon interneurons, many of which have inhibitory functions. These cells are probably among those that set the pace of the alpha rhythm and the spindle bursts of electroencephalograph (EEG) tracings at times when they have little to do (see Section 4.8). Their active function is, however, probably in the processing of information, but their exact role has not yet been discovered.

The main output of the posterior group of nuclei is also addressed to the neocortex. Its distribution has been mapped in the cat but is not accurately known in man. A small portion may project to the second somatic receiving area, and a large part possibly to adjacent "association" cortex.

7.7. The Somatosensory Areas of the Cerebral Cortex

The main (primary, or first) somatosensory receiving area (sometimes denoted as SI, sometimes as SMI) lies in human and other primate brains in the postcentral gyrus and in the posterior bank of the central fissure (Fig. 7.5). Neuroanatomists define it as coextensive with cytoarchitectonic areas 3-1-2, with area 3 lying in front of 1, and 2 lying behind it. This unusual sequence of numbers came about because of the orientation of the planes in which Brodmann, who pioneered cytoarchitectonic charting of the cortex, has cut his specimens.

If this area of the cerebral cortex is stimulated electrically in a conscious human patient, the subject reports "electric" or "vibrating" sensations in a region of the opposite side of his body. A regular relationship has been found between the cortical point stimulated and the body part in which the sensation is evoked. Stimulation of the most lateral part of the postcentral gyrus evokes paresthesias* in the face; as progressively more medial parts are stimulated, the sensation is projected into the hand, the arms and then the trunk, and closest to the midline but still on the lateral aspect of the hemisphere, the legs. On the medial aspect of the hemisphere, the foot and the sacral and coccygeal segments are represented (Fig. 7.6).

In experimental animals the projection of paresthesias cannot be determined, but it is possible to record the electrical responses evoked by stimulating peripheral nerves or, better yet, peripheral sensory receptors. Even in an anesthesized CNS, sensory pathways transmit impulses and evoked potentials can be recorded from the brain surface or the responses of individual neurons with the aid of microelectrodes. Electric recordings from the brains of subhuman primates correspond to a remarkable degree with the reports of human patients.

The sorting of input according to the type of adequate stimuli of

* Paresthesias are somatic sensations felt in the absence of an adequate stimulus.

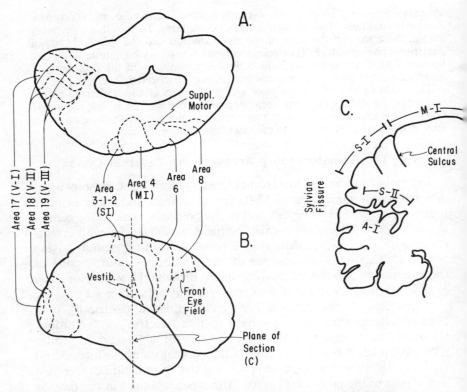

Figure 7.5. The location of some of the cerebral cortical receiving areas. *A*, medial aspect of hemisphere; *B*, lateral aspect of hemisphere; *C*, cross-section in the plane indicated by *straight vertical broken line* in *B*. *S-I* and *S-II*, somatosensory receiving areas I and II; *A-I*, auditory receiving area I; *V-I*, visual receiving area I; *M-I*, primary motor area; *Suppl. motor*, supplementary motor area; *Vestib.*, projection of vestibular organ.

peripheral sense organ that occurs in the dorsal column nuclei and in the sensory thalamus continues in the primary sensory receiving area of the cerebral cortex. Thus the orderly representation of body topography along a mediolateral axis is overlain by an ordering of afferent sensory signals by type along an anteroposterior axis. In other words, the primary receiving area consists of several modality-specific strips of cortex, one lying in front of the other. Each strip contains a representation of the parts of the body from head to tail (Fig. 7.6); the nature of the cortical "map," or somatotopic representation, is discussed later (see Section 7.8a). For example, input from proprioceptive stretch receptors projects to the most anterior (rostral) part of the somatic receiving area (sometimes designated 3a), which lies adjacent to the motor cortex of the anterior bank of the central fissure. Anticipating a later chapter (Section 18.1), we might add, that muscle stretch receptors also project into the motor area of the cortex (MI or, according to another notation MS I, or cytoarchitectonic area 4). Behind 3a there is a zone of cortex that receives input from slowly adapting cutaneous receptors, and behind that lies another zone to which rapidly adapting cutaneous input is relayed.

7.8. Columnar Organization

The cell population of the cerebral cortex is organized into 6 layers. The tip of a microelectrode inserted into the cortex encounters many cells on its way through the approximately 2.5 mm of gray matter. In the SI area a microelectrode traveling at right angles to the plane of the cortical surface will find cells of similar input, and of peripheral receptive fields which either overlap or are coextensive. If the electrode is withdrawn and then reinserted either medially or laterally, then the cells in the new track have inputs from another body region, but will respond to the same type of stimulation. If, however, the electrode is moved in an anterior or posterior direction, cells will be found with receptive fields in roughly the same body region, but the types of input will change (see above and Fig. 7.6).

The similar response properties of cells lying above and below one another reflect the so-called *columnar organization* of the cortex. Neuroanatomists first called attention to this feature of cortical architecture. They noticed that both the afferent fibers entering the cortex and the efferent axons of pyramidal cells leaving it run in the cortical gray matter at right angles to the surface. Moreover, the main dendritic trunks of pyramidal cells parallel the axons, being oriented normal to the surface. The mainstream of traffic flows vertically through the cortex, but this should not obscure the fact that there are also lateral connections. A plexus of fibers in the most superficial cortical layer lies parallel to the surface. However, these lateral connections span relatively short distances. The main connections between the cortex and the subcortical centers, as well as the U fibers which interconnect different cortical regions over longer distances, run normal to the surface.

The concept of columnar organization implies that vertical columns

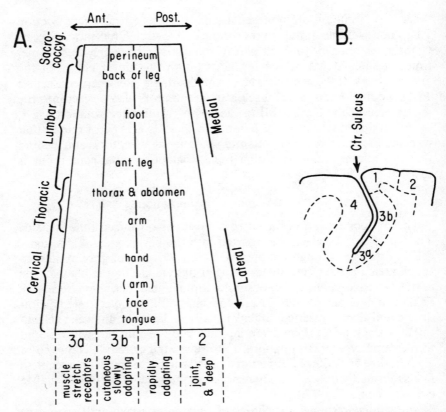

Figure 7.6. The intersecting representations of the topography of the body and of receptor types in the primary somatic sensory receiving area (SI) of the cerebral neocortex. *A*, the rectangular slab is an unfolded schematic representation of the surface of the SI area. The spinal segments (and hence body regions) are arranged in a mediolateral sequence. Different types of sensory receptors send signals to the different cytoarchitectonic strips (3a, 3b, 1 and 2). *B*, the boundaries of cytoarchitectonic areas of the banks of the central sulcus of a macaque monkey. Note that the primary motor area (4) lies anterior and adjacent to area 3a.

of cortical cells have some shared function. In a rough analogy, each column acts as a module or a computer chip consisting of several operational units wired together to perform a single operation. Such cortical circuits analyze input to *detect or extract specific features* of the stimulation.

Most, though not all, specific thalamic afferent axons end in the IVth cell layer of the cortex, from where intracortical, short-axon interneurons distribute the signals to the cells lying above and below. The main output from the cortex is conducted by the axons of the large cells in layers V and VI.

The responses of neurons in layer IV are the most similar to the input signals because they receive the input immediately, in raw form before it is modified by synaptic interconnections. Above and below the IVth layer, cells respond differently. For example, there may be neurons that respond maximally to the brushing of hairs in the receptive field in a distal direction and minimally or not at all to brushing in the proximal direction. Others will respond preferentially to a stimulus moving in the proximal direction. As mentioned already (Section 7.4) the only reliable test of damage to the dorsal columns of the spinal cord is a patient's ability to detect the direction of mechanical stimulation. It appears that the signals required for such detection travel along the dorsal columns and are then analyzed in the somatic sensory cortex, especially in those strips of cortex that receive the input of rapidly adapting mechanoreceptors.

Movement direction is but one of the features of cutaneous sensory input that may be analyzed in primary sensory cortex. Such properties as the roughness or the slipperiness of a surface, and many others, may also be detected here.

7.8a. NOTES ON TOPOGRAPHIC REPRESENTATION

We have met with several examples of the ordering of afferent units according to body topography. The main outline of such topographic ordering has been known for some time, but there has been much debate concerning the principles governing this anatomical organization, and the debate has not yet ended. For this reason, it is only possible to sum up the discussion as it stands today.

In most neuroscience textbooks one can find one, or several, illustrations showing a map of the body surface overlaid on a diagram of the cerebral cortex. On such diagrams the face lies laterally, the legs medially, the belly rostrally, and the back caudally. Facing this "sensory homunculus" across the central fissure, there is usually a "motor homunculus" (or siminculus, felinculus, etc. if a non-human cortex is depicted). These illustrations are not given here because there is considerable evidence that they may misrepresent the organizing principle of somatic projections.

The idea of body maps implies that the body surface is represented in the brain as a geographical projection, though not to a constant scale. The projections of the tongue and fingers are quite oversized and the trunk is disproportionately small in comparison. The relative size of the projection of a part was believed to be related to the density of its innervation and therefore to the finesse of tactile discrimination. Nevertheless, the relative position, if not the proportions, of body parts were believed preserved in the cortical projection. There has, however, been an alternative idea. Some investigators have thought that the cortex does not contain a surface map, but the representation of the sequence of dermatomes. This proposition may be closer to the truth. It certainly is more consistent with the discovery of multiple cortical strips, one for each type of sensory receptor. In each of these strips the body parts are represented in sequence, and it is easy to see how this could be a sequence of dermatomes, but not a true map of the body surface (Fig. 7.6). For example, the projection of the foot lies between the projections of the ventral and dorsal aspects of the leg. This is readily understood as a dermatomal sequence, since the anterior aspect of the leg is innervated mostly by L2–L4, the foot mostly by L5 and S1, and the posterior aspect of the leg by S1 and S2 spinal segments.

7.8b. CORTICAL REPRESENTATION AND BODY IMAGE

In our minds we all have an image of our bodies. It is based on visual, tactile, and proprioceptive information, integrated and organized into a whole and stored in memory. Excitation of somatic receptors is felt in one or other body part; in other words, we project the stimulus to a locus within the framework of our body image. The two main questions are: what cerebral mechanism enables us to form a body image? and, what mechanism places stimuli accurately within that image?

We do not know the answers, but we have some hints. If a pin pricks the skin, a blindfolded subject can find the injured spot literally with pinpoint accuracy. If an internal organ hurts, a patient's ability to localize the pain is far less accurate. As a previously injured peripheral nerve regenerates (see Section 6.8), the first to return is a diffuse pain sensibility without accurate localization. In general, a precise sense of body location is a property of myelinated fibers; it is missing from senses served by unmyelinated fibers.

Of course, the critical factor is not the myelination itself. Rather, it is that the afferent pathways retain, through several levels of signal processing in the spinal cord and brain stem, some manner of topographic ordering. It is not necessarily a "map," as long as there is a topographic system, perhaps along dermatomal lines. The pathways served by myelinated fibers have such organization. Where and how the brain constructs the neural basis for our experience of a three-dimensional space, and within it a solid image of our bodies, is not clear. The segmental ordering of mechanoreceptive afferent projections seems necessary to this computation, but it does not by itself explain it.

7.8c. SENSORY DEFICIT CAUSED BY LESIONS OF THE CORTICAL SOMATIC SENSORY RECEIVING AREAS

If SI and SII areas of the cerebral cortex are involved in the central processing of information furnished by somatic sensory receptors, then it is to be expected that somatic sensations should be abnormal in patients who suffered damage to these cortical areas. This is indeed the case. Surprisingly, however, sensory functions can recover some months after an accident destroyed an area of sensory cortex, especially if the lesion was small. The clinical rule must therefore be: if after brain injury somatic sensory function is disturbed, then there is reason to believe that the sensory cortex has been damaged, but if somatic sensory function seems intact, an old injury to this area cannot be ruled out.

The sensory deficit is worse if the lesion is large and, especially, if it is bilaterally symmetrical. Unilateral lesions impair the function of the contralateral limbs. The most impaired are functions requiring complex discrimination, such as the recognition of objects by touch. Two-point discrimination (see Section 7.10) and other tests of spatial discrimination are more affected than the psychophysical threshold for touch. Pain and temperature sensibility are not seriously affected by lesions to the somatic cortical receiving areas.

If monkeys are trained to recognize tactile stimuli and then their SI cortical areas are removed by surgery, they lose this ability; but then after a period of time they can re-learn the same task. The nature of the disability, while it exists, is similar to man's. Lesions limited to SII area have little effect, but combined lesions of SI and SII cause worse impairment than of SI alone.

When the cerebral cortex of a human patient is extensively damaged, it may be difficult to distinguish between true sensory loss and the disability typical of parietal lesion (unilateral neglect; see Section 21.2c). And the detailed testing of patients suffering with cognitive disabilities may prove almost impossible. Some of the controversy surrounding cortical function stems from the difficulties of testing. The functions of the so-called association areas of the cortex and the nature of the recovery of function after brain damage will be discussed in Chapter 21, but it must be admitted that much remains uncertain about these topics.

7.9. Comments on the Physiology of Pain Sensation

7.9a. DEFINITION

The literature concerning the physiology and psychology of pain is voluminous and, in part, needlessly contentious. Some of the disputes of the past century could have been avoided by a more careful choice of words. In English, and in most other languages, living and dead, the word *pain* has two quite distinct meanings. It denotes both a specific bodily sensation and the feelings of suffering, unhappiness, or of sorrow.

Now it is quite true that bodily pain is unpleasant to most, but it is equally clear that pain is not simply the opposite of pleasure. For one thing, some people, under certain special conditions, actually seek pain and seem to enjoy it. And equally clearly, one can be in the throes of deep anguish and yet be physically quite comfortable.

People's attitudes toward bodily pain, their level of acceptance, reactions to it, and the meaning they attribute to it, vary enormously. A discussion of these various reactions properly belongs in the provinces of normal and abnormal psychology. There can be little doubt, however, that, when anyone hammers his thumb instead of a nail, he experiences a bodily sensation which is the same in all, regardless of ethnic origin, upbringing, or religious conviction. Only the exclamation uttered is determined by social and psychological factors. It is this immediate bodily sensation that falls within the province of neurophysiology. If we limit our discussion to it, much of the arguments of the past become irrelevant.

It is the bodily sensation of pain that must be explored in the taking of medical histories. The physician must ask such questions as: "Show me: where does it hurt? What is it like—is it stabbing, or burning? Is it continuous, or does it come in waves?" When he does so, it is with the confidence born of experience that, by and large, patients can indeed give reliable answers to such questions. Admittedly, language is inadequate to describe all the qualities of pain, especially visceral pain. This inadequacy of language is because we cannot associate an external object with the stimulus giving rise to pain. We all can look at a patch of red paint, and all of us, except the color-blind, can agree to call that particular stimulus "red." But this is not possible with an intestinal colic or the ache of an ulcer. Imperfections of language notwithstanding, careful questioning of two people suffering a similar disease will reveal the similarity of their experience.

In summary: while bodily pain is unpleasant to most people most of the time, it is erroneous to define it as the "opposite of pleasure." More correctly, it should be defined as the sensation evoked by stimuli which either threaten or actually cause tissue damage. As with all sensation, the presence of such a stimulus is normally a necessary but not a sufficient condition to evoke it. To feel pain, the subject must be awake and attending. Usually, but not invariably, noxious stimuli are intensely attention-getting. And, as with other senses, under pathological conditions pain can arise in the absence of a peripheral stimulus (phantom pain and other pain states that originate in the CNS).

7.9b. STATES OF ANALGESIA

Occasionally children are born who cannot feel pain. Their life is full of hazard, and it takes an unusual effort on the part of those who care for them to bring them up without serious injury. More often than not, they develop serious deformities as a result of repeated burns and trauma. Such *congenital analgesia* is rare, and only a few cases have been studied adequately by neurologists and neuropathologists. In some, a deficiency of peripheral unmyelinated nerve fibers was found. These patients were also insensitive to temperature stimuli. However, in some analgetic children the spectrum of fiber sizes in peripheral nerves was normal; in these the deficiency is assumed to be an as yet undiscovered inborn error of the CNS. Usually these children had other deficiencies, such as mental retardation.

Another example that underscores the protective value of nociception is *tabes dorsalis*. In tabetic patients sensory fibers are destroyed by disease of dorsal root ganglion cells. The lumbosacral segments are usually maximally affected. One of several consequences of such sensory denervation can be the crippling deformity known as "*Charcot's joint*." This damage is not directly caused by the microorganism of the syphilitic infection, but, in essence, by the patient himself. Since he feels no pain, he causes repeated trauma to his own joints and continues to walk on them in spite of the damage.

These were examples of analgesia due to loss of input from sense organs. Pain may also be suppressed by inhibitory mechanisms. This can be normal physiological process. During a fight, pain is muted or absent. Bruises and wounds start to hurt when the excitement dies down. Doctors and psychologists who have witnessed battlefield casualties were often impressed by how much more stoically injuries were accepted by wounded soldiers than similar injuries would have been by civilians after an accident.

On a more trivial level, probably everyone discovers sooner or later that the pain of a bruise or of a hurting joint can be relieved somewhat by rubbing the overlying skin. Warming, massage, gentle moving of a limb, and the like can also provide relief to a varying degree. These phenomena can be described as a form of sensory *masking*, defined as one kind of sensory input preventing the action of another. In the examples given, tactile and proprioceptive inputs mask nociceptive input.

It is important to try to distinguish between true analgesia (the absence of pain) and increased tolerance to pain in which the patient does feel the pain, but does not mind or at least does not express distress. In practice this distinction is sometimes difficult. It seems very likely, though it is not definitely proven, that in either case it is some form of synaptic inhibition that brings relief, but at different levels of the CNS. We have learned earlier that the dorsal horns of the spinal cord receive inhibitory synaptic terminals from descending fiber tracts (Section 7.3 and Fig. 7.3). It has been shown that such inhibition can partly or wholly suppress the transmission of excitation from nociceptive and also from non-nociceptive peripheral afferent fibers. Either these inhibitory synapses or others in the thalamic nuclei may be responsible for the temporary suppression of pain sensation. Tolerance to pain on the other hand may be determined in the neuron circuits of the limbic system and of the frontal lobes (see Chapter 21).

Gate theory. In 1965 Melzack and Wall, a psychologist-physiologist team, proposed a theory by which they hoped to explain many seemingly contradictory observations concerning the perception of pain. They especially wanted to reconcile the arguments of the two camps favoring the *intensity theory* and the *specificity theory* of pain signals (see Section 6.7). According to their *gate theory*, there are no specific "pain fibers." Rather, whether pain is felt or not depends on a balance between input by high-threshold, fine-caliber and low-threshold, coarse-caliber afferent fibers. Ordinarily, large-diameter fibers would inhibit, and thereby keep in check, the effect of the small-diameter fibers. If the balance tilted in favor of the high-threshold small fibers, the spinal "gate" would open, the pattern of excitation of long-axon relay cells would change, and pain would be felt.

In its original form the gate theory has been rendered untenable by several recent observations, among them the discovery of specific nociceptive second-order afferent neurons (see Section 7.3). It was nevertheless necessary to summarize the theory here for several reasons: (1) because anyone interested in the clinical management of pain will sooner or later meet this theory in the literature; and (2) because several useful methods of treating chronically painful conditions have been inspired by it. The gate theory and Head's division of the senses into epicritic and protopathic classes (see Section 6.8) have in common the idea that there may be inhibitory interaction between the neural systems mediating the finely discriminating mechanoreceptive input and those mediating nociceptive input. This insight is based on sound observation even if the explanations offered so far are not accurate.

Electrotherapy of pain. Pain can be stilled by electrical stimulation in at least two different ways: (1) by stimulating non-nociceptive primary afferent fibers that cause the "masking" of pain (see above); and (2) by stimulating centers in the brain stem or diencephalon that give rise to the pathways inhibiting transmission of afferent nociceptive signals. The former approach is in clinical use at a number of neurosurgical centers.

The latter is, at the time of this writing, for the most part limited to the animal laboratory, although occasional attempts to apply it to human patients have already been reported.

It is possible to implant wire electrodes so that they encircle a major nerve. The wires are led under the skin to a subcutaneous receiving antenna. The broadcast antenna of an external radio stimulator is taped over the subcutaneous receiver. The arrangement is similar to a cardiac pacemaker, except that the patient controls his own stimulator. The nerve must be the one supplying the painful region, so that stimulation should cause a sensation irradiating into the painful part. The patient chooses a stimulus strength which causes a buzzing or vibrating feeling (paresthesia), but no pain. He can do so because the non-nociceptive mechanoreceptors are supplied by larger caliber fibers than the nociceptive sense organs (see Fig. 6.4) and the larger fibers have the lower electric threshold (see Section 3.1d). In successful cases the paresthesia masks the pain.

Stimulating a peripheral nerve to suppress pain is practical only in cases where the painful condition afflicts one limb. Pain in two limbs or in abdominal organs, when no single nerve could be selected for stimulation, can sometimes be masked by stimulating the dorsal columns of the spinal cord. The electrodes contact the spinal cord several segments above the entry of the sensory roots supplying the affected area. Sensation evoked by stimulating the spinal dorsal columns are projected into all the lower regions of the body, including those giving rise to the pain.

A similarity between the masking of pain by electrotherapy and the analgesia of acupuncture has been claimed. There are, however, important differences. For electrically evoked masking to be successful, mechanoreceptive fibers innervating the painful part must be stimulated, whereas the sites chosen for acupuncture are not neurologically related to the afflicted body parts. Moreover, in order to be effective, acupuncture must be moderately painful, but the masking stimulus must not. There have been a number of attempts to produce acupuncture analgesia in animals, with variable results in the hands of different investigators. When successful, the effect of acupuncture has been attributed to the release of enkephalin (see next section). Further discussion of acupuncture is better deferred until more experimental data will be available.

In experimental animals an apparent state of analgesia can also be achieved by electrical stimulation of a number of sites in the central nervous system. These include the periaqueductal gray matter of the midbrain; the raphe magnus nuclei of the pons and upper medulla; and some of the "self-stimulation" sites of the limbic system (see Section 21.6).

Comparing animal experiments with human experience is, obviously, not always possible. Analgesia is customarily gauged by the briskness of an animal's response to a noxious stimulus. It is, however, possible that an animal fails to make an escape movement, or responds more slowly or more feebly than usual, not because it does not feel pain, but because motor responses are inhibited. In general, the higher the center, the more difficult the interpretation of animal experiments.

As far as the raphe magnus nuclei are concerned, there are, however, independent reasons for believing that electric stimulation at this site may cause true analgesia. Cells in these nuclei give rise to axons that lead to the dorsal horns of the spinal cord—the raphe-spinal pathway (see Section 7.3). Input by nociceptive afferents is among those which have been shown to be suppressed by stimulation of the raphe-spinal pathway.

7.9c. ENKEPHALIN

The pain-quelling property of opium (laudanum) has been known since antiquity. Morphine was among the first alkaloids to be purified in crystalline form, and its chemical structure has been discovered several decades ago. It has more recently occurred to some investigators that the potent and specific actions of morphine and related drugs must be due to the existence of specific receptor molecules for a natural substance in the brain, whose action is mimicked by the opium alkaloids.

Once this idea was clearly formulated, specific binding sites for radioactively labeled morphine-like drugs were soon found in several brain regions. Shortly thereafter two classes of endogenous opioid peptides were extracted, first the endorphins and then the enkephalins. These peptides became known as "endogenous opioid ligands." The name is somewhat misleading, for it suggests that the natural brain substance imitates the effect of the poisons of the poppy, instead of the other way around.

Endorphins are relatively large molecules composed of 16–19 amino acids. They have been found in the posterior pituitary and in the hypothalamic region. Enkephalins are much smaller, consisting of five amino acid residues (Table 2.3). The met-enkephalin structure forms a part of α-endorphin, and the structure of the latter is a component of the lipotropin molecule.

Morphine, injected systemically, has many actions besides the suppression of pain. These are discussed in detail in all textbooks of pharmacology. When enkephalins are administered artificially, they produce most of the effects which morphine has on the central nervous system. The widespread presence of enkephalins and of their specific receptors in the brain suggests that they have many normal functions.

Even though enkephalins have been found in many parts of the gray matter, their concentration varies greatly. The highest concentrations (in the rat) are in the globus pallidus, followed by the caudate nucleus and nucleus accumbens. Most important to our present discussion is, however, their presence in the periaqueductal gray matter, in the raphe magnus nuclei, and in the substantia gelatinosa of the spinal cord. These are the sites where their effects may be related to their analgesic action. It will be remembered that electroanalgesia is also effective in the periaqueductal gray matter and raphe magnus. The possible interaction between enkephalin and serotonin in controlling transmission in the dorsal horns has not been clarified.

It seems then that the brain is equipped to produce its own "high." It is likely that brain-produced enkephalins have to do with the excitement that enables people to climb mountains, to win battles and Olympic medals, and to achieve other feats which, in the absence of such ecstasy, would cause severe discomfort.

When first discovered, there was hope that enkephalins would prove to be the ideal analgesics, free of the complications and drug-tolerance typical of opiates. It soon proved, however, that on repeated administration, enkephalins lose potency. The triple phenomena of desensitization, drug tolerance and drug dependence are just as marked for enkephalin as for morphine.

It may well be that the rapid loss of effectiveness of enkephalins is a natural protective device of the brain. Pain cannot be ignored forever without peril, or ecstasy long sustained without a dangerous disregard of realistic limits to human action. Healthy, natural rapture must be limited in duration and spaced at rare intervals. Those who abuse morphine and related drugs circumvent the limits imposed by drug tolerance by taking ever-increasing doses. The addict's enslavement soon takes effect, with inexorably diminishing returns of euphoria. To the calamities of addiction is then added the indignity of constipation, for morphine's effect on the gut (see Section 17.3c) is the one for which tolerance is the least pronounced.

7.9d. REFERRED PAIN

As mentioned earlier, surface pain, especially the kind involving stimulation of mechanoreceptive nociceptors, is accurately localized by the subject. Visceral pain is not. Pain caused by disease of the internal organs is felt "somewhere inside," but often it also radiates into superficial parts of the body, sometimes into one of the limbs. Pain felt in a part other than the injured one is *referred pain.*

The distribution of referred pain is not haphazard. As clues by which diseases of internal organs can be identified, medical students must learn the rules according to which visceral pain radiates. The most widely known example is angina pectoris, caused by ischemia of the heart muscle (see Section 6.7). The pain of angina is felt within the cavity of the chest but at the same time is usually also referred to the left side of the chest wall and sometimes the ulnar aspect of the left arm, along the distribution of the C8, T1 and T2 dermatomes.

Several theories have been proposed to explain referred pain. One has recently received support from neurophysiological experiments. Originally proposed by Ruch, it is known as the *convergent excitation* theory. It postulates that there are neurons in the spinal cord that can be excited by both nociceptive afferents of somatic nerves and nociceptive afferents innervating internal viscera. During most of the individual's life these neurons are excited only by stimulation in their peripheral receptive field, and the brain interprets their excitation as somatic pain. On the relatively rare occasion when an internal disease excites these same spinal neurons by their visceral input, the brain receives the same signal which it had been programmed to decode as peripheral pain. Neurons which behave as Ruch's theory predicted they should, have recently been found in the spinal cords of animals.

A final footnote: certain types of visceral pain are often described as having a "stabbing" quality. This usually means that the pain is of sudden onset, not that it is sharply localized. This is mentioned here only to illustrate how imprecise language can be when describing subjective experiences, which is not the same as saying that the experience itself is uncertain. The patient knows precisely what he feels; he just lacks the words to describe it.

7.9e. PAIN OF CENTRAL ORIGIN

Pain can arise without stimulation of sensory receptors; it is caused by the misfiring of neurons in the central nervous system. Such misfiring can be the result of an irritating lesion or of the loss of inhibitory restraint (release of function; see Section 4.10).

After amputation of a limb or of a finger, there may remain an illusion of the lost part still being there. This is called a *phantom* sensation. Such phantoms are often painful. A similar condition occurs when the dorsal roots are traumatically avulsed (pulled out) from their insertion into the spinal cord. In some cases the pain can be traced to irritation of cut or torn nerve fibers by scar tissue. In others it is assumed that the pain originates in the central nervous system, perhaps by denervation supersensitivity (see Section 3.4f) of central neurons which lost their synaptic input.

Facial pain syndrome or *trigeminal neuralgia* consists of brief spells of intense pain in the face. If associated with involuntary movements of the facial muscles, it is called *tic douloureux*. The mechanism is not understood, but it has been attributed to paroxysmal discharge of neurons in the trigeminal nuclei of the brain stem.

The rare *thalamic pain syndrome* is usually caused by cerebrovascular accident (stroke) involving the lateral nuclear group of the thalamus. The result is that the threshold to mechanical stimuli is raised in the skin of the contralateral body half (or part of it); but when threshold is reached, the sensation evoked has an abnormal quality and usually is painful. This *hyperpathia* is said to be similar to the abnormal feeling (dysesthesia) in denervated and partially reinnervated skin regions (see Section 6.8). Attacks of spontaneous pain may also occur as part of the thalamic syndrome and are thought to be caused by release from inhibitory restraint.

7.10. Clinical Testing of Skin Sensibility and Proprioception

Clinical examination of skin sensibility in the traditional way is simple, though time-consuming. The patient is usually asked to close his eyes, or his vision must be obscured in some other way. The equipment required is minimal.

1. *Superficial touch.* At irregular intervals the skin is touched with cotton wool. The patient is asked to indicate whenever he feels being touched. The skin is systematically explored and the boundaries of anesthetic areas marked with a pen.

2. *Pain.* A pin with a blunt head is used. The patient is touched at random either with the blunt head or with the point of the pin (no need to draw blood). He indicates whether he felt sharp or blunt.

3. *Vibration sense.* A tuning fork, usually of 128 Hz, is placed in contact with the skin, usually over a bone. Sometimes the fork is set into vibration, sometimes it is not. The patient indicates whether or not he feels vibration. With dissociated sensory loss (see Section 7.4a) he may be able to feel being touched, but not able to detect vibration. Auditory cues must be avoided.

4. *Kinesthesia.* The patient is asked to relax the muscles of the extremity tested. The examiner holds a toe, finger, arm or leg with a steady grip. He then gently moves the part either up or down (extension or flexion). The patient indicates which way the joint is being moved. Joint positions (to be distinguished from joint movement, see Section 6.5) are tested by the examiner slowly bringing a joint of the patient to a certain angle, and then asking the patient to bring the contralateral limb (that is left free to move) into the same position.

5. *Temperature sense.* A test tube or beaker filled either with warm or with cold water is brought in contact with the skin.

6. *Object recognition by touch.* Some everyday object, such as a key,

matchbook, pencil, or the like is placed in the patient's hand, and he is asked what it is. The patient is either allowed to explore the object by moving it in his hand; or the object is placed on his palm and his fingers are closed around it by the examiner. When tested in the latter way, object recognition is much more difficult. Object recognition is especially relevant as a test of brain damage, for example of the sensory cortex. It is in the province of the cortical processing of sensory signals to extract the specific features by which objects are recognized (see Section 7.8). Thus with cortical damage, sensory thresholds may be unaffected or only moderately elevated, when object recognition is markedly impaired.

It should be clear that all of these tests suffer two disadvantages. None is quantitative, and all require an attentive and cooperative patient. Ways have been devised to circumvent these disadvantages. These procedures are too elaborate for routine examination except in specialized clinics, but it is necessary for general physicians to know that they exist and to have an idea of what they accomplish. Quantitative psychophysical methods have been in use for some time. Other, much newer methods, rely on electronic equipment, some of it computer controlled, and are for the most part still experimental.

Examples of well-established quantitative psychophysical tests include *two-point discrimination* and the determination of tactile threshold with *Von Frey hairs.* Two-point discrimination is tested by touching the skin with the blunted points of a divider. It is essential that both points should touch the skin simultaneously since two successive touches are discriminated by a neural mechanism different from the mechanism detecting two that are simultaneous but spatially separate. If the two points are too close together, the subject feels them as one. The minimal separation that can be felt as two separate points is 2 mm on the fingertips, and more than 60 mm on the back, or the thighs. Standard charts are available for all skin areas.

Von Frey hairs are a kind of a single-bristle toothbrush. They come in sets of varying calibrated stiffnesses. The tip of the hair is placed on the skin and pressed down until it just bends. The threshold is determined by applying bristles of increasing stiffness until the patient feels that he is being touched. Two variables are relevant for touch threshold: surface area of contact, and the force exerted. In a variant method fine wires replace the bristles to determine the threshold of mechanical pain.

Another method to determine pain threshold uses radiant heat. The temperature of the skin is measured, and the level at which pain is reported is taken to be the threshold. Radiant heat tests nociceptors different from those examined with the Von Frey method (Chapter 6).

Electronic tests may rely on computer-assisted instrumentation. One method, developed in the Mayo Clinic, utilizes a mechanically moved fine-tipped mechanical probe. A 9-point (3 × 3) matrix is mapped on the skin, and the threshold determined at each point. The computer commands the motor moving the probe, and a gauge measures the pressure applied to the skin. This test must take the patient's word to determine threshold, but at least the physical stimulus is accurately controlled and measured.

Electric recording from sensory nerves or from sensory areas of the brain, can be substituted for the patient's verbal report. Measurements of conduction velocity of peripheral sensory nerves was briefly described in Section 3.3c. Sensory evoked potentials can be recorded from the scalp of human subjects with electrodes similar to those used for EEG recordings (Fig. 3.15). To evoke such potential waves, an electrically operated mechanical probe can stimulate mechanoreceptors, or an electric pulse is applied to the skin to stimulate sensory fibers directly. It usually is necessary to repeat the same stimulus many times and to obtain an electronically averaged recording of the response, because the stimulus-evoked waves are no greater and often much smaller in amplitude than the spontaneous waves of the EEG (see Fig. 21.1). On recordings obtained by averaging the responses to repeated stimulus presentations, the EEG waves cancel and the evoked responses are enhanced.

7.11. Chapter Summary

1. Spinal afferent pathways may be conveniently subdivided into the uncrossed and the crossed tracts. Uncrossed spinal afferent pathways include the dorsal columns and those in the dorsolateral white quadrant; crossed pathways the anterolateral spinothalamic tract and the spinoreticular tracts.

2. Lesion limited to the dorsal columns causes impairment of the ability to detect the direction in which a cutaneous mechanical stimulus is moving. Combined injury of dorsal and dorsolateral white matter (i.e. dorsal hemisection or dorsolateral quadrant lesion) causes loss of finely discriminating mechanical sensations below the segmental level of the lesion on the side of the lesion (dissociated sensory loss).

3. Lesion limited to the anterolateral quadrant of white matter causes loss of temperature and pain sensations below the segmental level of the lesion on the side of the body opposite to the lesion. One or several years after the lesion pain sensibility returns, but is then of an altered quality.

4. Neurons in layers I and II of Rexed (the marginal zone of Waldeyer and the substantia gelatinosa of Rolando) receive synaptic connections only from unmyelinated and finely myelinated (delta) primary afferent fibers; layers IV, V and VI receive direct and collateral input from coarser afferent myelinated fibers, plus input from fine fibers transmitted indirectly by way of neurons in layers I and II.

5. Spinal dorsal horns as well as the nuclei of the dorsal columns receive inhibitory input from descending tracts, including from fibers descending in the corticospinal tract.

6. Lateral inhibition operates in nuclei of the somatosensory pathways, especially in cell populations receiving input from low-threshold mechanoreceptors.

7. There is intersecting spatial ordering in the neuron populations of the dorsal column nuclei, of the somatosensory nuclei of the thalamus, and of the primary somatosensory receiving area of the cerebral cortex. Along one dimension these cell populations represent a topographic order, probably a dermatomal sequence; along an intersecting dimension there is ordering according to receptor type (modality). Thus neurons in one another's vicinity are likely to receive input from the same body region and from similar sensory receptor organs. In the cortex this ordering gives rise to the so-called cortical columns.

8. Neurons in segregated zones in the thalamus receive inputs from various types of mechanoreceptors, from thermoreceptors, and from nociceptors. Diverse types of mechanoreceptors are represented in parallel strips of tissue in the sensory cortex; cortical representation of nociceptors and of thermoreceptors is controversial and may not exist.

9. Pain sensation can be masked by stimulation of non-nociceptive afferent fibers innervating the same body area in which the painful stimulus acts.

10. Specific receptor molecules for morphine-like drugs have been discovered in many brain areas, including the periaqueductal gray matter, raphe magnus nuclei, and substantia gelatinosa of the spinal cord. These areas are also rich in enkephalin, an endogenous substance with morphine-like action. Electrical stimulation of these areas causes an apparent state of analgesia.

11. Pain of visceral origin may be referred to other body parts probably because of the convergence of nociceptive afferent fibers from visceral and from somatic nerves onto the same spinal neurons.

12. Clinical tests of cutaneous and proprioceptive sensibility are briefly described.

Further Reading for Chapters 6 and 7

Books and Reviews

Boivie JJC, Perl ER: Neural substrates of somatic sensation. In Hunt CC (ed): *Neurophysiology*, MTP International Review of Science, Physiology Series, vol 3. Baltimore, University Park Press, 1975, pp 303–411.

Brindley, GS (ed): Somatic and visceral sensory mechanism. *Br Med Bull* 1977, 33:89–177.

Carpenter MB: *Core Text of Neuroanatomy*, ed 2. Baltimore, Williams & Wilkins, 1978.

Mountcastle VB: The neural replication of sensory events in the somatic afferent system. In Eccles JC (ed): *Brain and Conscious Experience*. New York, Springer, 1966, pp 85–115.

Willis WD, Coggeshall RE: *Sensory Mechanisms of the Spinal Cord*. New York, Plenum Press, 1978.

Carpenter MB: *Core Text of Neuroanatomy*, ed 2. Baltimore, Williams & Wilkins, 1978.

Brindley, GS (ed): Somatic and visceral sensory mechanism. *Br Med Bull* 1977, 33:89–177.

Mountcastle VB: The neural replication of sensory events in the somatic afferent system. In Eccles JC (ed): *Brain and Conscious Experience* New York, Springer, 1966, pp 85–115.

Willis WD, Coggeshall RE: *Sensory Mechanisms of the Spinal Cord*. New York, Plenum Press, 1978.

Articles

Dykes RW, Rasmusson DD, Hoeltzell PB: Organization of primary somatosensory cortex in the cat. *J Neurophysiol* 1980, 43:1527–1546.

Perl ER: Sensitization of nociceptors and its relation to sensation. In Bonica JJ, Albe-Fessard D (eds): *Advances in Pain Research and Therapy*, vol 1. New York, Raven Press, 1976, pp 17–28.

Powell TPS, Mountcastle VB: Some aspects of the functional organization of the cortex of the postcentral gyrus of the monkey: a correlation of the findings obtained in single unit analysis with cytoarchitecture. *Bull Johns Hopkins Hosp* 1959, 105:133–162.

chapter 8

The Senses of Taste and Smell

How chemical stimuli from the environment are transduced.
How sensory information concerning such stimuli is processed.

8.1. Stimuli and Receptor Cells of the Special Chemical Senses

The chemoreceptors serving taste and smell are specialized epithelial receptor cells in the mucous membranes of tongue and nose. As in the receptors of other special senses, the transducing elements are appendages, cilia in this case, on the apical ends of the cells (Fig. 8.1). Olfactory cells are, however, unique in the mammalian organism in that even though their structure is that of epithelial cells and they are located in a layer of epithelial tissue, they have axons which conduct impulses. Such neuroepithelial cells are otherwise common only in the skin of certain simple animals, for example in coelenterates. Gustatory receptors are proper epithelial cells, and have no axon of their own but form synapses with the peripheral endings of taste nerve fibers.

Gases and vapors that stimulate the receptors of smell are carried into the nose with air currents. The substances acting on taste receptors are taken into the mouth with solids and liquids. In both cases, however, the stimulating compound must be in aqueous solution to interact with the receptor molecules in the cilia of the receptor cells. The olfactory cells are covered by a layer of mucus in which gases or vapors must dissolve before they can reach the receptive surface. The molecules that stimulate taste cells must similarly dissolve in saliva.

Excitation of olfactory and gustatory receptor cells occurs when stimulus molecules bind to receptor molecules in the sensory cilia. The bond is weak and rapidly reversible, so that decreasing concentration of the stimulus substance results in diminishing stimulation. The receptor cells respond to stimulation by depolarization—the receptor potential. The conductance change responsible for depolarization occurs across the part of the surface membrane that is surrounded by interstitial fluid and not exposed to the stimulus. Somehow the excitation of the cilia, which are at the apical end of the cell, must be transmitted to the

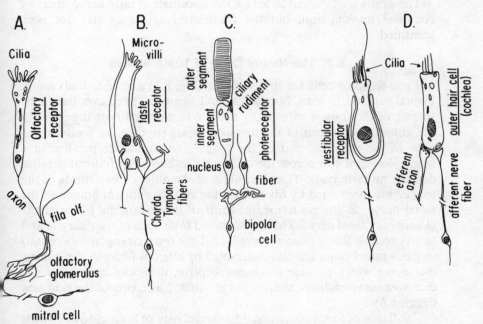

Figure 8.1.   Receptor cells of the special sense organs. *A*, olfactory neuroepithelial cell and its axon (see also Fig. 8.3). *B*, taste receptor cell (see also Fig. 8.2). *C*, photoreceptor cell of the vertebrate retina (see also Figs. 9.3, 9.4 and 9.8). *D*, the ciliated cells known as hair cells of the vestibular organ and of the cochlea (see also Figs. 11.3 and 11.8). (Reprinted with permission from G. Somjen: *Sensory Coding in the Mammalian Nervous System.* New York, Plenum Press, 1975.)

remainder of the cell membrane, and several theories have been proposed to explain this. One possibility is that an intracellular messenger substance carries the excitation from the ciliated end of the cell to the rest of the membrane. Another proposal postulates that molecules within the ciliary membrane change conformation and this change spreads over the surface, each molecule affecting its neighbor in turn. The conductance change responsible for depolarization could be directly related to this conformational change.

The receptor potential of olfactory cells directly triggers impulses in their axons. The olfactory nerve fibers are the thinnest, slowest conducting axons of mammals; their diameter is 0.2–0.3 μm. But the distance they cover is not very long and, besides, odor stimuli rarely demand a lightning-fast reaction.

Taste cells are believed to act on the terminals of taste nerve fibers by chemical transmission, but the transmitter substance has not been identified.

8.2. The Neural Code of Taste Stimuli

Taste receptor cells are in taste buds (Fig. 8.2) and taste buds are in lingual papillae. In man, fungiform papillae are scattered over the dorsal surface of the tongue with many being concentrated near the edges of the anterior two-thirds of the tongue. Foliate papillae are found at the edge of the posterior part of the tongue; circumvallate papillae in a single V-shaped row across the back near its base. The filiform papillae contain no taste buds. Taste receptors of the anterior two-thirds of the tongue are innervated by fibers from the chorda tympani branch of the facial nerve; in the posterior one-third of the tongue by fibers of the glossopharyngeal nerve. The few scattered taste buds of the pharynx and larynx receive fibers from the vagus. All the oropharyngeal (and nasal) mucous membranes are also innervated by afferent fibers of the trigeminal nerve which provide mechanoreceptive, thermoreceptive and nociceptive nerve endings, similar to the somatic afferents of the skin (see Chapter 6).

The flavor of foods is conveyed by the activity of both taste and smell receptors. After food has been taken into the mouth, its odor reaches the olfactory mucosa through the nasopharynx. The texture of food sensed by mechanoreceptors and the sometimes stinging quality sensed by mucosal nociceptors (see Section 6.7) also add to the appreciation of foods. Temperature also plays a part, as it may be noticed when a drink is chilled. Temperature may influence the response of taste receptor

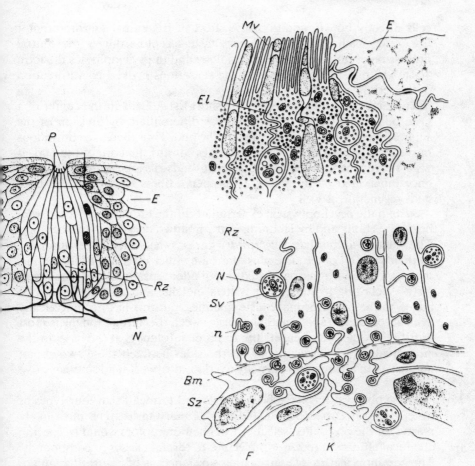

Figure 8.2. Taste receptor cells and their relationship to afferent nerve fibers. *Left,* a low-power view of a taste bud: *P,* taste pore; *E,* epithelium; *Rz,* receptor cell; *N,* nerve fiber. *Right,* details as revealed by electron microscopy: *top,* apical portion; *bottom,* basal portion of the taste bud; *Mv,* microvilli of taste receptor cells; *El,* terminal bars; *E,* detail of epithelial cell; *Rz,* receptor cell; *N,* large-caliber nerve fiber; *Sv,* synaptic vesicles (note that these vesicles are on the "wrong side" of the synapse and have unknown function); *n,* small nerve fiber; *Bm,* basal membrane; *Sz,* Schwann cell; *F,* fibroblast; *K,* collagen. (After A. J. DeLorenzo, in *Olfaction and Taste,* Oxford, Pergamon Press, 1963; modified by H. Hensel: *Allgemeine Sinnesphysiologie.* Berlin, Springer, 1966. Reprinted with permission.)

cells directly but, in addition, the effect of trigeminal thermoreceptor fibers may blend with signals from taste receptors during the central processing of information. In physiology and in psychophysics the term "taste" is, however, reserved for the sensations evoked by stimulation of the receptors in taste buds.

Taste receptor cells are relatively short-lived. Cells in the center of a taste bud die and are shed. New ones differentiate by division of the supporting cells that form the shell of the bud. Thus there is a continuous movement of cells from the outer zones toward the core of the bud. If taste nerve fibers degenerate, the taste buds disappear from the area once innervated by the fibers. If the nerve fibers regenerate, the taste buds regenerate as well.

Systematic psychophysical experiments of the human taste sense were begun by Hänig and by Henning in the first two decades of this century. They identified four basic or *primary tastes*: sweet, salty, bitter and sour. In their view all other taste sensations are either mixtures of these four, in various proportions, or admixtures of odor sensations that blend with taste. According to some later writers metallic and alkaline should be added to the list of primary taste qualities, but this has not universally been accepted. To substances that taste sweet, the human tongue is most sensitive on the sides near its tip; to bitter substances at the base, in the circumvallate papillae; to sour on the sides between these two zones; and to salt in an area that partially overlaps the sweet- and sour-sensitive areas.

These observations have been interpreted to mean that four types of taste receptors correspond to the four primary tastes. The most likely reason for the postulated selectivity of chemoreceptors would be specific chemical affinity of receptor molecules to certain classes of compounds. The common feature of sour-tasting substances is of course that all are acids, although not all acids taste equally sour. For example, at equal pH, dichloroacetic acid is more sour then acetic acid. All salts taste salty, but again some are saltier than others. Besides, KCl for example has a distinct taste quality (somewhat like licorice), quite different from NaCl. Such qualitative differences have been attributed to co-excitation of more than one of the primary taste receptors. The sensations of sweet and bitter are, of course, quite distinct and readily recognized, but each is evoked by a wide variety of substances. Certain requirements of molecular structure have been recognized that are typical of sweet, and others typical of bitter substances, but no unique characteristics identify compounds as such. Besides sugars, a series of sweet-tasting dipeptides and their derivatives have been studied, of which 1-aspartyl-1-phenyl-alanine methyl ester (aspartame) is the strongest tasting. Other classes of dipeptides taste bitter, yet others sour.

Substances have also been discovered that either enhance or suppress specific tastes. Their existence is also in agreement with the theory of specific taste receptors. For example, miraculine, a protein isolated from a Southwest African berry, enhances sweet taste; this effect is elicited at low pH only, and it can last for hours after eating the berry. On the other hand, gymnemic acid suppresses sweet taste.

It is possible to evoke sensations of taste by electrical stimulation of lingual papillae of human subjects. If the tip of the electrode is so fine and the intensity of the stimulus so near to threshold that just one papilla is stimulated, the sensation is similar to one of the four primary tastes. To be sure, these electrically evoked sensations were described as differing from any evoked by adequate, that is chemical, stimuli. The difference was explained by assuming that the electrically evoked sensation was the true primary taste because it excited one type of receptor exclusively, whereas chemical stimuli always caused some weak excitation of receptors of some of the other primary tastes as well. Stronger electric stimuli, or electrodes with a larger surface, evoke mixed or less well defined tastes. It has also been found possible to apply small drops of dilute solutions containing taste substances to just one papilla. To do so it was necessary to apply gentle suction to a taste papilla with a fine-tipped pipette until it stood erect. Individual buds again appeared to respond to just one taste, for example to solutions containing sweet-tasting substances. Furthermore it was difficult or impossible to evoke a sensation other than that to which the threshold was lowest, by applying any other solution, even if relatively concentrated, to that papilla.

All of these observations suggest that each taste receptor cell is sensitive to only one of the four primary taste stimuli and that all receptor cells in the taste buds of one papilla share specific sensitivity to the same primary taste stimulus. But electrophysiological experiments on taste buds of animals showed otherwise. Single taste cells were shown to produce receptor potentials when solutions of different taste substances were brought in contact with them. Moreover, receptor cells in the same taste bud showed different relative sensitivities to various substances. And no correlation has been detected among the sensitivities of taste buds located on the same papilla.

It could still be possible that there are four specific taste receptor molecules, one for each of the four primary tastes, but that the cilia of receptor cells contain several of these four basic receptor molecule types in varying proportions. It is however also possible that the number of receptor molecules is not four but greater, and that their affinities to various taste substances is graded according to rules not hitherto detected. From the available data it is not possible to distinguish between these two possibilities.

Each taste bud is innervated by several nerve fibers, and each fiber innervates several taste buds. To reconcile the contradictory observations just described, it could have been suggested that nerve fibers are connected to receptor cells in such a way that each fiber has its lowest threshold for one of the four primary taste stimuli, and high threshold to the other three. Experimental evidence again does not support this.

When a large number of taste fibers were tested for their responses to NaCl solutions of several concentrations, they did not fall into clear categories of high and low sensitivity. Instead, fibers could be ranked in a continuous series of subtly varying sensitivities. Each was also sensitive, to varying degrees, to other stimuli as well. The magnitudes of the responses of individual taste fibers to a series of different salts could not be predicted from the psychophysical ranking of the same taste stimuli by human observers. However, the statistically combined responses of many taste fibers to many stimuli matched rather well the judgment of human observers. For example, human tasters judge LiCl to be very similar to NaCl. The correlation of the response magnitudes of many fibers to NaCl and LiCl was high also.

From these electrophysiological observations a theory of neural processing emerged known as the *across-fiber pattern* coding of sensory quality. According to this theory there are neither "pure" primary taste stimuli, nor pure primary taste sensations. Instead, the quality of taste sensation is determined by the statistical distribution of excitation among the population of taste fibers, each of which has varying degrees of sensitivity to a wide range of taste stimuli.

At present, both the specificity theory and the across-fiber theory can explain certain of the experimental observations, and neither can explain them all. The solution to the riddle may be in the central processing of taste information, but investigation of the central nuclei to which taste signals are transmitted has so far yielded no clues. The target of taste fibers of both chorda tympani and glossopharyngeal nerves is the nucleus of the tractus solitarius. Cells in this nucleus respond when taste solutions are applied to the tongue much as the primary taste fibers do. Neurons that respond to taste stimuli have been found in the thalamus and also in the cerebral cortex, near the primary somatosensory receiving area of the tongue. Most of these higher level neurons respond not only to taste stimuli, but also to thermal and sometimes to mechanical stimulation of the tongue as well.

8.3. Olfaction

Odors are of paramount importance to many animals. Such *macrosmatic* species have more olfactory nerve fibers than they have of all other primary afferent fibers combined. People belong to the *microsmatic* species, but even so the accomplishments of a well-trained human nose can be impressive. Professionals evaluating wines or perfumes can recognize an amazing variety of scents, detecting many of them in very low concentrations indeed.

There have been several attempts to define primary odors, similar to the four primary tastes. Henning defined six: flowery, fruity, foul, spicy, burnt and resinous. Other investigators have come up with other lists, some containing as many as 30 separate primary odors. Several investigators believe, however, that primary odors do not exist at all. They do not think that the many different scents are composites of a small number of simple primaries. The very fact that there are such differences of opinion suggests that this may indeed be so. The controversy surrounding the problems of taste is different. There is disagreement whether primary tastes exist or not, but there is no argument about which ones they might be, if they do exist.

One method by which the nervous system could sort olfactory information would be if receptors of varying chemical affinities would be grouped over the surface of the olfactory mucosa in some orderly fashion. According to this *spatial theory* of olfactory coding, each odoriferous substance would activate a different spatial pattern so that different scents would be represented by different mosaics of excited receptor cells. Such zones of excitation of the olfactory mucosa would then be mapped first on the olfactory bulb and then in the central olfactory receiving nuclei. The quality of odors would thus be encoded in a manner similar to the topographic representation of touch and of the other somatic sensory modalities.

It has also been suggested that specific odoriferous molecules excite some receptors and not others because of their steric configuration. Certain shapes of odor molecules would fit the geometry of certain receptor molecules. The fit would not need to be exact, but the better the match the stronger the excitation. This hypothesis could account for the selectivity of excitation, and also for the fact that this selectivity is graded and not absolute.

Axons of the olfactory receptor cells are collected in bundles, the fila olfactoria (Fig. 8.1), which enter the skull through the holes in the cribriform plate. It then is but a short distance to the olfactory bulb which lies above this plate. In the olfactory bulb the olfactory nerve terminals enter synaptic glomeruli, where they come in synaptic contact with the dendrites of mitral cells. Mitral cells are the main projection neurons of the olfactory bulb, and they send their axons into the olfactory tract (Fig. 8.3). In all species that have been investigated, olfactory fibers greatly outnumber mitral cells.

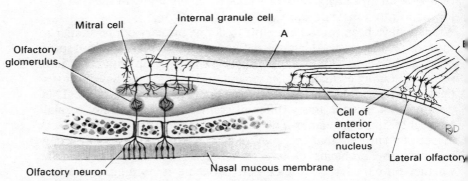

Figure 8.3. Main cell types of the olfactory bulb and their connections. The fiber labeled *A* is the axon of a cell in the contralateral anterior olfactory nucleus, arriving by way of the anterior commissure. The fibers labeled *B* are centrally projecting (third-order afferent) fibers of cells in the anterior olfactory nucleus. (Reprinted with permission from M. B. Carpenter: *Core Text of Neuroanatomy*, ed. 2. Baltimore, Williams & Wilkins, 1978.)

The olfactory bulbs are laminated structures, containing short-axon (intrinsic) interneurons besides projection cells. Each bulb is connected to its twin of the other side. Each bulb also receives efferent fibers from the brain, from olfactory nuclei of both ipsilateral and contralateral hemispheres. The axons of mitral cells give off recurrent collaterals before leaving the bulb, and these collaterals form synapses with some of the short-axon interneurons. The olfactory tract also contains the axons of tufted cells, which some consider to be miniature versions of the mitral cells.

The olfactory bulbs generate prominent rhythmic electric potential waves. These occur in bursts of 40–80 cps and are strongly modulated by respiration, being maximal while air currents blow over the olfactory mucosa. They are also influenced by the level of alertness of the animal, and they change both frequency and amplitude when an arousing scent reaches the mucosa. Models have been proposed to explain the generation of this wave activity by synaptic interaction between mitral cell collaterals and granule cells. Granule cells are interneurons that have no true axon; all their processes have the structure of dendrites, and they generate no impulses, only synaptic potentials (see Section 4.6). The proposed oscillatory mechanism is similar to but not identical with that of the burst generator of the thalamus believed to be responsible for sleep spindles and the alpha rhythm (Section 4.8)

It has also been suggested that the rhythm of the olfactory potential waves represents the coding of the quality of olfactory stimuli. There is however no simple relationship between the pattern of these waves and the nature of the olfactory stimulus. The theories relating some derivative property of the wave pattern to some aspect of the odor stimuli are complicated and, at present, controversial. Wave activity similar to and correlated with that of the olfactory bulb can also be recorded from piriform cortex and parts of the amygdala. This lends some credence to the idea that the wave pattern is in some way related to the processing of olfactory information.

The olfactory tubercle, the anterior olfactory nucleus, the prepyriform cortex (paleocortex) and the medial and cortical nuclei of the amygdala are the main targets of the output of the olfactory bulb. These structures have intimate connections with the so-called limbic system (see Chapter 21; Fig. 21.2) that have been invoked to explain the role of scents in instinctive behaviors. There are also connections to the dorsomedial nucleus of the thalamus and, indirectly, to the neocortex as well.

Loss of olfactory function (*anosmia*) may be the result of such trivial conditions as a common cold, but after trauma to the skull such a deficit may indicate fracture of the cribriform plate. Tumors affecting the olfactory pathways can also cause loss of the sense of smell, sometimes unilaterally.

So-called uncinate fits consist of seizures preceded by an olfactory aura. They suggest an epileptogenic trigger focus in the temporal lobe, near the olfactory structures.

8.4. Chapter Summary

1. Olfactory receptors are neuroepithelial cells with ultrafine axons and with cilia for transducing elements.
2. Taste receptors are epithelial cells that form synapses with the terminals of the gustatory fibers of the chorda tympani or of the glossopharyngeal nerve.
3. Molecules need to be dissolved in nasal mucus to stimulate olfactory receptors and in saliva to stimulate taste receptors.
4. By psychophysical experiments four primary tastes have been defined: sweet, salty, bitter and sour. There are several classes of compounds capable of eliciting each of these primary sensations.
5. There is no unanimity concerning either the identity or even the existence of primary odors. The simplest system names six: flowery, fruity, foul, spicy, burnt and resinous.
6. Individual taste receptor cells and individual gustatory nerve fibers almost always can be excited by more than one "primary" taste stimulus. The responsiveness of receptors does not conform to the four primary modalities.
7. Olfactory bulbs and olfactory receiving nuclei generate voltage oscillations of 40–80 cps.
8. A spatial theory of odor representation in the central nervous system has been proposed.

Further Reading

Books and Reviews

Paffmann C, Frank M, Norgren R: Neural mechanisms and behavioral aspects of taste. *Annu Rev Psychol* 30:283–325, 1979.

Sato T: Recent advances in the physiology of taste cells. *Prog Neurobiol* 14:25–67, 1980.

Wolstenholme GEW, Knight J (eds): *Taste and Smell in Vertebrates*: CIBA Foundation Symposium. London J & A Churchill, 1970.

chapter 9

The Eye

The optical equipment of the eye and the neural processes of the retina.

9.1. Image Formation

This chapter must begin with a brief summary of optics as applied to the eye. If any of the points raised is unclear, an introductory textbook on physics should be consulted.

Convex lenses with spherical surfaces collect incident light arriving in parallel rays in a point known as the *principal focus*. Its distance from the optical center of the lens is the principal focal distance. As a kind of shorthand, most authors write just *focal distance* or focal length. The shorter the radius of curvature of the lens, the shorter the focal distance. The other factor determining focal distance is the ratio of the refractive indices of lens and surrounding medium; a glass lens submerged in water has a longer focal distance than the same lens in air. Two convex lenses placed one behind the other have a combined focal distance shorter than either of them has alone.

If we take a box, place a convex lens in one of its walls, and replace the wall opposite the lens with light-sensitive film, we have a rudimentary camera. A small object, for instance the head of a pin, placed in front of the lens will cast its image on a small spot on the film, provided that it is "in focus." The closer the target is to the lens, the farther the film must be from the lens in order to form a focused image. To form sharp images of objects that are so far from the lens that light from them arrives in nearly parallel rays, the distance of the lens from the film must equal the principal focal distance. In the jargon of photography this is called "focusing at infinite distance." In photography, infinity is not very far away.

The image formed inside a camera is attenuated in size, inverted and real. Note that "real" in optics means the opposite of "virtual." A real image is formed on an opaque screen or on a photographic plate. A virtual image is seen by the human eye, but it cannot be focused on a screen or a film. When a convex lens is used as a magnifying glass the object to be viewed must be closer to the lens than the principal focal distance. The virtual image so formed is not inverted.

Concave lenses cause light rays to diverge (as opposed to convex lenses, which cause them to converge). A concave lens forms virtual images only, and has only a virtual focus (i.e. a point from which divergent rays seem to emanate but do not actually do so).

If a convex lens is used to cast an image on a flat surface (as it usually is in a camera), the entire surface of the film is not at equal distances from the optical center point of the lens. Consequently, with a simple spherical lens the peripheral portions of the image become progressively more blurred. This imperfection is called *spherical aberration*. To compensate for it, photographic lenses are not ground to spherical surfaces, but have continuously varying radii of curvature. In the eye, the problem is solved in a different manner: the retina is curved in such a way that all but the most peripheral points are optically equidistant from the lens system.

Light of different wavelengths (different spectral colors) is refracted to different degrees as it passes through the interface of optic media of different reflective indices. White light is a mixture of different spectral colors; consequently, images of white and grays cannot be focused precisely in a single plane. This is called *chromatic aberration* and is maximal around the edges of a lens and minimal near its center. Cameras and eyes are equipped with an iris diaphragm—an opaque disc with a central aperture of variable diameter. The smaller the aperture, the less chromatic aberration. Furthermore, the depth of focus or field (the range of distances within which objects form sharp images) also increases as the iris aperture decreases. Thus, the image sharpens as the aperture of the iris diaphragm is reduced for three reasons: (1) reduced spherical aberration; (2) reduced chromatic aberration; (3) increased depth of focus. However, by limiting the aperture, the total amount of light also diminishes. The best compromise is struck by choosing the smallest aperture compatible with external illumination. Another limitation is that with very small (pinhole) openings, diffraction degrades the sharpness of the image. Constriction of the pupil of the eye is limited, so that diffraction does not become a problem.

The refractive power of a lens is expressed in *diopters*, defined as the *inverse of the principal focal distance* measured in *meters*. Thus, a lens with focal distance of 10 cm is said to have a refractive power of 10 diopters; one with focal distance of 5 cm, of 20 diopters. The refraction of convex lenses has been defined as *positive*, that of concave lenses *negative*. If two lenses are placed in front of the other, their combined refractive power is calculated by adding or subtracting diopters.

9.1a. IMAGE FORMATION IN THE EYE

The eye contains several curved surfaces of different optical densities, and their refractive powers are summed. A special feature not usually found in man-made lens systems is that the medium in front of the eye is air, whereas inside it is filled with fluid. Consequently the anterior (external) focal distance of the eye's lens system is very different from the posterior (internal) focal distance. The highest refractive power is found where the curved surface of the cornea meets air. Relative to air, its refractive index is 1.37. For both aqueous and vitreous substance this figure is 1.33. The refractive index of the lens, 1.41, is the highest of all the optic media of the eye.

The unique feature of the crystalline lens, not yet duplicated by any man-made optical device, is its ability to change curvature and with it the refractive power. Focusing in cameras, projectors, telescopes and the like is achieved by moving the lens forward or backward. Such displacement is not necessary in mammalian eyes. With the crystalline lens at its flattest the eye is focused at "infinity," and the total refractive power of the eye's lens system is about 66.6 diopters (anterior focal distance of 1.5 cm). When the lens is maximally curved, it adds another 10 diopters to this total.

In the living eye, the shape of the lens is determined by the balance of three forces, two of them constant, the third adjustable. Removed from the eye and left to itself, the lens by its inherent elasticity assumes the maximally refractive shape. Pitted against this tendency is the elastic force of the radially arranged fibers of the suspensory ligament that holds the lens in place. The elastic force of the suspensory ligament is stronger than that of the lens, and if only these two forces are in action, the ligament keeps the lens maximally flattened. This, then, is the condition of the eye at rest. In this state, the eye is focused on objects at "infinite" distance, meaning objects at about 6 m and farther. In order to clearly see close objects, the circular fibers of the ciliary muscle must come into action (Fig. 9.1).

The increase of the refractive power of the lens achieved with the aid of the ciliary muscle is termed *accommodation* to near vision. The *near point* of clear vision during maximal accommodation in a healthy young individual is about 10 cm from the anterior surface of the cornea. Note that the near point of vision is *not* the principal anterior focal distance of the fully accommodated eye. The latter is about 1.3 cm.

It is important to realize that the ciliary muscle cannot actually squeeze the lens into the shape of a ball. All it can do is to counteract

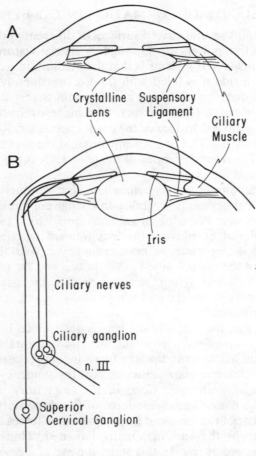

Figure 9.1. Accommodation of the crystalline lens. *A,* with the ciliary muscle relaxed, the suspensory ligament stretches the lens and vision is accommodated to distant objects. *B,* contraction of the ciliary muscle moves the anchorage of the suspensory ligament closer to the center, thereby diminishing the ligament's tension, and allowing the lens to assume a more curved shape. Parasympathetic fibers which originate in the ciliary ganglion innervate the ciliary muscle and also the constrictor muscle of the pupil. Sympathetic fibers originating in the superior cervical ganglion innervate the dilator muscle of the pupil.

the stretch exerted by the suspensory ligament, leaving the lens to assume its inherently curved shape. If the lens loses elasticity, focusing at near objects becomes increasingly difficult. This happens to all of us during the middle years of life, more rapidly to some than to others. Eventually, reading glasses become a necessity. The receding of the near point of clear vision with age is known as *presbyopia*. It is corrected by the wearing of convex eyeglasses. Convex lenses add diopters and so supplement the diminished power of accommodation (Fig. 9.2).

The ciliary muscle is composed of smooth muscle fibers. It is controlled by (parasympathetic) autonomic cholinergic nerve fibers. The preganglionic axons are contained in the IIIrd (oculomotor) cranial nerve, the postganglionic neurons are located in the ciliary ganglion, and their axons in the ciliary nerves. The reflex circuit adjusting the contraction of the ciliary muscle is controlled by input from the retina.

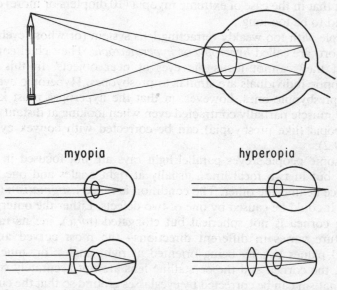

Figure 9.2. Image formation in the eye and the correction of anomalies of refraction. *Top,* when the eye is focused at an object, any point on that object casts the image of a point on the retina. (Note that the near point of vision is the limit of proper focusing: an object placed closer to the eye than the near point will cast a blurred image on the retina. By contrast, the principal anterior focus is a point, light rays emanating from which become parallel after having passed through the refracting media.) *Bottom,* in a myopic eye, focused at long distance, the principal posterior focal distance is shorter than the optic axis of the eye; consequently, distant objects cast blurred images on the retina. In a hyperopic eye the posterior focal distance is longer than the optic axis.

If the retinal image becomes blurred as one looks at objects at different distances, a correction signal is generated and the firing of the parasympathetic fibers innervating the ciliary muscle is adjusted.

People who cannot bring distant objects into clear focus are called nearsighted or *myopic*. Myopia can, in principle, be the consequence of either the front of the cornea being too curved, or of the eyeball being too long. In either case the result is that with the crystalline lens as flat as it can be (i.e. accommodated to distant vision), parallel rays are focused in front of the retina, not on it (Fig. 9.2). Since the error consists of too high a refractive power of the lens system, it can be corrected by wearing concave eyeglasses (recall that negative diopters subtract from refractive power). Measurements show that there is no consistent correlation between refraction errors and overall length of the eyeball, except that in the case of extreme myopia (10 diopters or more) eyeballs do tend to be too long.

People with too weakly refracting lens system (or whose eyeballs are too short) are called *hyperopic* or *hypermetropic*. Their chief complaint is that they cannot focus the eyes at near objects. In this respect hyperoptic individuals are similar to presbyopes. Hyperopic eyes differ from presbyopic ones, however, in that the hyperopes must keep the ciliary muscle partially contracted even when looking at distant objects. Hyperopia (like presbyopia) can be corrected with convex eyeglasses (Fig. 9.2).

In some people's eyes parallel light rays are not focused in a focal point, but in two focal lines, usually at right angles and one a slight distance behind the other. The condition is called *astigmatism* (*stigma*, spot). It could be caused by one of two defects. Either the outer surface of the cornea is not spherical but elongated (*toric*), i.e. its radius of curvature varies in different directions—the most curved and least curved planes usually being oriented at right angles; or, much more rarely, the cornea and the crystalline lens are not accurately centered. Astigmatism can be corrected by eyeglasses ground so that the curvature incorporates a toric or *cylindrical* component. In other words, the eyeglasses, too, must have an axis of maximal and another of minimal curvature. The glass must then be fixed in its frame so that its maximal curvature should coincide with the eye's minimal curvature and *vice versa*.

Infants are normally born hypermetropic. With age, emmetropization sets in (*emmetrope*, normal refraction), except in the cases where the process over- or undershoots the mark, and refraction anomaly develops.

Refraction anamolies are usually noticed around the age of 5 or 6, and they tend to get worse during the years of rapid growth. They then remain stationary during most of adult life. Many myopic elderly people believe their vision has improved. In fact this usually means that while their originally emmetropic contemporaries must put on reading glasses, elderly myopics can remove their everyday glasses when they want to read.

Astigmatism is more often than not associated with myopia. Not all myopic individuals are, however, astigmatic. Hypermetropia is much less common than myopia. The cause of these refraction anomalies is not known, but clearly heredity has much to do with it. Many lay people and a few ophthalmologists are convinced that children can "ruin their eyes" by reading, or by otherwise looking too close for long periods of time. The truth is that we do not know how the growth process of the eyes is regulated. In order to achieve the exact matching of the length of the eyeball and of the principal posterior focal distance (normally 2.2 cm for both) some form of feedback must be involved in the guiding of growth. Until we know more, we cannot absolutely deny the possibility that persistent close focusing might influence the manner in which growth sculpts the cornea and the eyeball.

9.1b. REFLEXES OF THE PUPILS

Looking near activates not only the reflex controlling the ciliary muscle, but two others. For one, the two eyeballs must turn inward (*converge*) in order to keep a near target in the line of straight vision of both eyes. In addition, the pupils constrict during accommodation for near vision. This reflex is also controlled by parasympathetic nerve fibers and is achieved by contraction of the circular (constrictor) fibers in the iris.

The pupils constrict, of course, whenever light falls into the eye. If light shines in one eye only, its pupil constricts (*direct light reflex*) as well as the unilluminated one (*consensual reflex*). Although activated by input from the retina and executed by parasympathetic efferents, nevertheless the light reflexes of the pupils are controlled by a different central circuit from the one coordinated with accommodation. A sign of tertiary syphilis of the central nervous system (CNS) is the so-called Argyll Robertson pupil, in which the pupils do constrict during near vision but not in response to light.

Constriction of the pupil improves the optic quality of the retinal image, as we have already seen. It has, however, another important function. Most school children play at one time or another with magnifying glasses and discover that they can burn holes in paper by focusing sunlight with such a glass. The retina would similarly be damaged if the pupil remained wide open in bright light. A few cases of retinal burn damage are usually seen after each total solar eclipse. During an eclipse the light of the sun is obscured, but the long-wavelength thermal infrared radiation is not screened. People looking directly at the darkening solar disk then run the risk of burn damage of the retina, for in the absence of a visible light stimulus the pupils widen and offer no protection against the invisible infrared waves.

At its smallest the diameter of the pupil is about 2 mm, at its largest 8 mm. The 4-fold change in diameter equals a 16-fold change in area, and therefore in radiant energy.

The iris also contains muscle fibers that widen the aperture of the pupil. The *dilator muscle* is innervated by noradrenergic sympathetic fibers, branches from the cervical sympathetic chain. In the steady state, both constrictor and dilator muscle are contracted and keep a balance. The adjustments related to near and far vision and to light intensity are made by variations in the discharge rate of the parasympathetic nerve fibers only. This varies the contraction of the constrictor muscle acting against the constant pull of the dilator muscle fibers. Active contraction of the dilator muscle occurs only under the influence of heightened emotion. This sympathetic effect is not specific for one affect: fright, anger and pleasure all seem to trigger widening of the pupil.

9.2. Photoreceptors

Photoreceptor cells are modified ependymal cells. This explains their peculiar orientation away from the light, with backs turned toward the source of stimulation. The business end of the photoreceptor is its outer segment, which is a single, greatly modified cilium. In early embryonic life the primitive retina is a vesicle, the cavity of which is connected by a hollow stalk with the cerebral ventricle. The vesicle is lined with ciliated ependymal cells. The vesicle then becomes flattened into a cup consisting of two layers of ciliated cells, with facing ciliated surfaces, and the cavity between them becomes obliterated. Ependymal cells in the layer that is farther from the brain divide and their offspring become the neurons and glial cells that populate the adult retina. The ependymal cells of this layer that remain in their place shed all but one cilium that grows enormously and acquires the photosensitive apparatus as it becomes the outer segment. In the process they become transformed into photoreceptor cells. The other original ependymal layer develops into the pigment epithelium. The hollow stalk that used to connect the optic vesicle with the brain becomes the optic nerve.

Notice that when talking about the eye, "in" and "inner" signify toward the center of the eyeball, not the center of the skull or of the brain. Thus at the back of the eye, moving "out" of the eye means moving toward the center of the skull and brain.

Light, then, must filter among blood vessels and through the inner layers of the retina before it reaches the outer segment of the photoreceptor cells (see Fig. 9.8C). The *fovea centralis* is a central depression in line with the visual axis of the eye, in the middle of the *macula lutea* (yellow spot) of the retina. The small depression is formed as cell layers and nerve fibers radiate away from this central spot. Light strikes the photoreceptors here the most directly. It is no coincidence that this is the site of the sharpest vision.

There are two types of photoreceptors: rods and cones. The names suggest that the former are long and slender, the latter short, stout at the base and pointed. Both types vary, however, in shape in different retinal regions and do not always conform very well to this description. There are morphological subclasses in each category. In their biochemistry and physiology rods and cones are, however, different enough to mandate distinct names. The outer segments of the photoreceptors contain pigments that absorb light and then undergo a series of photochemical transformations. Excitation of photoreceptors depends on these transformations.

The pigment epithelial cells that lie adjacent to the outer segments contain some of the common pigment melanin, but mainly the same photosensitive pigments as the photoreceptors. This dark layer of cells just beyond the photoreceptors minimizes the reflection and the scattering of light and therefore improves the sharpness of the retinal image. Carnivores have a reflecting layer, the tapetum, instead of the pigmented layer; they sacrifice some visual acuity in favor of improved night vision. Our pigment epithelium fulfills other important functions. From time to time the pigment cells "bite off" (by phagocytosis) the tip of the neighboring photoreceptor. The lost piece is replaced from below. In fact there is a continuous renewal of material, each protein molecule entering the base of the outer segment being shed at the tip in an average of 9 days. Servicing of photoreceptors by the pigment epithelium seems essential for the vitality of the outer segment. The underlying defect of *retinitis pigmentosa* is believed to be imperfect phagocytosis by the pigment cells, allowing the accumulation of spent photopigment at the tips of the photoreceptors, leading to their degeneration. Retinae sometimes become accidentally detached from the pigment layer. If they are re-attached in time, but not otherwise, they can regain function. Pigment epithelial cells are also believed to be a reservoir of pigment and of vitamin A for the use of photoreceptors.

9.2a. THE EXCITATION OF PHOTORECEPTORS

The photopigment of rods is *rhodopsin*. It was extracted from retinas of frogs shortly after the turn of this century and has been studied intensely ever since. It consists of a protein, called *opsin*, and a prosthetic group, a derivative of vitamin A, called *retinal*. Retinal is an aldehyde formed from vitamin A, which is the corresponding alcohol.

Cones contain three different photoreactive pigments. Their retinal is similar to that of rhodopsin, but the opsins are different, and each has a distinct absorption spectrum (see Fig. 9.7*A*). As a rule any one cone contains only one of these three pigments. This provides the basis for color vision, as we shall soon see.

A solution of rhodopsin absorbs light maximally at the 490-nm waveband, corresponding to the spectral band of green. Rhodopsin is also called visual purple because it reflects light of the two outer ends of the spectrum, red and blue, which when mixed appear purple. When exposed to light, the color of rhodopsin fades to pale yellow. This process is called *bleaching*.

In bleaching, retinal is cleaved from opsin by hydrolysis. The prelude to hydrolysis is an isomeric conversion of the retinal molecule from the bent (11-*cis*) to the straight (all-*trans*) configuration. It is believed that the 11-*cis* form fits snugly into a binding site on the opsin molecule, whereas the all-*trans* form does not. When retinal is straightened, but is still held fast to opsin at one end, the compound is called pre-lumirhodopsin. The reaction can literally be frozen in this stage at very low temperatures. At normal temperature, however, it proceeds rapidly through at least three more intermediate stages (lumirhodopsin and metarhodopsin I and II) to the final hydrolysis.

The very first step of the bleaching process, the unlocking of one end of retinal from its binding site, requires energy, and this energy is supplied by absorbed light. Once started, the reaction chain runs downhill, that is, without further addition of energy. In fact, the light energy required to trigger the reaction is less than the sum total of the energy liberated in the subsequent steps of the reaction chain. This is an example of chemical amplification.

If, after a period in darkness, a rod cell is exposed to a brief flash of light, then some of its rhodopsin is bleached and then it is re-formed from opsin and the liberated retinal. For these two components to be reunited, all-*trans*-retinal must first be bent into its 11-*cis* format. This requires an enzyme (retinal isomerase), metabolic energy, and a little time. The energy invested in reconstituting rhodopsin is then available for later release when light triggers the next bleaching reaction.

If illumination continues after bleaching, then retinal is reduced to vitamin A. Re-oxidation of the alcohol, vitamin A, to the aldehyde, retinal, demands more oxidative energy, and also more time, than does simple re-isomerization of retinal from all-*trans* to 11-*cis*. This fact should be remembered when we come to the discussion of adaptation to darkness and light (see Section 9.2c). The conversion of vitamin A to retinal can probably occur not only in the retina, but also in the pigment epithelium and in the liver.

We know more about rhodopsin than about the cone pigments. There is, however, good reason to believe that the bleaching process of the cone pigments is very similar to that of rhodopsin, except that in cones it requires more light energy.

The photochemical reaction initiates the excitation of photoreceptor cells. The exciting event probably comes early in the bleaching process: either the conversion to pre-lumirhodopsin or to lumirhodopsin. Pigment molecules form a mosaic on the disks that fill the photoreceptor outer segments. These disks begin as invaginations of the surface membrane of the outer segment near its base. As they form, the invaginated layers are flattened into disks, and as the tips of the photoreceptor are phagocytosed by the pigment epithelium (see above), the disks move upward. In rods but not in cones they lose continuity with the surface membrane and become flattened saccules, entirely contained within the interior of the cell.

A photon that entered the outer segment has a high probability of being captured by one of the pigment molecules that are tightly packed in many stacked disks. One captured quantum of light suffices to bleach the absorbing molecule. This initiates a cascading enzyme reaction chain, the analysis of which has only just begun. To excite the cell, the effect of the chemical reaction must be transmitted to the cell membrane. An internal messenger substance is believed to be responsible for this transmission. Cyclic guanosine monophosphate (GMP) and calcium ions, or a combination of the two, are the currently leading candidates for this role.

9.2b. ELECTROPHYSIOLOGY OF PHOTORECEPTORS

With care the retina can be removed from a vertebrate eye and kept alive *in vitro* in an oxygenated nutrient medium. A microelectrode can then be inserted into a single photoreceptor. If the photoreceptor is suddenly illuminated, a two-step electric change is detected. These two responses have been christened the *early receptor potential* and the *late receptor potential* (see Fig. 9.4A). When recorded by an intracellular electrode both steps are negative deflections, signaling an increased potential difference between inside and outside—a hyperpolarization of the membrane.

By cooling the isolated retina, or by depriving it of oxygen, or by changing the ionic composition of the bathing medium, it is possible to suppress the late receptor potential while the early potential remains preserved. The early receptor potential is then itself resolved to two phases, a negative followed by a positive deflection. Ordinarily the positive phase is obscured by the larger, late receptor potential. The negative phase of the early potential starts at the onset of a light flash without a measurable delay. The early receptor potential is thus resistant to a variety of manipulations which abolish the late potential, but the early potential is changed by anything that disrupts the ordering of the rhodopsin molecules within the layered membranes of the outer segment. From these and other observations it has been concluded that the early receptor potential is a photochemical electric event generated by conformational change of electrically charged components of the rhodopsin molecule.

The late receptor potential is, however, a true membrane potential change. It is exceptional among excitatory signals, because it is in the hyperpolarizing instead of the depolarizing direction. Associated with it is a decrease of the conductance (increased resistance) of the membrane of the outer segment.

In the tissue of the retina a continuous electric current flows between outer plexiform layer and the layer of the outer segments. Since this current is maximal when the retina is not illuminated, it was given the picturesque name *dark current* (Fig. 9.3*A*). Associated with the dark current is a standing gradient of extracellular potential, the layer of rods and cones being negative relative to the outer plexiform layer. Consequently the back of the eye is electronegative relative to the front (see Fig. 9.10*B*).

From these observations emerges the following picture: the membrane potential of photoreceptors is generated by a mechanism basically similar to that of other excitable cells. The membrane of the outer segment is, however, more permeable to sodium than that of the remainder of the cell. For this reason the membrane potential is lower at the outer segment than at the inner parts of the photoreceptor. The resulting gradient of potential between inner and outer segments drives a current, which returns through the interstitial space, and is detected there as the dark current (Fig. 9.3). As long as the retina lives, this current never ceases, but it does diminish when and where the retina is illuminated.

To summarize: Illumination of the outer segment triggers the photochemical reaction; then an internal messenger substance is released; the

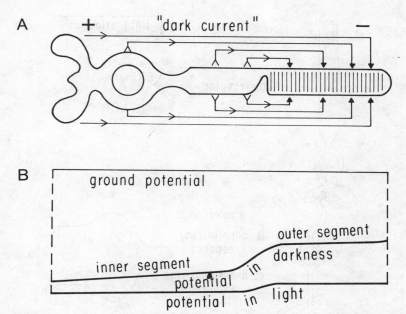

Figure 9.3. The dark current of the retina. *A*, current flow in the vicinity of a vertebrate photoreceptor kept in darkness; *B*, distribution of internal potential relative to ground potential at various points inside a photoreceptor, in darkness and during illumination of the retina. Note increased internal negativity (hyperpolarization) and decreased potential gradient during illumination.

messenger substance acts on the membrane to decrease sodium permeability; consequently the outer segment becomes more polarized (more internally negative); therefore the potential gradient and hence the dark current diminish (Figs. 9.3 and 9.4a).

Photoreceptors form synapses with dendrites of bipolar cells which, on electron microscopic examination, seem similar to other synapses between neurons. Since the interior of the photoreceptor cell is a continuous electric conductor of low resistance, the hyperpolarization of the outer segment spreads by electrotonus into the synaptic process of the cell (Fig. 9.3). At other synapses, depolarization of the presynaptic terminal by the presynaptic nerve impulse is the signal for the release of transmitter (see Section 3.2). Since the photoreceptor is relatively depolarized when it is in darkness and hyperpolarized when it is illuminated, it could be that in darkness the synaptic terminal releases the constant stream of transmitter and this output diminishes during illumination. This supposition is supported by the observation that adding an excess of Mg^{2+} to the solution bathing an isolated retina imitates the effect of illumination on

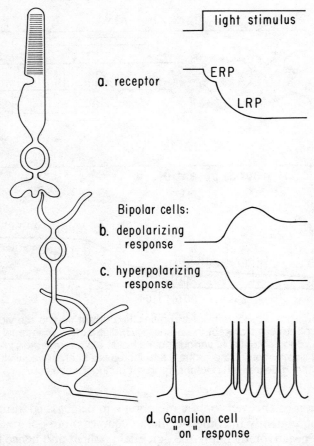

Figure 9.4. Potential responses of various cell types of the retina during illumination. *ERP,* early receptor potential; *LRP,* late receptor potential.

the second-order neurons (horizontal and bipolar cells). High $[Mg^{2+}]_o$ blocks the release of transmitter at other chemically operating synapses (see Section 3.2). Since Mg^{2+} and light have similar effects, it is likely that a light stimulus diminishes the output of transmitter from the synaptic terminals. An alternative but less likely hypothesis would be that at these terminals, unlike all others, hyperpolarization is the signal for transmitter release.

Before concluding that photoreceptors operate backwards by responding to stimulation with hyperpolarization, we should ask what a "stimulus" is in the visual world. A dark object on a bright background can be as interesting as a white outline against a dark field. Psychologically as well as physiologically, the darkening of the receptive field of a photoreceptor is just as much a stimulus as is its illumination. And, as we shall see shortly, it is *contrast* rather than total luminous flux *per se* that determines the response of most cells in most parts of the visual system.

9.2c. DARK ADAPTATION AND THE DIFFERENT FUNCTIONS OF RODS AND CONES

We all know that when we leave the sunshine to enter a dimly lit room it takes a while before we see anything. We say that we have to "get used to" the darkness. In visual physiology the process is called *dark adaptation.* Emerging from darkness into bright light, we are momentarily dazzled. Once more, it takes time for normal vision to be restored. *Light adaptation* is, however, faster than dark adaptation. Adjustments of the size of the pupils account for a small part of the adaptation process (see Section 9.1b); the retina is responsible for the rest.

Textbooks usually make the point that the eye is functional over an astonishing range of stimulus intensities. From a light intensity that is just perceptible in the fully dark-adapted state, to one that is the maximum tolerable when light-adapted, the energy flux reaching the retina varies over a 10^9-fold range. This is possible partly because the retina is not a single instrument, but consists of two distinct sets of sensors with different operating ranges.

What used to be called the *duplex* (sometimes ambiguously written as duplicity) *theory* of vision has now become a fully documented, accepted fact. In a dim environment most mammals, including man, use their rods (*scotopic vision*); in well-lit surroundings, the cones (*photopic vision*). Only the cones distinguish colors, and after dusk we all are color-blind.

The *threshold intensity* of a visual stimulus is the light energy that is just sufficient to be noticed. It is measured with some device that produces light flashes of graded intensities and, preferably, of variable durations and colors. To determine the time course of dark adaptation, visual threshold is determined first in a normally lighted room, and then the room is darkened. The threshold is again determined at set intervals and the results are plotted on a log scale as a function of time (Fig. 9.5). Such a plot reveals that threshold decreases during dark adaptation in two stages. The first, rapid phase represents dark adaptation of the cones and accounts for a gain in sensitivity (decrease of threshold) by a factor less than 100. The later phase of adaptation boosts

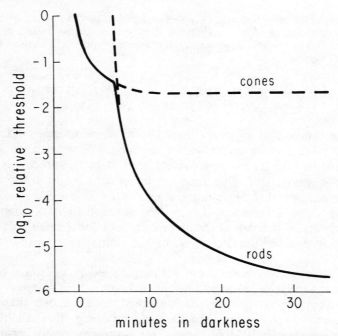

Figure 9.5. Dark adaptation of a human subject. *Abscissa,* time spent in darkness; *ordinate,* relative light intensity of minimal stimulus that is just perceived by subject.

sensitivity a lot more but takes more than half an hour to complete. In this phase the rods take over visual function.

If threshold is measured using red light instead of white, then only the early phase of dark adaptation is achieved (Fig. 9.5, curve marked *cones*). This is because rhodopsin, the pigment of the rods, does not absorb the longer wavelengths which we perceive as red so that rods are not stimulated by red light.

Figure 9.6 shows the so-called photopic and scotopic sensitivity curves, showing the relative sensitivity of the human eye to various bands of the visible spectrum. The scotopic (dark-adapted) curve is shifted toward the shorter wavelengths compared to the photopic curve; this is known as the Purkinje shift.

Purkinje (correctly spelled Purkyne and pronounced poorkinyah) was a Czech physiologist (also an anatomist, pharmacologist, patriot and poet) who became intrigued with color perception when one night in a hurry he pulled the wrong

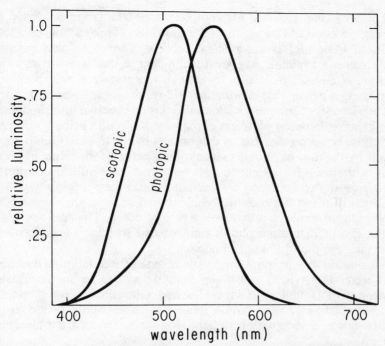

Figure 9.6. The relative sensitivities of a human eye in the dark-adapted (scotopic) and light-adapted (photopic) condition. *Abscissa,* wavelength of the light stimulus; *ordinate,* relative brightness of the stimulus as it appears to the observer, 1.0 being the maximum within each condition (scotopic and photopic).

coat out of a dark wardrobe. He wanted a red cloak, but when he arrived at the entrance hall of the theater, he noticed that what he took to be his red coat was actually black and quite unsuitable for the occasion. This experience was followed by deliberately planned observations in which he noted the gradual change of the apparent hue of flowers when the sun sets, as well as the loss of sensitivity to red, which in the dark-adapted state makes red objects indistinguishable from black.

The insensitivity of rod cells to light of long wavelength can be put to practical use in occupations such as darkroom work, or night piloting of aircraft, where dark adaptation is important yet personnel may temporarily be exposed to bright light. If, during periods of strong illumination red goggles are worn, the dark adaptation of the rods is preserved, because rhodopsin does not absorb light of long wavelength, and so to rods red illumination is as though there were no light present. Yet the subject can see, because the cones are excited by red light. Upon re-entering a dimly lit environment, the red goggles are removed, and the still dark-adapted rods can once more assume their function.

The long time required for complete dark adaptation is needed for the regeneration of rhodopsin in the rod cells. The bleaching of photo-pigment molecules is a statistical process. The more photopigment molecules are available, the greater the chance that one will absorb a photon. If enough molecules in enough receptor cells absorb enough light energy, perceptible stimulation will result. A bleached molecule is not available for further excitation until it is regenerated into rhodopsin. The balance, between numbers of pigment molecules being hydrolyzed and those being regenerated, is determined by the level of illumination, that is by the flow of photons reaching the retina. If the retina has been kept in darkness for a long enough time, rods contain a maximum of rhodopsin molecules ready for excitation, and their sensitivity will be maximal. If a rod has recently been exposed to light, then some of its rhodopsin molecules will have been broken down. This also applies to cones, except that more photons are needed to bleach a molecule of cone pigment than to bleach rhodopsin.

Adaptation to light is not simply the reverse of adaptation to darkness. If it were, then visual sensitivity would decrease in an illuminated environment as photopigment is bleached. Once most of the rhodopsin was bleached, rod vision would cease and cones would take over. In reality, however, adaptation to light is much faster than the bleaching process.

Several experiments have demonstrated quite convincingly that adaptation to bright light is a neuronal response in the first place and bleaching follows later. The basic principle of one such experiment was this: the subject was adapted fully to darkness. Part of his retina was then exposed to light, with care being taken to limit illumination by using sharply contrasting light patterns. Threshold was then measured in both the illuminated and non-illuminated areas of the retina. The threshold rose not only in the illuminated area (where rhodopsin has been bleached) but also in the non-illuminated area (where it has not been bleached). From this and many other experiments it was concluded that rod vision can be suppressed by an inhibitory process that is independent of the bleaching of rhodopsin. Such inhibition may operate at the synapses between rods and bipolar cells, but there is evidence that it in fact affects the rods themselves. It seems that if cones are stimulated, the receptor potentials of rods are suppressed.

Cone pigments are also bleached in the process of excitation, and in principle too much light could exhaust all pigment and blind the subject. Under ordinary circumstances, this does not occur because very strong light is quite unpleasant and is avoided. In anesthetized animals it can be shown that cone pigments can indeed be bleached so much that cone function temporarily ceases.

9.2d. THE ROLE OF CONES IN COLOR VISION

The absorption spectra of cone pigments were first determined by a complicated process of differential reflection spectrophotometry of the retina, using light shining through the pupils. Not much later the absorption spectra of individual cones in excised retinas were obtained. This was no mean technical feat, accomplished in the 1960s, first in retinas of goldfish, then of monkeys. The results are shown in Figure 9.7A.

The existence of three different color receptors in the retina had, however, been inferred for a long time before they were actually demonstrated. The trichromatic theory of color vision was first formulated by T. Young in 1801, and examined in great detail in phychophysical experiments by Helmholtz in the 1860s. It was Helmholtz who identified red, green and blue as the three primary colors. Some readers, especially if they are artistic, may at this point be perplexed, because the primary colors of painters are red, yellow and blue. The difference comes about because paints mix subtractively, while in physical and physiological experiments light of different wavelengths is mixed additively. Why this should matter can only be understood after opponent colors and color contrast have been explained, and for that we have to enter the realm of the processing of visual information in the central nervous system (see Section 10.2f).

Meanwhile, returning to Helmholtz, inspecting Figure 9.7 we can see that he was not far from the truth, even if not entirely right. When actual absorption spectra of cones were measured, two unexpected features were revealed. First, the three spectra overlap much more than had been suspected. Second, the pigment devoted to the longest waveband absorbs light maximally in the orange band, not in the red. It should, however, also be noted that only this cone absorbs light at the long-wave extremity of the visible spectrum (Fig. 9.7). This and other more indirect arguments suggest that excitation of this one long-wave receptor by itself alone would, in fact, evoke the sensation of redness, although some investigators might disagree with this conclusion.

Although this and a few other theoretical points remain in dispute, there is general agreement that under conditions of ordinary illumination and normal vision, most color sensations arise by the simultaneous excitation of either two or all three cone types (Fig. 9.7,B and C). The perceived hue is determined by the relative contributions of the three. We shall have more to say about the central processing of wavelength information later (Section 10.2f).

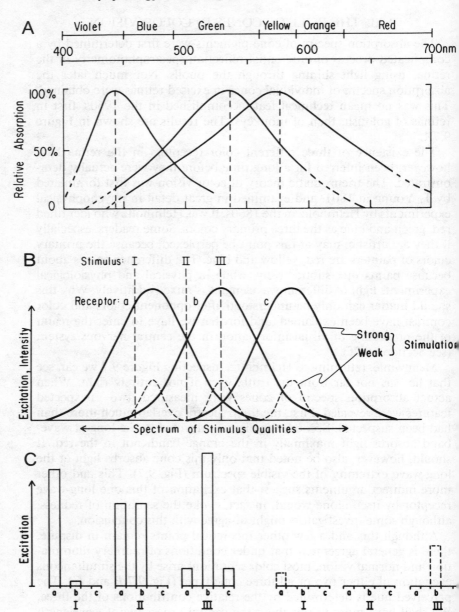

There are as yet no generally accepted names for the three cone pigments. *Cyanolabe, chlorolabe* and *erythrolabe* have been suggested, which translate into "blue-catching," "green-catching" and "red-catching." There are fewer blue-catching cones than either red-catching or green-catching ones; and correspondingly there is less blue-catching pigment in the retina than there is of each of the other two cone pigments.

9.2e. SENSITIVITY AND ACUITY OF VISION

Different species of animals rely on vision to different degrees. Most primates including man are diurnal in habit, and vision provides them with more information than any of their other senses.

At night, vision can detect that "something is there," perceive the direction of movement and perhaps define the vague outline of a shadow. When light is scarce, its mere detection may be critical and the *sensitivity* of the eye is its limiting parameter. In daylight, when photic energy is abundant, sensitivity is not critical. In its stead, *acuity* becomes the most significant measure of the eye's usefulness. Visual acuity (sharpness) is the ability to resolve fine details. It depends in part on the quality of the optical image cast on the retina and in part on the detection of contrast by the circuits of visual neurons. Not all species of animals are able to distinguish wavelengths (color). Those that do have an important advantage in detecting details in what they see.

The faintest light flash that a completely dark-adapted healthy young adult can perceive has an energy content of 50–150 photons. It has been calculated that of these 150 photons only about 15 actually reach the retina, the remainder being scattered and absorbed in the optic media of the eye. Since these 15 photons are distributed over a finite area of the retina, the chance that several

Figure 9.7. Trichromatic vision. *A,* normalized absorption spectra of cones in the retina of monkeys. Abscissal scale shows wavelength of light. (After data of W. B. Marks, W. H. Dobelle, and E. F. MacNicholl: *Science* 143:1181–1183, 1964.) *B,* hypothetical response curves of three receptors of different response spectra to strong and to weak stimulation. For the sake of simplification the three response curves are constructed identically and displaced equal distances along the stimulus spectrum (i.e. wavelength). *C,* relative response magnitudes of three hypothetical receptors (*a, b,* and *c* of diagram *B*), when stimulated by stimuli of "wavelengths" *I, II* and *III* (indicated on *B*), either strongly (*three bar graphs to the left*) or weakly (*bar graphs to the right*). (Reprinted with permission from G. Somjen: *Sensory Coding in the Mammalian Nervous System.* New York, Plenum Press, 1975.)

of them will hit the same rod are vanishingly small. It follows that one photon absorbed by one rod is enough to trigger a signal which is detected by a bipolar cell; and furthermore that the simultaneous excitation of 15 rods is the minimum that is perceived as a faint flash.

Vitamin A deficiency causes loss of visual sensitivity. Vitamin A is required for the functioning of both rods and cones. Deteriorating night vision is the first symptom of such deficiency, because a moderate change in visual sensitivity interferes with vision only when light is scarce. Severe Vitamin A deficiency causes deterioration of day vision as well, but then the disease affects the integrity of the skin and cornea too.

Under optimum conditions of illumination, a healthy young eye can distinguish details such as a white gap in a thick black line if they subtend one minute of arc of *visual angle*. The visual angle is formed by two straight lines connecting the edges of the object viewed to the optical center of the eye. In clinical practice visual acuity is measured with the aid of the familiar *Snellen charts*, consisting of black letters of different standardized sizes on a white background. The test is taken so that the subject sits 20 feet (6 m) from the chart so that accommodation is not required. To have 20/20 vision (metric scale 6/6) means that the subject is just able to read those letters that the average normal eye also just can read. These are the letters that subtend 5' of visual angle, and the strokes of the letters 1' or arc. If the subject can resolve only larger letters, then the denominator increases. Thus 20/40 vision means that the subject who is sitting 20 feet from the chart is able to read only the letters whose strokes would subtend 1' of arc if he would move to 40 instead of the 20 feet.

The most frequent cause of less than normal visual acuity is error of refraction, but this is by no means the only possible reason. Diseases of the retina, the visual pathway, and of the visual centers of the brain can each impair acuity as well.

In the line of the visual axis of the eye lies the fovea centralis where all the photoreceptors are cones. In the very periphery of the retina there are only rods, no cones. In between there is a mixed population of photoreceptors of gradually varying composition. This distribution has several practical consequences. First, while in daylight (photopic conditions), acuity is greatest at the center of gaze, in dim light the center of the visual field becomes blind (no rods). Second, a small lesion in the fovea centralis devastates visual acuity, whereas a lesion of similar size in the periphery of the retina may go almost unnoticed. Third, the periphery of the visual field is color-blind (no cones).

Where the optic nerve leaves the retina there are no photoreceptors at all. Consequently, we all have a *blind spot*, or physiological *scotoma*. Few people notice it until they learn of it in class. For the physician examining a patient's retina with the aid of an ophthalmoscope, the site of exit of the optic nerve (the *optic disc*) and the macula lutea are the two most important landmarks.

9.2f. CRITICAL FUSION FREQUENCY

A light flashing on and off at a sufficiently high frequency appears continuous and steady to the eye. Motion pictures and television images are made possible by this peculiarity of visual perception: in the case of both, discontinuous visual events appear to the viewer as though they were continuously changing. The lowest frequency at which intermittent illumination becomes apparently steady is the critical fusion frequency (CFF). This is much higher for cones than for rods, and the difference has been related to the duration of the late receptor potential. The receptor potential of rods outlasts a brief flash stimulus, much more so than the receptor potential of cones does. In other words, cones resolve temporal sequential stimuli more finely than do rods.

The critical fusion frequency is, however, not constant either for rods or for cones, but varies according to the intensity of illumination. For rods, the range is between 10 and 20 Hz, for cones between 20 and 60 Hz. Thus home movies can be viewed at a lower number of frames per second than professional ones, because the lamp of home projectors is weaker.

9.2g. COLOR BLINDNESS

Some individuals cannot distinguish colors at all. Such total color blindness is quite rare. One of its possible causes is absence of cones (*rod monochromats*) in which case acuity is also very deficient. There is another form of total color blindness, even rarer, in which the retina contains besides rods but one type of cone (*cone monochromats*). In these cases the acuity of vision is better than in pure-rod retinas. The world of the totally color blind consists of shades of gray, as in a black-and-white film.

Much more common than total color blindness is an inability or a weakness of distinguishing some but not all colors. When this condition is fully developed, the patient lacks one of the three cone pigments: *dichromats.* We speak of *protanopia* (missing the first, *protos*, the red-catching pigment); of *deuteranopia* (missing the second, the green-catching pigment) and of *tritanopia* (missing the third, blue-catching pigment).

Total lack of one pigment (total protanopia and deuteranopia) is less common than a partial deficiency (color weakness; protanomaly and deuteranomaly). One in 13 men and one in 200 women have some degree of inherited deficiency of either the red or of the green-catching pigment. Other forms of disturbed color vision also exist, caused either by abnormal absorption spectra or the mixing of two pigments in the same cones. Many color-blind people are unaware of their defect until it is discovered, for example, during screening for the military or for a driving license. In fact, the condition had not been described in the scientific literature until 1794, when the chemist, John Dalton, himself color-blind, discovered that he saw colors differently from the way in which his friends described them.

The (totally) protanope misses the red experience and sees the world in shades of yellow, green and blue. The proverbial protanope is the one who goes to a funeral wearing a red tie, believing it to be black. (Perhaps this never really happened, but it is a good paradigm of protanopia). The protanope also has difficulty in distinguishing orange from green. To the deuteranope shades of green are indistinguishable from yellows. The more common color-weak patients can see strong red and green colors as such but have difficulty in picking out unsaturated red and green hues from an assortment of other colors. (Saturation means the spectral purity of a color. Unsaturation may be achieved by admixing white to a spectrally pure color). The typical error made by both protanomalous and deuteranomalous patients is to confuse red and green hues.

Protanopia and deuteranopia are separately inherited, recessive, sex-linked, Mendelian traits. Women are usually carriers, and have a rare chance to manifest the disease if their father was color-blind, and their mother a carrier of the same defective gene.

Tritanopia as an inherited disease is exceedingly rare and is not sex-linked. Color-blindness, including blue-yellow blindness, can also be acquired by chronic poisoning with methanol and certain other toxic agents and by avitaminosis.

9.3. Neuronal Responses in the Retina

The retina is a piece of displaced central gray matter. It develops during embryonic life as an outcropping of the brain (see Section 9.2), and it eventually acquires a neuronal circuit every bit as intricate as many parts of the CNS of similar dimensions. The output pathway of the retina, the optic nerve, is more like a tract in the white matter than a peripheral nerve. Its fibers have the fine structure of central axons, and their satellite cells are oligocytes, not Schwann cells.

The fibers in the optic nerve are the axons of the ganglion cells of the retina. The chain of transmission runs from photoreceptors by way of bipolar cells to ganglion cells. Horizontal cells and the amacrine cells are additional interneurons of the retina (Figs. 9.4 and 9.8C).

9.3a. BIPOLAR AND HORIZONTAL CELLS

Neither bipolar nor horizontal cells generate all-or-none impulses. They respond to synaptic input with graded depolarizing and hyperpolarizing transient potentials, resembling excitatory postsynaptic potentials (EPSPs) and inhibitory postsynaptic potentials (IPSPs) of other central neurons (Fig. 9.4B). The axons of these cells are very short, and potential changes generated in their dendrites are conducted electrotonically into their axon terminals; hence there is no need for propagated action potentials. Bipolar cells receive input from photoreceptors not only directly, but also indirectly, mediated by the horizontal cells. The polarities of the effects of direct and indirect input appear to be opposites. Many bipolar cells are depolarized when light shines on a small group of receptors that are in immediate contact with them, but hyperpolarized when light shines on the receptors surrounding the former group. Many other bipolar cells respond the other way; by hyperpolarization when light shines on the center of the receptive field and depolarization when it falls on the encircling ring-shaped area. The responses to diffuse illumination are like those evoked by illumination of the center, but weaker. Whatever the response to light being turned on, it usually is followed by the opposite response (rebound) when light is turned off.

What the synaptic mechanisms are that mediate these responses is not quite clear. Electron microscopy of the outer plexiform layer has revealed synaptic junctions between the following elements: from photoreceptors to bipolars cells; from photoreceptors to horizontal cells; from bipolar cells to photoreceptors; from horizontal cells to bipolar cells. In addition there are apparent functional junctions between the synaptic processes of certain classes of photoreceptors and not between certain others. How all these interact to produce the observed physiological responses remains to be discovered.

Some bipolar cells receive input from cones only, some from rods only, and some, the so-called flat bipolars, from both rods and cones. (Only the dendritic expanse of these cells is "flat," not the cell itself.) Those bipolar cells that are connected only to cones have the smallest

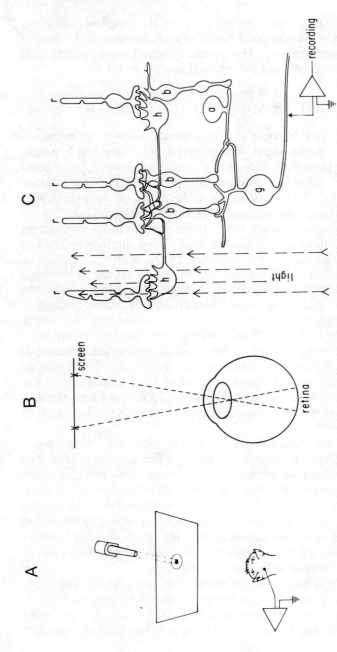

Figure 9.8. Experimental arrangement for recording the firing of retinal ganglion cells. *A*, the experimental animal faces a screen, upon which moving or stationary stimuli in the form of light-and-dark or colored patterns can be projected. Computer-generated images on a TV screen can take the place of the slide projector. *B*, the image on the screen forms an image on the retina. *C*, the light from the stimulus reaches the photoreceptors by penetrating through the layers of ganglion cell axons, and the cell layers of the retina. Signals from the photoreceptors are then transmitted to the ganglion cells as indicated in Figure 9.4. The impulses of the ganglion cells can be recorded either within the retina itself or in the optic nerve. *r*, photoreceptors; *b*, bipolar cells; *h*, horizontal cells; *a*, amacrine cells; *g*, ganglion cells.

and most compact receptive fields, but even flat bipolars have receptive fields which cover only a small fraction of the total surface of the retina.

The transmitter substances of the retina have not been identified, but there are several candidate compounds which may have such a function. Nor has it been determined whether all photoreceptors release the same transmitter or whether different transmitters are used at different receptor-bipolar cell synapses.

9.3b. REMARKS CONCERNING VISUAL AND RECEPTIVE FIELDS

By *visual field* we mean the entire field of vision of an individual. In clinical practice it is customarily mapped in a procedure termed *optic perimetry*. Pathological restrictions of the visual field occur when the retina, the optic pathway, or the visual cortex are damaged.

Receptive field has two linked but distinct meanings in visual physiology: first, the area of the retina within which stimulation can evoke a response (excitatory or inhibitory) of a particular neuron; or, it can mean the portion of the visual field "out there" within which photic stimulation (light, shadow, images) can influence a neuron. Since the one depends on the other, the use of a single expression to define both concepts is permissible.

The limits of the visual field of a patient, as well as the limits (diameter) of receptive fields of neurons studied in animal experiments are usually given in degrees of visual angle. The use of degrees, instead of centimeters or inches, makes the measurement independent of distance from the eye.

9.3c. GANGLION CELLS OF THE RETINA

Ganglion cells receive signals from photoreceptors by way of bipolar cells. They also receive input from amacrine cells. Unlike bipolar and horizontal cells, ganglion cells fire proper, conducted action potentials. Indeed they need to do so, for they must send signals to the brain through long axons which form the optic nerve.

Ganglion cells respond to stimulation of their receptive fields in many and varied ways. The properties of the photoreceptors and of the connecting cells, and their interactions in the networks of inner and outer plexiform layers, determine their behavior. By response types, ganglion cells have been classified from several points of view. It is neither necessary nor possible to catalog here all types that have been described, but some of the principal classes will be described by way of illustration.

In common with the bipolar cells that feed input to them, most ganglion cells in the retina of monkeys have concentric antagonistic receptive fields (Figs. 9.8 and 9.9) and may be divided into two classes. *On-center* ganglion cells are excited when light shines at the center of their receptive field. These same cells are inhibited when light shines on the (concentric) surround zone of their receptive field. When the stimulating light is turned off, a rebound occurs: when light that had been shining at the center is turned off, on-center cells fall silent; when illumination of the surround ceases, there is rebound from inhibition and the cell actually fires a burst of impulses in response to light-off. *Off-center* cells behave in exactly the reverse way. Receptive fields of ganglion cells are usually larger than those of the bipolar cells, indicating that input from several bipolars converges on each ganglion cell.

Some ganglion cells receive input from cones only, others from both rod and cone cells. Pure-cone-input ganglion cells have smaller receptive

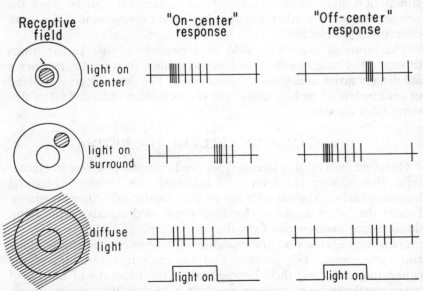

Figure 9.9. Response types of retinal ganglion cells. Receptive fields are mapped in experiments arranged as shown in Figure 9.8. For further description see text.

fields than rod-and-cone-input ganglion cells. At the fovea centralis where there are only cones, receptive fields are smallest. The ratios of receptor to bipolar cells, and bipolar to ganglion cells, are lowest here, approaching unity at times. Toward the periphery of the retina, where there are only rods, hundreds of receptors may supply a single bipolar, and many bipolars are in turn connected to a single ganglion cell. In cases where input from both rods and cones is channeled to a ganglion cell, transmission will be dominated by the cones under photopic conditions, and by the rods under scotopic conditions but never simultaneously by both (see Section 9.2c).

The majority of the ganglion cells of mammalian retinas show incessant low-level activity when the eye is in darkness or in semi-darkness.

There is yet another classification of retinal ganglion cells, embracing on-center and off-center cells, as well as others with no concentrically antagonistic fields. This classification is based in part on axonal conduction velocity and in part on the degree of response adaptation. Some investigators speak of *transient* (fast-adapting) and *sustained* (slow-adapting) response types. Others use the designations *W, X* and *Y cells.*

Y cells are the largest, and have the fastest conducting axons. X cells are intermediate, and W cells have the thinnest, slowest conducting axons. Y cells have larger receptive fields than X cells, and they give only brief, transient responses, be it excitation or inhibition. X cells have the smallest receptive fields of the three. Both X and W cells respond in sustained fashion as long as a stimulus is acting on their receptive field. All X and Y and some W cells have circular antagonistic receptive fields: they are either on-center or off-center types. Among the W cells there are many that have no antagonistic zones in the receptive fields, but respond uniformly to illumination anywhere within the field, either by increasing or by decreasing firing.

From all three types, X, Y and W, signals are transmitted to the cerebral cortex by way of the lateral geniculate nucleus. W and Y cells, but not X cells, also send axon branches through the retinotectal pathway to the superior colliculi of the midbrain. Most investigators believe that these three cell types furnish different categories of information. Signals of fast-conducting, fast-adapting Y cells enable the cortex to determine the velocity and direction of the movements of visual stimuli. X cells with their small receptive field and sustained discharge resolve the fine detail in visual pattern. W cells, especially those whose receptive fields contain no antagonist zones, tell the cortex and the tectum mainly about overall light intensity. Neither X nor Y cells can signal overall light levels very well, since diffuse illumination of their receptive field evokes only weak responses (Fig. 9.9).

We shall meet the X, Y and W systems again as we discuss the central processing of visual information (see Sections 10.1 and 10.3). Discussion of the opponent color responses of neurons is also best deferred to the next chapter (Section 10.2f).

9.4. Diagnostic Electrophysiology of the Eyes

9.4a. ELECTRORETINOGRAM (ERG)

Illumination of the retina evokes a series of electrical potential changes that can be recorded at some distance from the retina itself. In clinical practice the "active lead" is an electrode in a contact lens in contact with the cornea, and the "indifferent lead" is attached to a convenient distant point on the head (Fig. 9.10). It should be realized that a positive deflection of potential at the cornea usually corresponds to a negative deflection at the outer layers of the retina.

Shortly after the onset of illumination three conspicuous waves are generated, conventionally labeled a, b and c (Fig. 9.10C). The a wave is brief and has negative polarity at the cornea (positive at the outer segments of the photoreceptors). The b wave is longer and of larger amplitude; it is corneo-positive. The c wave is the slowest in onset and longest in duration, and is also positive at the cornea. When light is turned off, the d wave is registered, but in people it is small and sometimes absent.

The mechanism by which the waves of the electroretinogram are generated is only partly understood. The a wave is caused by the late receptor potential (see Section 9.2b). The early receptor potential is not detected by ERG leads attached to the outside of the eye. The b wave is believed by some but not by all investigators to be generated by depolarization of the Müller (glial) cells of the retina. It is a fact that in the retina, as in other CNS tissues, glial cells are depolarized by K^+ ions accumulating an interstitial fluid during the excitatory process (see Section 5.9b). The dispute concerns only whether glial depolarization is registered in the ERG. The c wave is probably generated by the pigment epithelium.

One of the clinical uses of the ERG is the examination of retinal function after eye injury. After an accident the ocular fluids may be discolored. This obscures vision of the patient; it also obscures the view of an examining physician

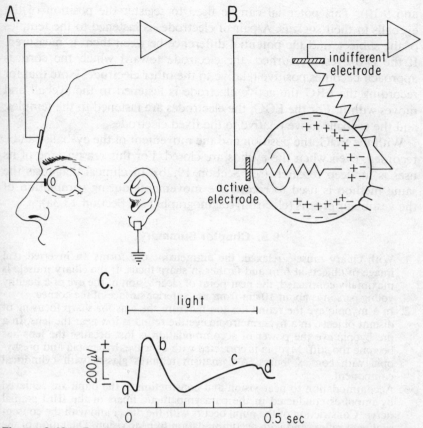

A.

B.

indifferent
electrode

active
electrode

C.

light

200 μV

a   b   c   d

0   0.5 sec

Figure 9.10. Recording human electroretinograms. *A* and *B* show the arrangement of recording and ground electrodes, *C* the main components of the potential waves so recorded.

who attempts to see the retina with an ophthalmoscope. It can be important for the planning of therapy to know whether the retina is viable. A clouded vitreous admits enough light to evoke an ERG, provided that the retina is still functioning.

9.4b. ELECTRO-OCULOGRAM (EOG) AND ELECTRONYSTAGROGRAM

The steady radial current flowing in the retina makes the back of the eye electrically negative relative to its front (see Section 9.2b; Figs. 9.3

and 9.10). This potential can be used to register the position of the eyeballs in their sockets. A pair of electrodes is fastened to the temples of the subject, and the potential difference between them is measured. If the two eyes are turned, the electrode toward which the corneas approach becomes positive relative to the other electrode. Note that for recording the ERG the active electrode is fastened to the eyeball and moves with it. For the EOG, the electrodes are fastened to the temples, and the eyeballs move relative to the fixed electrodes.

With the EOG, the position and the movement of the eyeballs can be recorded, even when the eyelids are closed. For this reason, one of its uses is in sleep research (see Section 19.2b). In clinical diagnosis the same method is used to record eye movements during stimulation of the vestibular organs (electronystagmography: see Section 13.3a).

9.5. Chapter Summary

1. With ciliary muscle relaxed, the emmetrope eye forms an inverted real image of objects at 6 m and farther in sharp focus. If the ciliary muscle is maximally contracted, the near point of clear vision of the eye of a healthy young person is about 10 cm from the anterior surface of the cornea.

2. In a myopic eye the retina lies too far from the lens for sharp focusing of distant objects; in a hypermetropic eye the retina is too near the lens. In a presbyopic eye the power of accommodation is lost because the lens has become too stiff. Myopia is corrected with concave, hyperopia and presbyopia with convex lenses. Astigmatism requires glasses with cylindrical component.

3. Accommodation to near vision and constriction of the pupil are achieved by impulses conducted in the parasympathetic fibers of the IIIrd cranial nerve. Constriction of the pupil occurs with the direct and with the consensual light reflex, and with accommodation to near vision. Dilatation of the pupil in response to darkening is achieved by relaxation of parasympathetic tone; dilatation of the pupil due to emotional excitement by the action of sympathetic dilator fibers from the superior cervical ganglion.

4. The photopigment of rods is rhodopsin, consisting of retinal combined with opsin. Cones contain three different photopigments with partly overlapping absorption spectra, with absorption maxima in the orange, green and blue bands of the visible spectrum. The cone pigments contain the same retinal as rhodopsin, but their opsins differ.

5. In rods as well as cones illumination causes bleaching of the photopigment. In the course of bleaching retinal undergoes isomeric transformation and then becomes detached from opsin. The initial step in the bleaching process excites the photoreceptor cell membrane through mediation by an as yet unidentified internal messenger substance.

6. When illuminated, photoreceptors generate two successive electric responses. The early receptor potential is due to charge displacement associ-

ated with the photochemical reaction of the photopigment. The late receptor potential consists of a hyperpolarization of the photoreceptor membrane; it causes the *a* wave of the electroretinogram.

7. Dark-adapted rods require much less light for excitation than do cones. When light is scarce, the fovea contralis is inactive because it contains no rods, only cones. Impaired night vision is an early sign of vitamin A deficiency, because elevation of the threshold of rod vision is noticed before elevation of the threshold of cone vision.

8. Under photopic (as opposed to scotopic) conditions, vision is most acute in the center of the visual field, corresponding to foveal vision.

9. When moving from a dim into a brightly lit environment, the retina adapts by inhibiting synaptic transmission from rods, thus allowing cone function to take over. Adaptation to darkness requires regeneration of bleached photopigment, because bleached molecules are not available to mediate excitation. Adaptation to darkness takes place in two phases: first cones come to maximal sensitivity, then rods. Adaptation to darkness takes longer than adaptation to light.

10. The maximal sensitivity of a dark-adapted eye is at a shorter wavelength than the maximal sensitivity of a light-adapted eye (Purkinje shift). Rods are insensitive to red light.

11. Discrimination of all hues of color is made possible at the level of the retina by excitation of the three cone types in various proportions.

12. Red-green color blindness can be the consequence of missing either the red-catching or the green-catching cone pigment (protanopia and deuteranopia).

13. Snellen charts are used to determine visual acuity clinically.

14. Photopic vision has a higher critical fusion frequency than scotopic rod vision.

15. Photoreceptor cells, horizontal cells and bipolar cells generate no all-or-none nerve impulses; some amacrine cells, and all ganglion cells, do.

16. In on-center ganglion cells illumination of the receptive field center causes increased firing at light-on and decreased firing at light-off; illumination of the receptive field surround causes decreased firing at light-on and increased firing at light-off. Off-center cells also have reciprocally antagonistic receptive field zones; in off-center cells the effect of illumination is the reverse of that seen in on-center cells.

17. Y cells have relatively large receptive fields and respond only transiently (dynamic response) to changing levels of illumination. X cells have small receptive fields and their response adapts only partially (dynamic plus static response). W cells give sustained responses either in direct or in inverse proportion to illumination. All X and Y cells have concentric antagonistic receptive fields (either on-center or off-center); many W cells have uniform receptive fields (either excitatory or inhibitory). X, Y and W cells project to visual cortex; only Y and W cells project to the superior colliculi.

18. The electroretinogram consists of the corneo-negative *a* wave, and the

positive b and c waves. The d wave at light-off is small or is not seen in human subjects.

Further Reading

See at end of Chapter 10.

Visual Functions of the Central Nervous System

How the brain processes the information it receives from the optic nerves.

10.1. The Dorsal Lateral Geniculate Nucleus

The lateral geniculate nucleus (LGN) is the principal way station in the pathway from retina to visual cortex. The location and the function of the LGN can be compared to those of the ventroposterolateral (VPL) nucleus in the somatosensory pathway.

The right lateral geniculate receives input from the temporal half of the right retina and from the nasal half of the left retina. In other words, the right geniculate receives input from the right half of the retinas of both eyes; the reverse is true for the left lateral geniculate nucleus. Each lateral geniculate nucleus sends fibers only to the cortex of its own hemisphere. Thus signals received from the right side of both retinas remain in the right brain (see Fig. 10.3; also Carpenter, Figs. 9.18 and 9.21). Since the optical system of the eye reverses the image of the visual field, the right hemisphere "looks out" on the left side of the world. Exceptions are the very centers of each retina, which are represented bilaterally: both central foveas project to both hemispheres.

It will be remembered that the VPL nucleus of the thalamus and the

279

primary somatic sensory area of the cortex receive input only from the contralateral half of the body. Thus the right brain is informed about the state of the left side of the body, and also about the left half of the visual world. Later we will see that this principle extends to the motor cortex, where the right hemisphere controls the musculature of the left side of the body (see Section 18.1) and *vice versa*.

In primates, including man, the lateral geniculate nucleus contains 6 cell layers. Optic nerve fibers from the contralateral eyes have terminals in layers 1, 4 and 6, those from the ipsilateral eye in layers 2, 3 and 5. Since the different layers are not interconnected, the LGN projection cells that send axons to the visual cortex receive input from either the one or from the other retina, but not both. Convergence of input from the two eyes does occur in the cortex, as we shall see presently.

Another significance of lamination in LGN is that input from W, X and Y cells is addressed to different layers. Thus the different kinds of visual information handled by these three ganglion cell types (see Section 9.3c) are processed by distinct neuronal circuits in the LGN. For this reason the labels W, X and Y are used to designate not only the ganglion cells of the retina, but also the neurons connecting LGN to cortex.

Concentrically arranged antagonistic (either on-center or off-center) receptive fields are common (cf. Section 9.3c) in the LGN nucleus but other types have been also found. Differences exist between the behavior of LGN cells and ganglion cells, but are not very striking.

10.2. The Visual Receiving Areas of the Cerebral Cortex

The striate cortex (Brodmann's area 17), most of which is in primates located in the calcarine fissure of the occipital lobe, is the primary visual receiving area (V-I). The axons of the LGN projection cells form the optic radiations which bring the visual input to the cerebral cortex. Adjacent to the striate cortex, three additional areas of cortex are dominated by visual input. They are variously labeled as prestriate or peristriate areas, and are divided into areas V-II, V-III and V-IV. In man all four visual receiving areas are located in the occipital lobe (Fig. 7.5).

The extent to which the V-II, V-III and V-IV areas receive signals directly from the LGN, or get them "second-hand" after they have first been processed in V-I, seems to vary with species. In primates V-II, V-III and V-IV seem more dependent on V-I (that is receive less direct input from LGN) than in some other mammals.

Electrical stimulation of the primary visual cortex in a conscious patient evokes a visual sensation. If the stimulus is kept at the minimum

effective level, the sensation is that of a small white luminous spot, like
a star. This elementary electrically evoked sensation has been named a
phosphene. If the same point on the cortex is stimulated repeatedly, the
phosphene is always perceived in the same place of the visual field
contralateral to the stimulated hemisphere. If the electrode is moved in
the cortex, the phosphene moves in a predictable manner.

The outline of the orderly representation of the retina in the LGN, in
the optic radiation and in the visual cortex was discovered in anatomical
tracings and from clinical experience before the introduction of electrical
stimulation and recording. This topographic order is known as *retinotopic organization* of the visual pathway.

The retinotopic representation in area 17 is not a scale map of the
retina or of the visual field, for a disproportionately large area of cortex
is reserved from the representation of the central area of the retina, the
fovea and macula lutea. For this, and for other reasons which will soon
become obvious, it would be wrong to compare the visual cortex to a
movie screen.

The retinotopic organization of the cortex has, nevertheless, inspired a serious,
if futuristic, suggestion that blind people be provided with an electroprosthetic
device based on electric stimulation of the cortex. A TV camera is to be used as
substitute eye; it is to be wired to a computer programmed to deliver stimulus
pulses through an array of stimulating electrodes implanted in the cortex. Even
if the images so evoked were lacking in detail, just outlining objects would
greatly help blind people. It will be appreciated that the technical problems that
must be overcome are great. Translating the TV image into the topography
valid in the cerebral cortex, difficult as it is, is by no means the worst of the
obstacles. Attempts at realizing this concept have had so far limited success.

Electric stimuli stronger than necessary to evoke phosphenes evoke
larger, more complex sensations of visual shapes, flashes and sometimes
colored patterns. Color sensation may be due to conduction of excitation
to the adjacent pre- or peristriate areas.

10.2a. SIMPLE AND COMPLEX RECEPTIVE FIELDS

Most fibers of the geniculocortical projetion terminate in layer IV of
the striate cortex. In this layer some neurons have receptive fields of
circular shape. Many cells in layer IV, and practically all those in the
layers above and below, do not have circular receptive fields, but
elongated rectangular ones. They differ also from LGN cells and from
retinal ganglion cells in that the stimulus optimal for their excitation (or
inhibition, as the case might be) is neither a circular spot nor an anulus

of light, but a straight-edge image of high contrast: either a white line on a black background, or a black line on a white field, or a straight boundary between a bright and a dark field. In all cases the line or edge must be within the receptive field of the neuron. Furthermore, to be maximally exciting, the line, or edge, must have a particular orientation in visual space that could be vertical for one neuron, horizontal for another, and any angle in between for yet others. Whatever the optimal stimulus orientation, it is a constant for that one cell. Images oriented at right angles to the optimal stimulus evoke either no response or a very feeble one; this is sometimes defined as the null orientation. Moreover, most cortical cells respond more vigorously to stimuli moving across their receptive fields than to stationary images. Many prefer stimuli moving in one direction over those moving in the opposite direction (Fig. 10.1).

The preference for straight-edged contrast is characteristic of the great majority of neurons in the 1st and 2nd visual areas (V-I and V-II, or

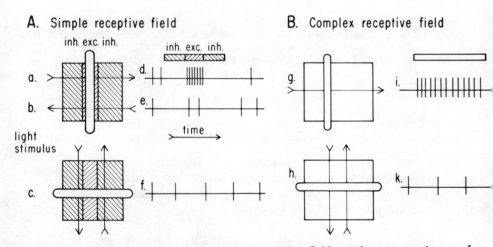

Figure 10.1. Some of the typical receptive fields and response types of neurons in V-I and V-II areas (areas 17 and 18) of the cerebral cortex. *A*, a simple receptive field consisting of an excitatory zone flanked by two inhibitory zones. *a*, a stimulus (an illuminated line) is moved in the optimum orientation and in the optimum direction across the receptive field; it then evokes the firing pattern shown in *d*. *b*, a stimulus moved in the direction opposite to the optimum one evokes a feeble response (*e*). *c*, a stimulus oriented at an angle at 90° to the optimum orientation evokes no change in firing (*i*). *B*, stimulation (*g* and *h*) and responses (*i* and *k*) of a neuron with a complex receptive field.

areas 17 and 18 of Brodmann). These cells can further be subdivided into two large groups according to the repertory of their responses: The *simple* and *complex cells*, distinguished by simple and complex receptive fields.

A simple receptive field is composed of excitatory and inhibitory zones, which may lie side by side in the visual field, or two inhibitory zones may flank a single excitatory zone. Other combinations have been found, but in all cases the boundary between excitatory and inhibitory areas is a straight line.

A complex receptive field has no separate zones for excitation and inhibition. The optimal stimulus of different complex cells may be a black line, or a white line, or an edge between a bright and a dark area. Whichever it is, the cell responds with equal vigor whenever and wherever the stimulus appears within its receptive field, provided that the stimulus retains the optimal orientation.

It is an almost inescapable assumption that the receptive fields of cortical neurons reflect the arrangement, the "wiring diagram," of their excitatory and inhibitory connections. For example, it has been suggested that a simple receptive field, which consists of an excitatory strip flanked by two inhibitory zones, could be constructed as follows. The cortical cell would receive convergent input from several on-center LGN cells, provided the receptive fields of the LGN cells lie in a straight line in visual space. The excitatory centers of the LGN cells would then coalesce into a straight strip, and the inhibitory surrounds into the flanking inhibitory zones (Fig. 10.2). Other, more intricate receptive fields require more complex synaptic interactions in which cortical interneurons must play a part.

There are indications that input to complex cells is dominated by the Y system (fast-conducting axons, transiently excited) and input to the simple cells by the X system (slow-conducting axons, sustained excitation and smaller receptive fields). This conclusion cannot yet be considered firmly established but it is supported by several observations, including the one that simple cells are more readily excited by stationary and by slowly moving stimuli than are complex cells.

10.2b. COLUMNAR ORGANIZATION IN THE VISUAL CORTEX

A microelectrode inserted into the primary visual cortex perpendicular to the surface will encounter many cells on its way through the cortical gray matter. These cells may respond to various test stimuli in

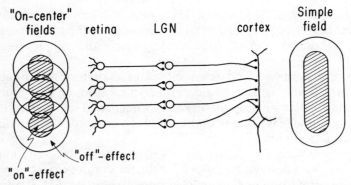

Figure 10.2.   The simplest possible hypothetical connections by which synaptic excitation from several on-center cells converging on a single cell in visual cortex could result in a simple receptive field; *LGN*, lateral geniculate nucleus.

a variety of ways. Some will have simple, others complex receptive fields. All, however, will have certain features in common. All neurons within one cortical column have overlapping receptive fields and all have the same optimal stimulus orientation. The common orientation preference cuts across the classes of simple and complex cells and their variants.

If the electrode is withdrawn and then reinserted some 0.05 to 0.1 mm from the previous point, the chances are it will find a column of cells the optimal stimulus orientation of which will be somewhat tilted compared to the previous column's optimal stimulus orientation. Moving further in the same direction, the best stimulus will be tilted yet further in the same direction. The entire visual cortex seems organized into slabs, or imaginary slices of tissue, each representing another optimal stimulus orientation. These are the *orientation* columns of the visual cortex (Fig. 10.3).

While many neurons in the visual cortex receive input from corresponding points of both retinas, the input from the two eyes is in most cases not equal. In layer IV of the striate cortex, where most of the fibers of the projection cells of the LGN terminate, most cells are influenced by input from one eye only, just as the LGN cells are, from which these cortical cells receive their input. Above and below layer IV, cortical neurons may receive convergent input from both eyes (Fig. 10.3), but the effect conveyed from one of the two eyes usually dominates. Cells above and below one another are dominated by the same eye, forming

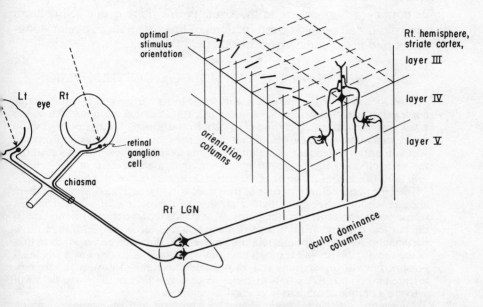

Figure 10.3.   Columnar organization of the striate cortex (V-I area). The striate cortex is organized into intersecting sheets of cells, one set of sheets representing progressively changing optimum stimulus orientation, and the other an alternation of dominance of input of left and right eyes. *Rt LGN,* right lateral geniculate nucleus. Note that the right half of the retinae of both eyes projects to the right hemisphere, and inputs from corresponding points of the two retinae converge on single cells within the striate cortex. The width of ocular dominance columns is about 0.5 mm, of orientation columns about 0.05 mm (in macaque monkeys). (In part modified and redrawn after T. N. Wiesel and D. H. Hubel: *Journal of Comparative Neurology* 146:421–450, 1972.)

ocular dominance columns. Dominance alternates between input from the left and right eye at intervals of about 0.5 mm, and the boundaries of these columns of ocular dominance intersect the columns of optimal stimulus orientation. This is illustrated diagrammatically in Figure 10.3, but in reality the boundaries between the columns (or sheets of cells) are not straight but swirling, and the intersections are not orthogonal.

In summary: the primary visual cortex (V-I) is parceled according to three different organizing principles: retinotopic representation; optimal stimulus orientation; and ocular dominance. In any one column of cells the information processed concerns a single locus in visual space, a particular angle of stimulus orientation, and input from one, the other, or both eyes. Somewhere in the visual cortex there is one cell column reserved for all possible combinations of line orientation, ocular dominance and place in the visual world.

10.2c. NOTES ON THE PHYSIOLOGY OF FORM VISION

If we look at an object, we perceive its shape by its outline and by conspicuous contrasting lines that define its various parts. It is thus that cartoons sketched in a few lines are accepted as images of people and things, no matter how spare the representation. When we look at real scenes, our brain excerpts from the vast amount of redundant visual information reaching it those features essential for recognition. *Feature detection* may in mammals be one of the unique functions of the sensory areas of the cerebral neocortex (see also Section 7.8).

It seems that a column of cells in the visual cortex is activated whenever there appears within its receptive field a portion of the outline of a visual image, whose geometric tangent at the point corresponds to the optimal orientation of the cortical column. If the image is moving across the visual field, then those particular cells whose optimal stimulus-movement direction corresponds to that of the moving object will respond maximally. Since in the cortex as a whole all possible tangent orientations and all possible directions of movement are represented for all possible points in visual space, any object in the visual field will activate a unique combination of cortical columns.

Of course, when one object changes its position and orientation in visual space, it will excite a different combination of cortical columns. Yet we perceive it as identical with itself although we realize that it has moved. The perceived identity of an upside-down letter A with a right side-up letter A, and of a small-sized letter A with a large one, is defined in psychology as *form constancy*. This concept presupposes a brain mechanism that detects interrelationships between points and lines independently of their orientation and their absolute size. We do not yet know how this is achieved, but patently it cannot be a function of the primary visual cortex. This insight underscores that what happens in the V-I area of the cortex is but an early phase in the analysis of visual information. Final recognition of objects and people must depend on matching the perceived image to a specific item among a vast amount of visual information stored in memory (cf. Chapter 20).

10.2d. STABILIZED IMAGES

Our eyes are never still, not even when we fixate our gaze on a single point. The small, involuntary, and nearly imperceptible oscillations of the eyeballs are clearly visible when the eye is observed under low-power magnification (e.g. under the so-called slit-lamp microscope of the ophthalmologist). It follows that the retinal images cast by visual targets are never still either, but dance around in random directions. It is possible to prevent this incessant, random dance by the technique of *stabilizing the image*. To achieve this, the eye is fitted with a contact lens to which is attached a light support for some visual stimulus. This can be a small card with a pattern, or a lightweight lens system with which patterned images are focused on the retina, so that the target pattern moves with the eyeballs. Subjects in these experiments report that stabilized line patterns— letters, and the like—are not constantly perceived but tend to fade, reappear, then fade again. It seems likely that the fading of stabilized images has to do with the transient nature of the excitation of neurons in the retinogeniculocortical projection system. The involuntary random eye movements normally counteract adaptation, since they constantly shift the stimulus from one receptor to another, from one cortical column to another. The brilliance of the background, and its color, do not disappear when stabilized on the retina. This may be the result of the ability of the W system to sustain excitation.

10.2e. BINOCULAR AND DEPTH VISION

Why have two eyes instead of just one? The brain fuses the images produced by the two retinas into a single visual experience, a function termed "cyclopean vision" by some. To achieve fusion, corresponding points of the two retinas must be "wired" to single cortical columns during embryonal development. Moreover, the movements of the two eyes must be coordinated exactly (see Section 10.4a) to keep the two eyes' gaze directed at the same target. Could not all the cost of this complicated machinery have been saved by having, in truly cyclopean manner, just one eye in the middle of the face?

Having a spare eye has some advantage, of course, when one of the two is out of action. Besides, the combined field of vision of two eyes is larger than that of one eye alone. As far as that is concerned, most birds and also rabbits, horses, and other mammals with laterally placed eyes are much better off than are primates and carnivores. What, then, is the main advantage of our two frontally placed eyes?

The answer is depth vision. Our paired eyes view objects from slightly different angles (parallax). The brain fuses the two, slightly disparate, two-dimensional images into a single, three-dimensional visual experience. This is especially well demonstrated by the illusion of depth created in a stereoscope (for example Viewmaster pictures). Stereoscopic photos are produced by using a dual lens photographic camera, which makes two pictures of the same object from different angles, imitating our two eyes. The two pictures are then viewed so that the left picture is seen by the left eye only and the right picture by the right eye. This creates the illusion of three dimensions.

Of course if we close one eye, scenery seen by the open eye does not seem to collapse into a flat image. The brain can construct a three-dimensional experience even from the two-dimensional image of one retina. In this it must rely in part on such clues as the perceived relative size of objects; shadows of one object falling on another; and apparent relative movement of objects as we move our head. Distances can however be judged much more accurately when both eyes are used than with one eye alone.

In summary: while it is not essential to have two eyes to experience visual depth, depth vision is much more accurate with binocular than with monocular vision.

If one looks at an object at a given distance, then other objects in line with the target either in front or behind it cast images which do not occupy exactly corresponding points in the two retinas, but are shifted: they occupy laterally disparate points (Fig. 10.4). Objects closer than the target have images displaced somewhat outward (toward the temporal side), those farther will cast retinal images shifted inward (nasally). We do not see such objects as double images but as being far or near.

Neurons have been found in the visual cortex whose two receptive fields in the two retinas do not occupy exactly corresponding positions but are somewhat shifted. To achieve simultaneous stimulation of such disparate receptive fields, the stimulus must be located either farther or nearer than the main target of the gaze. (The distance toward which the

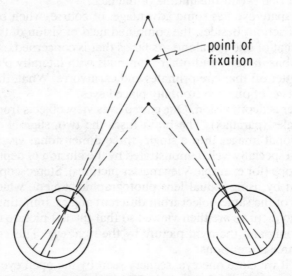

Figure 10.4. Binocular parallax. Objects in front and behind the one at which we are looking cast images at disparate (non-corresponding) points of the two retinae.

two eyes are directed is determined by the degree of convergence of the eyeballs (Fig. 10.4); if the two eyes are parallel, the gaze is directed at "infinite" distance). Such cells, the optimal excitation of which is influenced by the distance of the stimulus, are of course found only among those that receive input from both eyes. These cells seem not only to detect the distance of visual targets, but also to ensure fused vision, instead of double vision, of objects at different distances from the eye.

10.2f. COLOR CODING IN THE VISUAL CENTERS

Toward the end of the 18th century, Hering proposed a theory of color vision that for several decades was considered the chief rival of the Young-Helmholtz trichromatic theory (cf. Section 9.2d). Hering agreed with Helmholtz that there are three distinct receptor types in the retina. In his opinion, however, each was capable of evoking one of a pair of distinct sensations. He regarded such pairs as opposites and mutually exclusive. Hering's three opponent stimulus pairs were green and red, blue and yellow, and white and black.

Earlier we saw that the essential features of the Young-Helmholtz trichromatic theory have been confirmed by the discovery of the three cone pigments. It turns out, however, that Hering was also on the right track. His error lay in assuming that the receptors of the retina were responsible for opponent color effects. As it turned out, opponent color effects are brought about by reciprocal inhibitory synaptic interactions in the central visual pathway.

In the lateral geniculate nucleus of monkeys, cells have been found that are excited by a flash of red light and inhibited by green light. Others respond the other way around. A smaller number of cells show blue-yellow antagonism. There are also cells that do not discriminate between wavelengths; they are either excited by turning light on, regardless of wavelength; or they are inhibited by illumination and then discharge at light-off. The latter are usually called broad-spectral-band (broad-band for short) or broadly "tuned" cells and, in a sense, they correspond to Hering's postulated white-black antagonistic units.

These opponent color responses were evoked by stimulating the eyes with diffuse light flashes. When the details of the receptive fields of these cells were explored, many were found to have concentrically antagonistic receptive fields. Thus among the broad-band, white-black antagonists units there are on-center and off-center cells (Fig. 9.9). More intriguing are the receptive fields of red-green antagonist LGN cells. Some of these are excited when red light is turned on at the receptive field center and inhibited by green light shining on the receptive field surround. These cells cease firing when red light in the receptive field center is dimmed, but respond with a burst of impulses when green light illuminating the surround zone is turned off. Such neurons were categorized as "red-on-center-green-off-surround" cells. Four meaningful permutations are possibly by rearranging this name and all four have actually been found as receptive fields of LGN cells. Examination of the receptive fields of blue-yellow opponent color cells revealed in some cases similar, in others different principles of organization.

It would not be useful to catalog all color-coded response types here. It is instead worth mentioning that the behavior of these color-coded cells may well be responsible for certain visual effects produced in psychophysical experiments. These phenomena include color contrast effects, both simultaneous and successive, and colored after-images.

Color-coded cells have also been found in the visual cortex. In the striate area (V-I) these are a minority of the cell population. In the peristriate areas more cells respond differentially to wavelength. In the 4th visual area (V-IV) they may be the majority; this claim has however become the subject of controversy. Most of the cells in V-IV are said to respond only to a limited portion of the visible spectrum. They have been called narrow-band or narrowly tuned cells. Some are excited, some inhibited by their characteristic wave band, and neither type respond to stimulation by light of any other color. No color antagonism of the kind described for LGN and V-I cells has been found here. The response of narrow-band cells is nevertheless enhanced when a small patch of the preferred color is presented on a background of contrasting color. The response maxima of different cells occur at seven or eight distinct wavelengths, roughly corresponding to those hues for which the human languages have separate words (the seven colors of the rainbow). Cells in V-IV area have large receptive fields without preference for spatial orientation or for the direction of movement of the stimulus.

If the functioning of the area V-I seems to be essential for form vision, V-IV seems to have a key role in the analysis of wavelength information. How the three types of cones of the retina with their widely overlapping absorption spectra (Fig. 9.7) are wired to the LGN cells to produce the complex opponent color receptive fields, and how the color antagonistic responses of LGN cells are converted to the seven or eight narrow-band response spectra of the cortical neurons in V-IV area, is left for future research.

10.3. Visual Responses in the Superior Colliculi

The optic tectum is the principal visual center in the brain of lower vertebrates. Its main function in mammals is believed to be the coordination of the reflexes guiding involuntary *eye movements*. The *pupil-*

lary light reflex was once considered also to be regulated here, but is today believed to depend on the adjacent *pretectal area*. Reflex eye movements are elicited by, among other stimuli, targets moving in the visual field. The Y system of optic nerve fibers mediates the kind of information that could most readily be decoded to detect movements. The size of the pupils is governed by the total amount of light reaching the retina. The W system is the best suited for metering light intensity. It is thus, as one might expect, that the tectal and the pretectal areas receive fibers from Y and W ganglion cells, but not from X cells.

In the most superficial (dorsal) cell layer of the superior colliculus there are neurons that respond to visual input and only visual input. Their receptive fields map visual space; that is, the superior colliculus has a retinotopic organization. A variety of response repertories have been described, but virtually all these cells have one characteristic in common: they respond maximally to stimuli moving in a particular direction. And, for most, the preferred plane of movement is horizontal, the optimal direction either from left to right or from right to left.

Deeper (more ventrally) in the tissue, cells have been found that receive convergent input from both visual and auditory pathways. In the cat and rat, some have also been found that receive in addition also tactile input mainly from the whiskers of the face. What is more, if a cell's optimal visual stimulus is an image moving from left to right, its optimal auditory stimulus will be a sound source moving in the same direction (cf. Section 12.7). If there is tactile input as well, then the preferred stimulus will be bending of the whisker, also to the right.

The neurons in the deepest layer of the superior colliculus are the output cells. Electric microstimulation in this layer causes the eyes to move toward that part of the visual field where the receptive fields of the overlying more superficial neurons are located. With an indwelling microelectrode in this layer it is possible to record the discharge of these cells while the animal moves about. The output of cells deep in a given column of the superior colliculus discharge whenever the animal turns his gaze or head toward the part of his visual field from which that column receives its input.

Thus the superior colliculus seemed programmed to alert the animal toward objects moving in his visual (and auditory) space, and then to turn toward that target. If an animal's superior colliculi are destroyed by an experimental lesion, it loses the ability to fixate his gaze at a target. It also becomes severely handicapped in using vision to guide its movements, or to learn to solve the kinds of visual riddles experimental psychologists like to pose for their animal subjects.

Much of the output of the superior colliculus is conducted to the oculomotor nuclei, consistent with its function in guiding eye movements. That the superior colliculus has other functions also is suggested by the numerous efferent fibers connecting it to the pulvinar nucleus of the thalamus. The latter is connected to the prestriate components of the visual cortex, and also to the so-called visual association areas of the inferior aspect of the temporal lobe. Input to the superior colliculus comes not only from the retina but also from the visual cortex. There are thus two-way connections between the tectum and cerebral cortex. This and other experimental data have suggested that the optic tectum may have retained some visual sensory function even in mammals. We shall return to this point when discussing the consequences for visual function of damage to the occipital lobe (see Section 10.6).

10.4. Eye Movements

The origins, insertions and innervations of the six pairs of external eye muscles are topics for anatomy courses. This information will not be repeated here.

Usually the two eyes are moved as if yoked together, in *conjunction*. Common and normal exceptions are the *vergence* movements, (convergence and divergence) necessary to look at near or at far objects. Eye movements can be smooth or sudden (*saccadic*). Eyes follow conjointly a fixated moving target in *smooth pursuit*. They jump in saccades when fixation is shifted from one target to another.

Nystagmus consists of a smooth pursuit movement in one direction, followed by a quick saccade in the opposite direction, with the two phases repeated in oscillatory fashion. Nystagmus can be evoked by movement of the visual scene, as when looking out of the window of a moving vehicle (*optokinetic* nystagmus). First the eyes follow the moving scene, then when they can go no further, the saccade brings them back to start another pursuit movement. Nystagmus can also be evoked by stimulation of the semicircular canals of the vestibular organ (see Section 13.3). When the head is being turned, optokinetic and vestibular stimulation reinforce one another.

It may be necessary to emphasize here that eye and head movements can be coordinated for two opposite purposes. When *orienting* towards a stimulus that appears in the peripheral visual field, the eyes and head turn in the same direction, both moving toward the target. When, on the other hand, the head is turned but the eyes remain fixated on a stationary target, the eyes turn in a direction opposite to the movement of the head (*compensatory eye movement*).

In addition to the just discussed types of eye movements, the eye undergoes small, barely perceptible oscillations mentioned earlier (see Section 10.2d).

It is interesting and puzzling that while the eye is moved in a saccade, vision does not become blurred. Yet if a visual target is moved in front of the eye at the same relative velocity as a saccade, a blurred image is perceived. Moreover, if a subject is making an eye movement in darkness, but a brief flash of light illuminates the scene just as he makes a saccadic eye movement, he sees a blurred image. If, however, the flash is continued for a brief time after he has completed the saccade, the perceived image is sharp, not blurred. It seems, then, that some mechanism of the central nervous system (CNS) retroactively extinguishes the blurred image before it becomes conscious, and substitutes the clear, stable image that in fact was seen only after the eyes have come to rest.

In experiments on animals, stimulation of an area rostral to the motor cortex, area 8 of Broadmann, evokes conjugate eye movements away from the stimulated side. This part of the cortex has been called the *frontal eye field* (Fig. 7.5*B*) and is considered by many to be the main coordinating area for voluntary (as opposed to reflex) eye movements.

Keeping the two eyes moving together requires delicate adjustment, guided mostly by the retinal image. For the brain to fuse the two images, visual targets have to be projected to *corresponding points* of the two retinas. The fusion process itself seems to provide the correction signals necessary for accurate conjugate movement. Thus when the two images fall out of alignment, a correction signal is apparently sent to the oculomotor system, which brings the two eyes back in line. If one eye is closed, or if it is blind, it no longer follows its sighted partner. This underscores the importance of visual input for guiding conjugate movements.

10.4a. STRABISMUS (SQUINT)*

In some people the neural mechanism yoking the two eyes fails and one of the two eyes comes to rest either turned out (*strabismus divergens*) or inward (*strabismus convergens*, or cross-eyed). Minor misalignment of the two eyes leads to minor blurring of binocular vision (heterophoria). Gross misalignment results in double vision. After a while double vision ceases because the brain suppresses the image transmitted by one of the two eyes. Usually the eye with the suppressed function is the one that becomes motionless. Some squinting individuals use alter-

* The words "to squint" have come to mean in everyday American usage to narrow the eyelids, as in "squinting against the sun." Its original meaning was "to look out of the corner of the eye," and in medical terminology it denotes misalignment of the two eyes.

nately the left and right eye, but more often one eye becomes permanently active, and the other remains permanently fixed in position with its image suppressed (the "lazy eye").

10.5. Visual Deprivation Syndromes

If vision is suppressed in a squinting eye, in the long run it deteriorates irreversibly. This condition used to be known as *amblyopia ex anopsia*, literally "dim sight from not looking." The name implies that the loss of acuity is the consequence of disuse. It has become clear recently that the two conditions, image suppression and lasting loss of visual acuity, are not directly or causally related. The neuroanatomical site and the mechanism of image suppression are not known, but we have begun to learn something about the mechanism of amblyopia.

Besides strabismus, amblyopia can be the consequence of congenital cataract and of severe refraction errors in children. If these conditions are not corrected in early childhood (by removal of the cataract or prescribing eyeglasses) visual acuity is irreversibly damaged and later treatment will fail to bring improvement. The same conditions, for example cataract, do not cause the same loss of visual acuity if the disease begins later in life. Surgical correction of late-onset cataract can be very satisfactory.

Much research has been devoted to experimental amblyopia. Kittens have been made to squint in surgical operations and the neurophysiology of their visual system was examined at variable time intervals. In another series of experiments, the eyelids of young kittens were sutured shut before they had a chance to open their eyes, or translucent shields were implanted to cover one or both eyes. In this manner the eye received diffuse light stimulation, but image formation was prevented.

No matter which method was used to prevent sharp images from being cast upon the retina, the outcome was similar. When the obstacle to vision was removed, the cats showed signs of poor visual acuity. The functions of retinal ganglion cells and of neurons in the visual cortex were also drastically altered. In the retina, the X cells of the foveal region were most affected. In the eyes that previously have been made to squint the responses of X cells to moving visual stimuli consisting of contrast patterns were degraded compared to normal eyes. Eyelid closure at an early age also caused loss of responsiveness and of stimulus discrimination by simple and by complex cells in the cerebral cortex. Such cells in visually deprived animals did not show the usual preference to a particular stimulus orientation, and their responses were feeble compared to the normals. The boundaries of the receptive fields were also less sharp than in normal cats.

The factor common to squinting and to visually deprived kittens is that the foveal region of their eyes receives no stimulation by sharply focused images. In the case of strabismus, this is because the immobile eye does not focus. Now we should add that in a squinting eye of a human patient visual acuity deteriorates mostly in the center of the visual field. In the visual periphery where acuity is poor even in normal eyes, it is not worse in squinting eyes. In the artificially squinting kittens, resolution of ganglion cells is also maximally affected in the foveal region and almost unchanged elsewhere.

When only one eye is visually deprived, the consequences for the cerebral cortex are different from those of bilateral deprivation. After monocular lid closure, the great majority of the cortical cell columns is dominated by the intact eye. Input from the deprived eye is disconnected, while input from the other eye has normal receptive field properties.

In newborn kittens who have not yet opened their eyes, there already are functioning synaptic connections from the two eyes to the cortex. The beginnings of ocular dominance columns and of the receptive field properties can be discerned, albeit in imperfect form. Visual deprivation not only prevents the normal maturation of connections but it destroys even those synaptic functions which are there at birth. In adult cats the eyes can be closed surgically for prolonged periods, and if they are opened later visual function returns to normal. In kittens the sensitive period in which disuse can permanently damage sight lasts only 12 weeks after birth. In humans the age limit until which therapeutic intervention is helpful is less precisely determined, although it obviously is longer than in kittens.

An especially striking change of visual function has been produced as follows. Kittens were reared from birth in darkness, except for set periods each day when they were placed in an illuminated drum. The walls of this drum were painted in black and white stripes, vertical for one, horizontal for another group of animals. A harness prevented the kittens from tilting their heads. Thus the visual world of these young animals consisted of nothing but vertical (or horizontal) stripes. After some months, their visual cortices were examined. The majority of cortical neurons in cats exposed to vertical stripes were optimally stimulated by vertically oriented visual stimuli, in the cats exposed to horizontal stripes, by horizontal stimuli. We should add, that the same experiment had different outcomes when other species of animals were tested. The interpretation of the data has also become controversial. Nevertheless it was an important study, because it stimulated renewed interest in the plasticity of the nervous system (see also Section 20.3).

10.6. Functional Consequences of Lesions in the Visual Pathway

If parts of the retina, optic nerve, or optic tract are destroyed the patient will not see objects in part of his visual field. If a patch of retina is missing, the resulting blind area in the visual field of one eye is called a *scotoma*. If one optic nerve is severed, then, obviously, one eye will be totally blind. If one optic tract suffers similar damage, then the vision will be lost in one half of the visual field of both eyes: *contralateral homonymous hemianopsia* (cf. Carpenter, Figs. 9.18, 9.21 and 9.22).

The deterioration of visual function that results from destruction of the occipital cortex has been well known in clinical neurology for many years. The precise nature of the visual deficit has, however, recently become controversial. The *visual agnosia* caused by damage to cortical regions other than the occipital visual receiving areas will be described elsewhere (see Section 21.2b).

Experimental lesions of the visual receiving areas have been inflicted on many animals and later these were tested in a variety of ways. Cortical damage affects different species of animals to different degrees and for this reason much caution is needed in drawing inferences from such animal experiments for human pathology. Interviewing cortically damaged human patients is not easy either. Vision is rarely the only function affected after penetrating head injuries or other conditions causing cortical damage. There seems to be a peculiar tendency on the part of some cortically injured patients either to deny their visual (and other) disabilities or to speak in vague and evasive terms about them.

A lesion in one occipital lobe affects vision in the contralateral visual field of both eyes (cf. Fig. 10.3). A small lesion will affect a small part of the visual field; total destruction of one occipital lobe will cause homonymous hemianopsia. A frequent feature of cortical hemianopia is *macular sparing*: vision in the center of the visual field often remains relatively intact. This is one reason why patients may be unaware of their defect or tend to minimize it, since they indeed may have relatively intact vision in the most important part of their visual field. The representation of the central part of the retina in the cortex is bilateral and disproportionately large, and moreover it is buried in a relatively protected position in the calcarine fissure. This explains the sparing of central vision in many patients, but in some cases the reason for it is obscure.

Cortical defects do not cause total blindness. Light, and the movement of objects, are apparently perceived, but fine details in visual stimuli are not resolved and objects are not recognized when presented within the impaired zone of the visual field. Monkeys with large bilateral occipital cortical lesions will, with much patient training, relearn to reach with precision for small objects, such as peanuts, offered within the "blinded" part of the visual field, and to perform certain other tasks for which visual guidance is needed. They will fail, however, in tasks requiring recognition of more intricate visual patterns.

One peculiarity about patients with occipital cortical injury is that they sometimes can point to, or grasp, objects they claim they cannot see. Recently such a patient on the Neurology Service of Duke University accurately threw a paper ball into a waste basket from a considerable distance. From other tests this man was judged to be nearly totally blind, and later computer-assisted tomography revealed a massive infarction of his occipital lobe that had destroyed virtually all of his visual receiving area (recounted by Dr. J. McNamara). The ability to sometimes use visual guidance in active motion by patients who do not consciously see was termed *blind sight* by Weiskrantz, the British neuro-psychologist who has defined the phenomenon. (See also Weiskrantz' paper quoted at the end of Chapter 21.)

To explain the residual visual abilities of patients and of animals who have suffered extensive damage to the occipital visual areas, some investigators suggest that visual information may reach the forebrain through a pathway other than the geniculocortical radiation. The phy-logenetically more ancient retinotectopulvinar pathway may provide this secondary input (see Section 10.3). From parts of the pulvinar nucleus there are projections to the cortical association areas of both temporal and parietal lobes. The existence of the connections linking the geniculostriate and tectopulvinar systems (see Section 10.3) under-scores this supposition. If the total visual input to the brain is inter-rupted, as is the case when an eye or an optic nerve is destroyed, then all visual functions served by that eye cease, but if only one of the two main pathways of central visual information processing and control is destroyed, either the occipital cortex or the tectum, then the deficit, though severe, is not total.

10.7. Visual Evoked Potentials (VEPs)

Potential waves evoked by sensory stimuli can be recorded from the exposed cortical surface in animals or from the scalp of patients. The electrophysiology of these electric waves was discussed in Section 2.2. To determine the waveform of VEPs, it is necessary to use computerized electronic averaging of the responses to repeated stimulation, otherwise they would be buried among EEG waves.

The visual evoked potential is, as may be expected, of maximal amplitude in the EEG leads placed over the occipital lobe of the cerebral hemisphere. A flashing light source has often been used as a visual stimulus, but an image of contrasting light and dark areas evokes a stronger cortical response. A checkerboard pattern with light and dark squares alternately illuminated (contrast reversal) is becoming the stand-ard in clinical laboratories. That patterned contrast is the best stimulus for the visual cortex should be clear from what has been said about the response properties of neurons in V-I and V-II areas (see Section 10.2a).

The amplitude of the evoked potential, as measured in recordings made from the scalp, is influenced by too many extraneous and incidental factors to be of much diagnostic significance by itself. Its latency (time from the onset of the visual stimulus until the onset of the evoked potential) and the degree of similarity of the waves recorded over the two hemispheres are, however, of clinical interest. So is any change of amplitude seen in the same patient over a period of time.

In an awake and cooperating patient, sectors of the visual field can be tested separately, provided that the patient is able to fixate an illuminated spot. The alternating checkerboard stimulus pattern may be presented to one half, a quadrant, or an octant of the visual field of either one eye or the other. Stimuli presented to left and right halves of the visual field evoke maximal responses in right and left hemispheres. If the VEP is recorded differentially between two electrodes, one placed in front of the other but both over the occipital region of the brain, then the polarity of the evoked waves is determined by whether the upper or the lower half of the visual field is stimulated. In this way the various parts of the visual pathway, representing different sectors of the visual fields, can be examined. Such a study is more objective, though less detailed, than the plotting of the visual field by perimetry. The two methods complement one another.

10.8. Chapter Summary

1. Each lateral geniculate nucleus receives input from the temporal half of the retina of the ipsilateral side and from the nasal half retina of the contralateral side. The output of each LGN is addressed to the visual cortex of the ipsilateral brain half. Thus each brain half receives visual information from the contralateral half of the visual field.
2. Most LGN cells have receptive fields that differ only in minor ways from those of retinal ganglion cells.
3. Retinotopic organization of visual input is preserved through LGN to visual cortex. The retina is mapped multiply on V-I, V-II, V-III and V-IV cortical areas, as well as on the superior colliculi.
4. Receptive fields of simple cortical cells are elongated and rectangular and are composed of excitatory and inhibitory (on and off) areas. Complex cells respond in a uniform manner to stimuli of the correct orientation falling within their receptive field.
5. Some cortical cells respond predominantly to stimulation of the ipsilateral eye, some to the contralateral eye, and some to stimulation of either eye.
6. Columnar organization of the visual cortex is the result of intersecting progressions of regularly changing ocular dominance and of optimal stimulus orientation, both superimposed on a retinopic map.

7. Depth vision is more precise when both eyes are used than when only one is.
8. Red-green and blue-yellow opponent color pairs arise as a consequence of synaptic interaction between neurons of the visual pathway. For instance, some cells that are excited by blue light falling on their receptive field are inhibited by yellow light in their receptive field; some cells that are excited by red being turned on in the receptive field center are also excited by green-off in the receptive field surround; and many other combinations of color contrast response types have been described. They can explain the psychophysical reciprocal antagonism of opponent colors. Color coded cells are found among retinal ganglion cells, LGN cells and cells of the visual cortex, in largest numbers in V-IV area.
9. Cells in the superficial layers of the superior colliculi (optic tectum) are selectively excited by visual stimuli moving in one direction. Intermediate layers contain cells on which visual, auditory, and sometimes tactile input may converge, all coded for the same direction of stimulus movement. Output cells in the deep layers seem to initiate eye movements in a given direction, in response to input reaching them via the more superficial layers.
10. Optokinetic nystagmus consists of a compensatory smooth pursuit movement by which the eyes follow a moving fixation target, followed by a saccade in the opposite direction that resets the eyes when the limit of their excursion has been reached.
11. Amblyopia may be the consequence of any affliction occurring at a young age for an extended period of time due to which the fovea centralis of one retina receives no clear image, only poorly focused or diffuse stimulation.
12. Destruction of the visual cortex of a human patient causes severe visual deficit in the contralateral half of the visual field, often with macular sparing, but does not cause total blindness in the impaired sector of the visual field.

Further Reading: Chapters 9 and 10

Books and Reviews

Bishop PO: Beginning of form vision and binocular depth discrimination in cortex. In Schmitt FO (ed): *The Neurosciences: The Second Study Program* New York, Rockefeller University Press, 1970, pp. 471–485.

Bownds MD: Molecular mechanisms of visual transduction. *Trends in Neuroscience* 4:214–217, 1981.

Carpenter MB: *Core Text of Neuroanatomy.* Baltimore, Williams & Wilkins, 1978.

Cone RA, Pak WL: The early receptor potential. In Lowenstein WR (ed): *Principles of Receptor Physiology: Handbook of Sensory Physiology,* vol 1. Berlin, Springer, 1971, pp. 345–365.

Helmholtz HLF von: *Handbuch der Physiologischen Optik,* 1856–1866. Translated: *Helmholtz's Treatise on Physiological Optics.* New York, Dover, 1962.

Ikeda H: Visual acuity. Its development and amblyopia. *J Roy Soc Med* 73:546–555, 1980.

Ratliff F: *Mach Bands: Quantitative Studies On Neural Networks in the Retina.* San Francisco, Holden-Day, 1965.

The retina and the visual system. In: Watson, JD: *The Synapse, Cold Spring Harbor Symposia on Quantitative Biology*, vol 40, pp. 521–618, 1976.

Articles

Hubel DH, Wiesel TN: Receptive fields, binocular interaction and functional architecture in the cat's visual cortex. *J Physiol Lond* 160:106–154, 1962.

Kuffler SW: Discharge patterns and functional organization of mammalian retina. *J Neurophysiol* 16:37–68, 1953.

Weiskrantz L, Warrington EK, Sanders MD et al: Visual capacity in the hemianopic field following restricted cortical ablations. *Brain* 97:709–728, 1974.

Wiesel TN, Hubel DH: Spatial and chromatic interactions in the lateral geniculate body of the rhesus monkey. *J Neurophysiol* 29:1115–1156, 1966.

Zeki S: The representation of colours in the cerebral cortex. *Nature* 284:412–418, 1980.

chapter 11

The Ear

The properties of sound waves; how sound waves set into motion the structures of middle and inner ear; how sound waves are transduced into electric signals; clinical measurement of electric signals of the cochlea.

11.1. The Properties of Sound

The reader might find it helpful to review the properties of sound waves, as discussed in any elementary college physics text, before proceeding with this chapter. The objective of your review should be to gain a clear understanding of the following points.

1. Sound waves are longitudinal vibrations. This means that the axis of translation of vibrating molecules is aligned with the direction of propagation of the sound waves. Sound waves in air consist of moving fronts of alternating compression and rarefaction. By contrast, ripples on the surface of a pond are transverse waves.

2. As sound propagates, there is no net movement of matter, particles just oscillate to and fro. The waves propagate, nevertheless, because each oscillating particle sets its neighbor into motion which, in its turn, causes its neighbor to vibrate, and so on. Where there is net movement of mass, we speak of a current, or of streaming, or of wind.

3. The velocity of sound is independent of its wavelength but is influenced by the medium within which it propagates. The denser the medium, the faster the velocity of propagation. In air at sea level sound is conducted at a rate of 340 m/sec (in round numbers); in water about four times faster. Currents in the

medium alter the apparent velocity. (Sound is carried by wind.) Movement of the sound source alters the frequency perceived by a stationary observer (Doppler effect), but not the velocity of propagation.

4. Energy is required to initiate sound waves. As it propagates, sound dissipates energy as heat. Eventually sound waves "die out" or, in technical language, are damped. Heat energy resides in matter in the form of Brownian motion, which differs from sound vibration in that each particle moves about at random, and independently of its neighbors. The amplitude of sound waves is moreover, generally greater than that of Brownian motion, although this need not always be the case, as we shall see later.

5. The wavelength of sound waves is given by the velocity of propagation divided by the frequency: $\lambda = v/f$.

6. When sound waves reach a solid object, they set it into oscillation; this is *resonance*. To the degree that an object is elastic, it will also tend to oscillate when struck by another solid object (think of drums, bells, wine glasses). The frequency at which an object tends to oscillate is called its *resonant frequency*. Objects resonate at the greatest amplitude when sound waves of their own resonant frequency reach them. Note that all solid objects resonate to some degree, but only some have a particularly well-defined characteristic resonant frequency.

7. If sound waves in air reach the surface of a fluid or solid, part of the energy is absorbed and part is reflected (*echo*). Transmission of sound energy from one medium to another is resisted, and this resistance is expressed as the ratio of the impedances of the two media.

11.2. Psychophysics of Hearing

A vast amount of literature deals with man's perception of sound, which is reviewed in college textbooks of psychology. Here only those aspects of this topic can be summarized which pertain most directly to auditory physiology.

Sounds that can be described by a simple sine wave function are rare. All sounds can, however, be considered to be the composite of a number of different frequencies. *Tones* are sounds composed of sine waves of a single *fundamental frequency* and of its simple arithmetic multiples called *harmonics*. Mixtures of harmonically unrelated frequencies are called *noises*. Human speech is always noise.

The perceived pitch, or height, of a tone is determined mainly, though not entirely, by its fundamental frequency. The perceived loudness of a tone of given frequency is determined by the amplitude of the sound waves as they reach the hearing organ. If, however, two tones differing in both amplitude and frequency are compared, then perceived loudness becomes a joint function of both amplitude and frequency. This is because the sensitivity of the ear varies for different frequencies (Fig. 11.1). Of two tones equal in amplitude but different in frequency, the

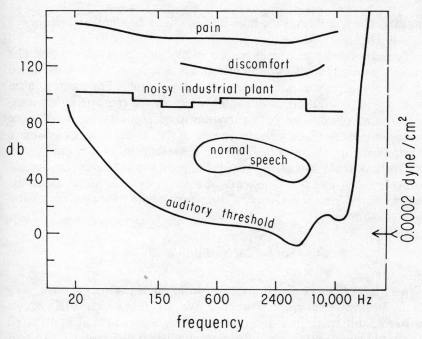

Figure 11.1. Auditory thresholds as function of sound frequency. Note that both *abscissa* and *ordinate* are scaled logarithmically. (Compiled from various sources.) The threshold of "discomfort" is highly variable, but the threshold of pain, that is of a pricking sensation felt in the eardrum, can be determined rather precisely.

one to which the ear is more sensitive will be heard louder. The human ear is most sensitive to tones of about 3000 Hz (hertz = cycles per second).

For man the audible spectrum ranges from about 20 to about 20,000 Hz. It must be said, however, that these are the outer limits, and many people, especially those not so young, have difficulty hearing any sound of frequency higher than 10,000 or 15,000 Hz. Dogs, on the other hand, hear well up to about 40,000 Hz and some bats over 100,000 Hz. Vibrations of frequencies higher than the human audible spectrum are termed *ultrasonic*.

In music if the frequency of one tone is the double of another, the two are said to be one octave apart. Tones separated by an octave sound similar not only to musically trained people but also, to a lesser degree, to cats. The A4 note on the musical scale has a fundamental frequency of 440 Hz.

Sound intensity can be expressed in absolute or relative units. The most commonly used absolute measure is the pressure variation caused by the sound waves, ΔP, expressed in dynes$\cdot$cm^{-2}. For most medical and psychophysical applications, however, sound pressure is not measured in absolute terms but in relation to an arbitrary standard. Since sound energy declines with the square of the distance, it is customary to indicate its intensity as it is at the eardrum of the subject. A logarithmic scale is used. A 10-fold change in sound energy (i.e. one log unit) is called one *bel*. One-tenth of a bel is a *decibel* (db). Since the energy varies with the square of the pressure, the following expression is obtained:

$$\text{Relative sound energy in db} = 20 \log_{10} \frac{\Delta P}{\Delta P_{st}}$$

Where ΔP is the measured pressure variation of the sound wave, ΔP_{st} is the arbitrary standard, or reference level. In other words, 20 db equals a 10-fold difference in sound pressure level, abbreviated SPL; 40 db (2 log units) equal a 100-fold difference; and 10 db (0.5 units) a 3.16-fold difference in sound pressure. The standard may be the "threshold" intensity for human hearing, in which case the reference varies with the tone frequency (see Fig. 11.14). In other cases, a fixed reference may be chosen, for instance of 1.0 dyne$\cdot$cm^{-2}, or any other arbitrary level (Fig. 11.1). When comparing audiological data from different publications, it is advisable to read the small print because the reference levels need not be the same, and thus the same numbers of decibels may mean different absolute intensities.

Harmonic mixtures make up musical tones, as already mentioned. The "quality" or "color" of the tones produced by musical instruments depends, in part, on the admixture of harmonics and, in part, on the envelope of intensity transients, in other words on the way the tone builds and then dies down. From these characteristics it is possible to recognize a particular musical instrument and still identify the same tone produced by two different instruments as having the same height.

Even though noises are not composed of harmonics, they can have a characteristic "height" if one particular frequency dominates. Noise of random composition and a wide frequency band is called "white."

11.3. Functions of the Middle Ear

Man's outer ears (pinnae) have often been belittled as being of little real use and faintly comical in appearance. Certainly the ears of cats and horses (for example) are far more efficient funnels of sound. Recent measurements and calculations have, however, restored some dignity to our own external ears. If not the pinna, then at least the outer auditory meatus apparently has just the right proportions to aid sound waves in setting the tympanic membrane in motion. The major credit for making hearing possible must go, however, to the middle ear, not to the outer ear.

The different impedances of air and of the fluids filling the cochlea poses a problem. Air is rare and the aqueous solutions of the inner ear are dense by comparison. If the two media were in direct contact, 99.9% of the incident sound energy would be reflected from the liquid surface (cf. Section 11.1, point 7).

The middle ear is a small air-filled chamber between the eardrum (tympanic membrane) and the inner ear, which houses the three auditory ossicles (Fig. 11.2). In it we also find two tiny muscles, the tensor tympani which pulls the tympanic membrane inward, and the musculus stapedius which pulls the stapes sideways and slightly outward. Therefore, contractions of the stapedius muscle partially counteract those of the tensor tympani. In some species the two middle ear muscles always contract simultaneously. In man, it is mainly the stapedius that contracts

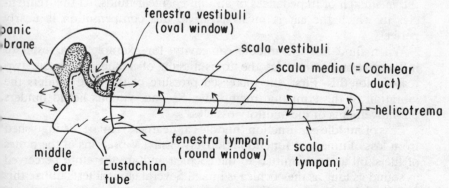

Figure 11.2. The transmission of vibrations through the middle and inner ear. The cochlea is depicted as though it were straight. (The scala vestibuli is separated from the scala media by Reissner's membrane, the scala media from scala tympani by the basilar membrane; see also Fig. 11.3.)

when the stimulus is a loud noise; but both muscles contract during generalized muscle tension, as in alerting or emotional excitement. In any case, contraction of either or both middle ear muscles stiffens the sound-transmitting system, attenuating its vibration. This has a protective function, which is more effective against low-frequency vibrations than against high frequencies.

It is well worth remembering that the tensor tympani is innervated by the Vth cranial nerve, the stapedius by the VIIth nerve. If one of the two nerves is injured, the unopposed muscle with intact innervation will cause the tympanic membrane to bulge or to sink, as the case might be. This causes some hearing loss, especially for low tones.

As sound is transmitted from tympanic membrane to the membrane of the oval window by the three auditory ossicles, its pressure is amplified for several reasons. First, the surface area of the tympanic membrane is some 26 times larger than that of the oval window: the same force concentrated on a smaller surface yields more pressure. Since, however, the entire surface of the tympanic membrane does not vibrate uniformly, the gain is somewhat less than would be expected from the ratio of surface areas. Second, there is leverage, because the movement of the long handle of the malleus is transmitted to the shorter arm of the incus, yielding an additional gain by a factor of about 1.3. Besides, because the tympanic membrane is curved, intricate patterns of vibrations are generated, distributing energy so that the maximum is imparted to the malleus. All this amplification of pressure is required to compensate for the mismatch of impedances of air and cochlear fluids. At the frequencies to which the ear is most sensitive, this compensation is nearly perfect.

When fluid fills the middle ear cavity, for example as a result of inflammation, it impedes the transmission of sound. There are two reasons for this. First, the increased pressure of the fluid hinders the vibration of the tympanic membrane. Second, viscous liquid hinders the movements of the auditory ossicles.

Loss of middle ear function (middle ear deafness) can be distinguished from loss of inner ear function relatively easily. Vibrations of the bones of the skull are transmitted to the cochlea and are therefore perceived as sound as long as the cochlea is intact. Several clinical tests utilize this fact. For example, to examine unilateral deafness, a tuning fork is placed in contact with the center of the forehead of the patient (Weber's test). If the deafness is caused by a defect of the cochlea, the patient perceives the sound as coming from the "good" ear (lateralization); if it is caused by a defect of the middle ear, the patient lateralizes the sound to the "bad" ear (which is favored by bone conduction).

Preserved *bone conduction* of sound can also be exploited with hearing aids for chronically damaged middle ears. For this purpose the sound-emitting device of the hearing aid must vibrate the skull at or near the temporal bone.

11.4. The Cochlea

The bony cochlea is coiled in the manner of a snail's shell. In man it has 2½ turns and a total length of 35 mm. This bony canal encloses three parallel membranous channels which follow the 2½ turns. The two outer channels, the *scala vestibuli* and *scala tympani*, communicate with each other at the tip of the snail's shell, the *helicotrema*. The middle channel, the *scala media* or *cochlear duct* ends there blindly (Fig. 11.2). Scala vestibuli and scala tympani are filled with perilymph, a fluid similar in composition to extracellular fluid elsewhere in the body, and having the attributes of a filtrate of plasma. There is, however, a narrow channel between the perilymphatic space and cerebrospinal fluid (CSF): the cochlear aqueduct. In autopsy specimens it is patent to varying degrees. If it is open during life, then some limited exchange between CSF and perilymph must occur, but not enough to allow equilibration of solutes.

The scala media contains endolymph which, unlike all other extracellular fluids, is rich in K^+ and poor in Na^+. Endolymph is believed to be secreted by epithelial cells lining the *stria vascularis* and to be absorbed into the bloodstream in the endolymphatic sac. An alternative theory proposes that endolymph is secreted through the Reissner membrane, utilizing perilymph as raw material, and is absorbed in the stria vascularis.

Reissner's membrane separates the scala media from the scala vestibuli; the basilar membrane separates scala media and scala tympani (Fig. 11.3). The former is quite thin, but the latter is a substantial ribbon of tissue. One edge of the basilar membrane is attached to a bony shelf, the spiral lamina, that follows the turns of the cochlea. On the opposite side, the spiral ligament attaches the basilar membrane to the wall of the bony cochlea. Even though the bony canal is widest in the first,

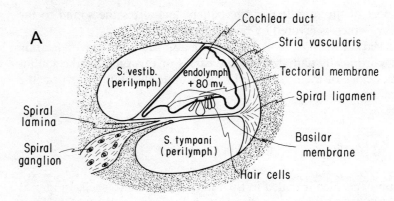

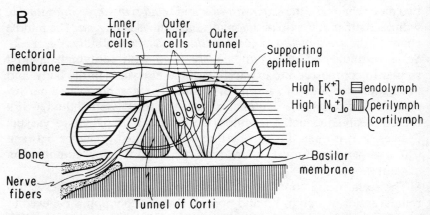

Figure 11.3. Fluid spaces, receptor cells and nerve fibers in the cochlea. *A*, cross-section of the cochlea; *B*, enlarged portion of *A*, showing the organ of Corti and associated structures. The boundary of the endolymphatic space is indicated by the *heavy line* in *A* and *B*.

most basal* turn, the basilar membrane is narrower near the base than at the apex of the cochlea. This is so because the bony spiral lamina narrows from base toward apex so that more room is left for the membranous basilar membrane near the top.

* A source of much confusion is this: the *base* of the cochlea is the widest part of the snail's shell where the first turn abuts the middle ear. Its apex is its narrow tip. The *basilar* membrane does *not* derive its name from *base*; it is a narrow ribbon running the entire length of the cochlea from base to apex (Figs. 11.2 and 11.3).

The sensitive elements, the transducers of sound, are the so-called hair cells. These ciliated cells are attached to the basilar membrane embedded among supporting cells of several types, the name of each commemorating a distinguished histologist. There is also a narrow canal-within-a-canal, the tunnel of Corti (Fig. 11.3B). Some investigators believe that the tunnel is filled with perilymph, others that it has its own fluid, cortilymph. It generally is assumed, however, that the tunnel does *not* contain endolymph. Why this needs emphasis will become clear soon.

The hair cells form a single inner and three outer rows on the two sides of the tunnel of Corti. Covering them is the thick tectorial membrane, which either rests on or actually is embedding the tips of the cilia. Hair cells form synaptic contacts with the nerve endings of the fibers of the VIIIth nerve (see Figs. 11.3 and 11.8).

11.4a. MECHANICS OF COCHLEAR VIBRATION

Ever since it was realized (1) that sound is sensed in the inner ear and (2) that sound consists of vibration, scientists have searched for resonant structures in the inner ear. Speculation about the role of resonance began more than 300 years ago, but it was in the 19th century that the first realistic scientific theory of cochlear function was formulated. Ohm (the same man who gave us the law of electric current) suggested that the essence of auditory function is Fourier analysis of the complex waveforms of natural sounds. By this he meant that the ear extracts from complex sound waves the component frequencies. Helmholtz thought of a way in which the structures of the inner ear could do this. He saw the basilar membrane as a series of transversely stretched bands, similar to the strings of a piano, each with its own characteristic resonant frequency. The resonant frequency would be high at the base of the cochlea, where the basilar membrane is taut and narrow, and low where it is broad and slack near the apex. Wherever the basilar membrane vibrates maximally, the hair cells attached to it would be maximally excited. The hair cells in turn stimulate the endings of the VIIIth nerve. Consequently the fibers of the VIIIth nerve with terminals at the base of the cochlea would be maximally stimulated by high-frequency sound waves, those with endings in the apical portion of the basilar membrane, by low frequencies.

Actual measurements of the vibratory motion of the basilar membrane by Békésy proved Helmholtz right in essence, but wrong in certain important details. What follows is a simplified summary of the current consensus concerning the mechanical behavior of the organ of Corti.

When sound pressure pushes the tympanic membrane inward, the motion is transmitted through the middle ear, and the stapes presses on the membrane of the oval window. Pressure then rises in the fluid filling the scala tympani and is transmitted through both Reissner's membrane and the basilar membrane (and to a lesser degree through the helico-trema) to the fluid in the scala tympani. Consequently, to the extent that the membrane of the oval window moves inward, the membrane of the round window (at the end of the scala tympani) moves outward (bulges into the middle ear cavity) (Fig. 11.2). Inward-outward motion of these membranes repeats itself at the same frequency as that of the sound stimulus.

As a consequence, oscillatory pressure waves act on the basilar membrane. The basilar membrane is elastic and has inertia and hence momentum, so it will, under the influence of oscillating pressure, begin to vibrate also. Since the basilar membrane is stiffer at its narrow, basal end than at its wide, apical end, ripples will run from its base to its apex (Fig. 11.4). This is so even when, in an experiment, a vibrating micro-stylus is applied to the apical end of the basilar membrane. The *traveling*

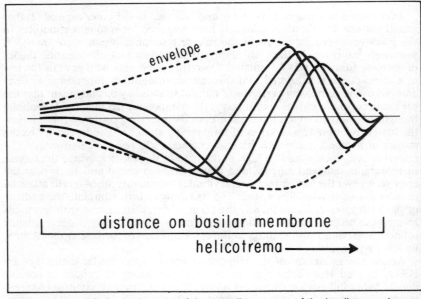

Figure 11.4. Békésy's diagram of the traveling waves of the basilar membrane. The four *solid lines* show the positions of the vibrating basilar membrane as though frozen at four successive moments in time. The *dashed lines* plot the points of maximal excursion of the vibrating membrane. This diagram is not drawn to scale; vertical distances (vibration amplitudes) are vastly exaggerated in comparison to horizontal distances (positions on basilar membrane).

waves stubbornly move from base to apex, in this experiment toward the vibrating stylus which set the membrane in motion in the first place.

Under normal conditions, traveling waves are, of course, started by the motions of the footplate of the stapes, and they would run from base to apex even if there were no gradient of stiffness at all. The strictly one-way traffic does become important, however, when the middle ear is put out of commission and hearing must depend on bone conduction. Even then, without benefit of a moving stapes, the cochlea receives auditory stimulation patterned in the usual way.

The stability of the pattern of traveling waves was also exploited in the surgical treatment for *otosclerosis*. In this condition the footplate of the stapes is fixed to the rim of the oval window by excess connective tissue. Instead of transmitting sound, the stapes then acts as a brake, preventing vibrations in the cochlea. In the operation called *fenestration*, the surgeon makes a new, artificial window between the cochlea and middle ear, at the level of the second turn, and covers it with a membrane transplant. The rationale of this operation was that the round window can substitute for the oval window, provided that there is "give" at some point in the hydraulic system. In these patients transmission from tympanic membrane to the round window is through the air (*the aerotympanic effect*) which is much less efficient than through the normal route of the auditory ossicles, but better than no transmission at all. Fenestration has been largely supplanted by the more modern technique of replacing the stapes with a prosthesis. It has been mentioned here only to illustrate the mechanical principles involved.

That the basilar membrane is stiffer at one end than at the other has yet one even more important consequence. The membrane is stiffest at the point nearest to the oval window, where it is also the narrowest, therefore has the least mass per unit length. Low mass and high stiffness combine so that here the membrane vibrates by preference at high frequencies. Thus high-frequency vibrations will have their maximal amplitude near where the waves start to travel, will soon dissipate most of their energy, and then die out on the way, never to reach the apex. Low-frequency vibrations, on the contrary, will start small and increase in amplitude on their way to the apex (Fig. 11.5*A*).

Three points must be clarified here. First, traveling waves are to be distinguished from standing waves. In standing waves, adjacent points oscillate *in phase* except at points of phase reversal (so called nodal points) and these points of phase reversal remain stationary. Vibrations of violin strings are standing waves. In the case of traveling waves (such as the ripples on the surface of a

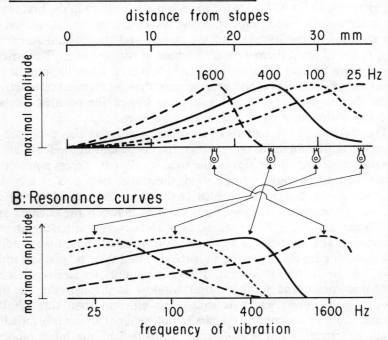

Figure 11.5. The vibrations acting on hair cells at different points along the basilar membrane. *A*, half-envelopes of maximal vibrations (cf. Fig. 11.4) during stimulation with pure tones of four different frequencies. *B*, relative amplitudes of vibration as functions of auditory frequency, plotted for hair cells located at four different points along the basilar membrane. (Compare these idealized curves with one based on actual measurement, shown as line *1* of Fig. 11.12.)

pond) there is a continuous phase shift of the motion of adjacent points; this is the very reason that the waves appear to travel (Fig. 11.6).

The next point in need of clarification: there is a difference between the velocity of the pressure wave imparted to the fluids of the inner ear by the thrust of the stapes and the velocity of the wave traveling on the basilar membrane. The pressure wave moves with the speed of sound in water and reaches the apex in microseconds. The peaks and troughs of the oscillations of the basilar membrane travel much more slowly and cover the distance from base to apex in 2–5 msec.

Finally, one more point: the waves traveling on the basilar membrane do not cause a net displacement of fluid between scala media and scala tympani. As much as the peaks of a traveling wave move fluid in one direction, the valleys

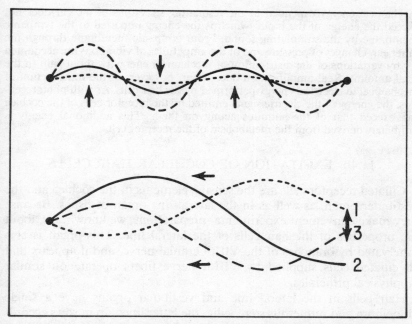

Figure 11.6. Comparing the motions of a string vibrating in a standing-wave pattern (*top*) and in traveling-wave pattern (*bottom*). In both diagrams, the three lines (*dotted*, *solid* and *dashed*) represent three successive moments in time.

move it in the other (Fig. 11.4). To be sure, the movements of stapes do cause some net displacement of fluid: from scala vestibuli into scala tympani when the membrane of the oval window moves inward, and in the reverse direction when it moves outward (Fig. 11.2). These displacements involve the basilar membrane and are added to the movements caused by the traveling waves. Since, however, the surface area of the oval window is many times smaller than the surface area of the basilar (and Reissner's) membrane (Fig. 11.2), these net displacements are minute, much smaller than the amplitudes of the traveling waves. Since, moreover, the net displacements are driven by the pressure waves, and since the pressure waves are conducted much faster than the traveling waves, the net displacements occur virtually in phase over the entire surface of the basilar membrane.

The traveling waves of the basilar membrane are thus not hydraulically driven as are the pistons in the brakes of an automobile. Rather, the motions of the basilar membrane are resonant motions whose frequency is set by the input frequency (the stimulating sound); their amplitude and pattern of distribution is determined by the mechanical properties of the membrane itself: its mass, elasticity and stiffness.

At the peril of stressing the obvious, I should add that the sum total of the mechanical energy expended in the resonating structures of the ear does not exceed the energy of the input, which is the energy imparted to the tympanic membrane by the stimulating sound. From tympanic membrane through the inner ear, changes of pressure and of the amplitudes of vibrations are accounted for by variations of the distribution of mechanical energy, without gain in the total amount. Real amplification does occur, however, in the transduction of mechanical to electrical energy performed by the hair cells. As with photoreceptors, the energy of the electric signal emitted by the receptor cells of the cochlea can exceed that of the stimulus acting on them. This additional energy is ultimately derived from the metabolism of the receptor cell.

11.4b. EXCITATION OF COCHLEAR HAIR CELLS

Ciliated receptor cells are the sensing elements in the cochlea and the vestibular organ, as well as in the lateral line organ of fishes. Because they make convenient experimental preparations, we know most about the properties of the hair cells of the lateral line. This organ is also innervated by branches of the VIIIth cranial nerve, and it appears that all ciliated cells supplied by VIIIth nerve fibers operate on similar biophysical principles.

Hair cells in the lateral line and vestibular organs have a single kinocilium and numerous stereocilia, the latter lined up in rows according to size. The hair cells of the cochlea, however, lack the kinocilium; only the basal body can be found where the kinocilium should be (Fig. 8.1D). In all hair cells the bending of the stereocilia causes a change in membrane potential: bending toward the kinocilium (or basal body) causes depolarization; bending in the opposite direction, hyperpolarization.

In the cochlea the cilia of hair cells are bent when the upper surface of the hair cells slides relative to the tectorial membrane. Two models have been proposed to explain this. One is based on the assumption that the tectorial membrane is fastened at one edge and free at the other. When the basilar membrane vibrates, the underside of the tectorial membrane rubs on the upper surface of the hair cells (Fig. 11.7). This relative motion may be visualized with the help of a soft-cover book. When such a book is bent, the pages slide one upon the other. Like the basilar membrane, the pages of the book are held fast on one side by the binding and are free on the other.

Some anatomists hold, however, that the tectorial membrane is anchored at both sides. If so, then the tectorial membrane can slide over the cilia of the hair cells only if the vibrating tissue is alternately stretched and compressed.

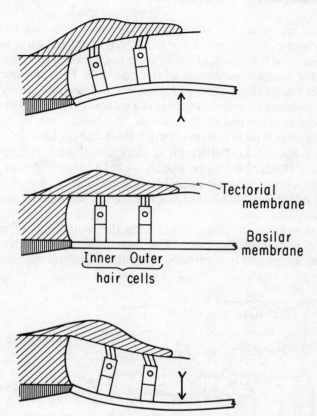

Figure 11.7. How the vibrations of the basilar membrane cause shearing motion between tectorial membrane and the upper surface of the hair cells. Note that outer hair cells are exposed to more intense stimulation than inner hair cells. (Modified and redrawn after R. Klinke: Physiology of hearing. In *Fundamentals of Sensory Physiology*, edited by R. F. Schmidt. New York, Springer, 1978, pp. 180–204.)

Until recently, the resonance of the tectorial membrane and of the cilia themselves have been largely neglected in theoretical treatment of the cochlea. Reasons are now emerging that suggest that these may be quite important for determining the excitation of hair cells.

11.4c. ELECTROPHYSIOLOGY OF THE COCHLEA

Intracellular recordings from individual hair cells have shown that during auditory stimulation the membrane potential undergoes oscillations which reproduce the vibrations of the sound stimulus. In addition to these electric oscillations, there is a steady depolarization and, associated with it, a reduction in membrane resistance. These are components of the receptor potentials of the hair cells. How the movements of the cilia causes these electric changes has not been determined.

In the inner ear of mammals there is a standing potential between the scala media and the rest of the cochlea, the endolymph being electropositive by 80 mV relative to perilymph; this is the *cochlear DC potential* (Figs. 11.3 and 11.8). Perilymph is isopotential with the rest of the extracellular fluids of the body. The cochlear DC potential is an example of a secretory potential; it probably is generated by the electrogenic transport of K^+ ions that maintains the high K^+ activity in endolymph (see Section 2.4a).

There is some uncertainty concerning the boundaries of endolymphatic and perilymphatic spaces. The interstitial spaces of the tectorial membrane are probably permeated by endolymph, and the cilia and the

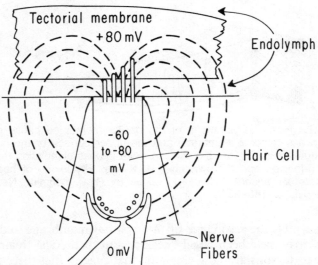

Figure 11.8. Current flow around an excited hair cell. Bending of the cilia caused by the shearing motions of the tectorial membrane (Fig. 11.7) cause variations of the electric resistance of the ciliated surface of the hair cell. These variations of resistance cause variations of current flow between the body of the hair cell and its ciliated upper surface. The currents flow along the *dashed lines* of the diagram, traversing the VIIIth nerve terminals.

upper surface of the hair cells are bathed in endolymph (Figs. 11.3B and 11.8). The remainder of each hair cell is probably surrounded by either perilymph or cortilymph, but in any event by a fluid rich in Na^+ and poor in K^+. Otherwise it would be hard to understand how hair cells and nerve fiber terminals sustain a normal membrane potential. Other excitable cells lose resting potential when submerged in a medium containing too much K^+ (see Sections 2.4b and 3.4a).

The boundary between endolymphatic and perilymphatic spaces is thus apparently level with the upper end of the hair cells at the reticular lamina. One then must expect a diffusion barrier to exist here, as well as in Reissner's membrane. The structure, permeability and transport properties of these barriers are not completely understood.

Since the intracellular potential of the hair cells is 70–90 mV negative relative to perilymph, and since endolymph is 60–80 mV positive, the total potential drop across the cilia-bearing membrane at the upper end of the hair cells is some 160 mV. This unusually steep potential gradient may have some significance for the transducing function of the hair cells. If so, this is not an essential factor, for in birds the endocochlear potential is only 4 or 5 mV and they nevertheless hear well. In birds, however, as in mammals, the endolymph contains more K^+ than Na^+.

Unlike the positive potential, the high K^+ content of the endolymph is essential for the well-being of the tissues of the organ of Corti and also of the vestibular sensory epithelia. If, in an experiment, a hole is made in Reissner's membrane so that perilymph contaminates the fluid in the cochlear duct, hair cells lose their function and become visibly damaged. The same happens if the endolymph is replaced by Ringer's solution.

During stimulation by sound, the living cochlea generates oscillating electric potentials. With proper amplification these oscillations can be recorded at some distance, for example, from the outer surface of the eardrum (Fig. 11.9), but optimally they are picked up by differential recording between two electrodes, one in the scala vestibuli, the other in the scala tympani. These alternating potentials reproduce precisely the waveform of the stimulating sound, and have, therefore, been called *cochlear microphonic potentials* (see Fig. 11.10).

The cochlear microphonic is the extracellularly recorded counterpart of the oscillating receptor potential of the hair cells. The mechanical equipment of the cochlea also generates electric oscillations by a kind of piezoelectric effect, but these are much weaker than the cochlear microphonic.

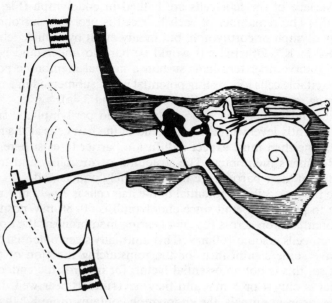

Figure 11.9. The method of clinical electrocochleography. The electric responses of the cochlea may be recorded either with an electrode in contact with the tympanic membrane, or with a needle electrode inserted through the tympanic membrane until it makes contact with the promontory in the wall of the middle ear. (Reprinted with permission from J. J. Eggermont and D. W. Odenthal: *Acta Otolaryngologica, Supplement (Stockholm)* 316:17–24, 1974.)

If the cochlear microphonic is recorded from within the cochlea (rather than from the middle ear or outer ear canal), then its amplitude will vary with the sound frequency and with the position of the electrode. In the first (basal) turn of the cochlea high tones evoke maximal microphonics, in the third (apical) turn, low tones. There is also a phase difference: the basal turn leads (is phase-advanced) relative to the apical turn. Thus the cochlear microphonic follows the motions of the basilar membrane, as it should if what we have said so far about the excitation of hair cells is true.

With appropriate (DC-coupled) amplifiers, the cochlear microphonic oscillations appear to "ride" on a sustained shift of electric potential. This shift has been called the *summating potential* (see Fig. 11.10). It, too, is generated by the hair cells, presumably by the sustained component of the receptor potential.

Recorded response

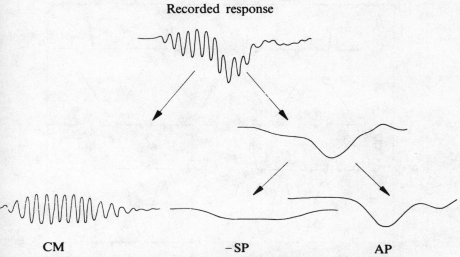

CM   −SP   AP

Figure 11.10. Potentials recorded by the method illustrated in Figure 11.9. The cochlear microphonic (*CM*), summating potential (*SP*) and auditory nerve action potential (*AP*) can be derived from analysis of the recorded response. (Reprinted with permission from J. J. Eggermont: *Acta Otolaryngologica, Supplement (Stockholm)* 316:7–16, 1974.)

Recording cochlear potentials in human patients for clinical diagnosis is a relatively recent innovation (Figs. 11.9 and 11.10) gradually gaining acceptance. It should prove invaluable in the diagnosis of hearing impairment in infants. Using brief stimuli, the action potential of the VIIIth nerve can also be recorded separately from the cochlear microphonic. This is a help in differentiating the deafness caused by degeneration of VIIIth nerve terminals from deafness caused by damage to hair cells.

11.4d. TRANSMISSION OF EXCITATION FROM HAIR CELLS TO VIIITH NERVE ENDINGS

As shown in Figures 11.3*B* and 11.8, hair cells form synaptic contacts with the afferent terminals of the auditory nerve fibers. The morphology of these synapses suggests the operation of a chemical transmitter substance.

In the absence of any sound, many fibers of the auditory nerve fire impulses at a low frequency and irregular intervals. Under the influence of sound, the

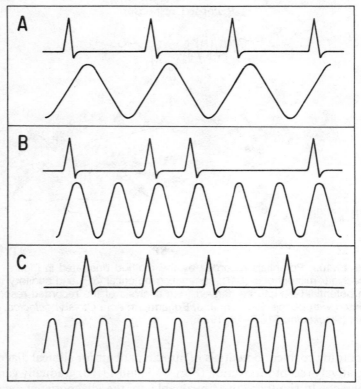

Figure 11.11. Comparing entrainment (*A*) with phase locking (*B*) and independent firing (*C*). In each diagram the *upper tracing* represents nerve impulses, the *lower tracing* the vibrations of the stimulus, and the *abscissa* is time.

frequency of discharge increases. Not all auditory nerve fibers respond, however, to all audible sound frequencies. The "tuning" of VIIIth nerve units is the subject of the next section.

With low-frequency, high-intensity tones, the discharge of auditory nerve fibers can follow the frequency of the stimulating sound in a manner similar to the response of the Pacinian corpuscles to vibrating mechanical stimuli (Fig. 6.8). This is called *entrainment*. With frequencies of the middle range of the audible spectrum (roughly 200–2000 Hz) the impulses are no longer entrained by the input, but impulses can still be *locked to* a particular *phase* of the vibration. At yet higher frequencies phase locking is lost, and impulses are fired without a constant relationship to the phase of the input sound (Fig. 11.11). It was mentioned earlier (see Section 11.4b) that cochlear hair cells are depolarized when their cilia are bent toward the basal body. The fact that impulses in auditory nerve fibers are phase-locked to the auditory stimulus suggests that the transmission of excitation from hair cell to nerve fibers is closely linked to the waves of depolarization of the hair cells. The question is, what is the mechanism of transmission between hair cells and nerve endings?

All known chemically transmitting synaptic terminals require calcium for the release of transmitter, and all can be blocked by excess Mg^{2+} or Mn^{2+} (see Section 3.2). Experiments have been performed in which perilymph of the scala tympani was replaced by fluid deficient of Ca^{2+}, or enriched with Mg^{2+} or Mn^{2+}. This treatment abolished the "spontaneous" ("resting") discharge of nerve impulses in auditory nerve fibers, and it also blocked the transmission of excitation in response to high-frequency tones. Low-frequency input was still able to excite the nerve fibers, albeit more weakly than in the normal condition.

From these experiments the following picture emerges. The "resting" discharge of auditory fibers can no longer be considered spontaneous, rather it seems to be the consequence of a continuous low-level release of excitatory transmitter in the absence of auditory stimulation. During auditory stimulation, the steady (non-oscillating) depolarization of hair cells may be the signal for the influx of Ca^{2+} into hair cells, and hence for the increased release of excitatory transmitter. While chemical transmission is the only mechanism that is effective during high-frequency stimulation, with low-frequency tones, chemical transmission is supplemented by electric current. The current is supplied by the oscillating receptor potential of the hair cells, and the same alternating current is registered by recording electrodes as the cochlear microphonic potential. As it flows through the nerve endings (Fig. 11.8) this alternating current will now add to, and then subtract from, the depolarization caused by the chemical transmitter. Impulses are likely to be fired when the microphonic current is in the depolarizing direction, hence phase locking.

11.4e. THE TUNING OF AUDITORY RECEPTORS AND NERVE FIBERS

The excitation of a hair cell is, in large measure, determined by the excursions of the basilar membrane. Because, as we have seen, at different points the amplitude of the vibrations of the basilar membrane varies with the stimulus frequency, the degree to which a given hair cell is excited is a joint function of its position on the membrane and the sound frequency. For example, never in a lifetime will a hair cell near the apex of the cochlea experience a high-frequency vibration, because high-frequency waves do not travel that far (see Section 11.4a and Fig. 11.5). A hair cell in the first turn of the cochlea will, however, receive both high and low frequencies, but high frequencies will excite it more vigorously than low frequencies.

The maximal excursions of the basilar membrane have been plotted as a function of distance from the stapes, for tones of equal intensity but varying frequency. Such plots are termed the *envelopes* of the traveling wave. Fig. 11.5 shows examples. Using the data needed for the construction of such envelopes, one can also plot the relative amplitudes of the excursions for given points on the basilar membrane as a function of input frequency. These are the mechanical tuning curves (or resonance curves) of points on the basilar membrane (Fig. 11.5).

The resonance curve of the basilar membrane would accurately describe the excitation of hair cells as a function of frequency, if it were the only factor influencing the vibration of the cilia. In reality, however, as we have already hinted, the mechanical properties of the cilia and of the tectorial membrane covering them also enter into the equation. For example, the stiffness of the cilia varies from one end of the basilar membrane to the other. The mass and elasticity of the tectorial membrane also vary. The resonance of the hair cell-tectorial membrane complex has the effect of limiting the "tuning" of hair cells to a narrower band width of frequencies than that of the point of the basilar membrane to which the cell is attached (Fig. 11.12).

The fibers of the auditory division of the VIIIth nerve have been divided by anatomists into two classes. The so-called radial fibers are in synaptic contact with the inner hair cells. The ratio of inner hair cells to radial nerve fibers is less than 1: each nerve fiber contacts but one hair cell, but each hair cell is innervated by endings of more than one nerve fiber. The spiral fibers cross the floor of the tunnel of Corti and innervate the outer hair cells. There are many more outer hair cells than spiral fibers. These nerve fibers run some distance following the curvature of the cochlea (hence the name "spiral"), and on their way divide into branches, each axon making contact with numerous hair cells.

Outer hair cells are located farther from the attachment of the basilar membrane to the bony spiral lamina than the inner hair cells. Outer hair cells are, therefore, subjected to larger excursions of the membrane than the inner ones (Fig. 11.7).

These anatomical arrangements seemed to suggest two conclusions: (1) that spiral nerve fibers should be more "broadly tuned" than radial fibers because they receive excitation from a wide expanse of the basilar membrane, whereas radial fibers are influenced only from the point occupied by one hair cell; and (2) that spiral fibers should have a lower threshold than radial fibers, since outer hair cells receive more energetic vibrations than inner hair cells (Fig. 11.7).

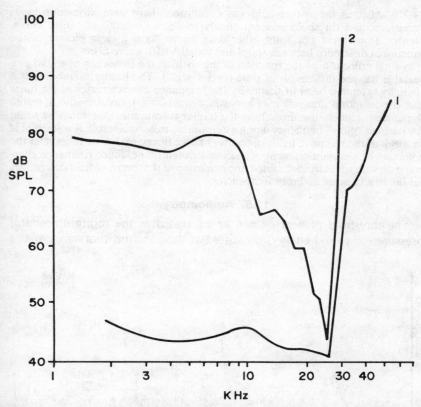

Figure 11.12.   The resonance curve of a point on the basilar membrane (*1*) and the tuning curve of a nerve fiber innervating a hair cell at that point (*2*). The resonance curve (*1*) shows the relative sound pressure levels (*SPL*) required to vibrate the membrane at that point to a given amplitude at various frequencies of sound; the tuning curve (*2*) shows the threshold of the nerve fiber to sound stimuli of varying frequency. Note that curves *1* and *2* have similar high-frequency cutoffs, but on the low-frequency side curve *2* is much steeper than curve *1*. (Reprinted with permission from J. R. Johnstone: *Trends in Neuroscience* 4:106–109, 1981.)

Examination of the physiological properties of a great many auditory nerve fibers by numerous teams of investigators has so far not found two such clearly distinct classes of nerve fibers. Generally the fibers with high "best frequencies" had narrower tuning curves than those with low best frequencies. But while some fibers did have quite narrow tuning curves and others were relatively broadly tuned, there were also some that behaved in intermediate ways (Fig.

11.13). Also, as far as threshold was concerned, there were wide continuous variations, and threshold was not clearly related to breadth of tuning curve. Neither from these nor from other data do we have a clear picture of the functional difference between spiral and radial VIIIth nerve fibers.

A final reflection on the function of the cochlea: the frequency of sound as a variable has the dimension of time (cycles·sec⁻¹). The basilar membrane is a spatially extended band of tissue. By the resonance characteristics of the inner ear, the temporal dimension of acoustic frequency is translated into a spatial dimension, namely distance along the basilar membrane. One might say that the cochlea "plots" frequency along a curvilinear axis. As a result, it is justifiable to speak of the receptive fields of auditory nerve fibers: each fiber innervates the receptors of a certain segment of the basilar membrane. Since resonance characteristics are spatially distributed, the extension of the receptive field determines tuning to a band of auditory frequencies.

11.5. Audiometry

The threshold of hearing can be expressed as the minimum sound pressure (or sound energy) measured at the eardrum that can evoke a

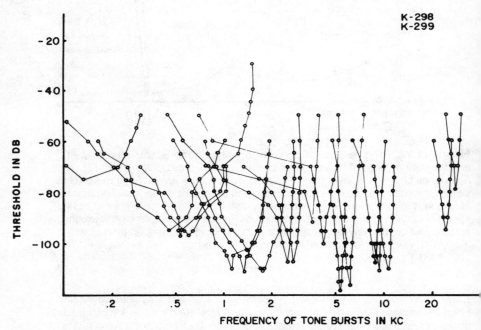

Figure 11.13. Tuning curves of auditory units. (Reprinted with permission from N. Y. S. Kiang, T. Watanabe, E. C. Thomas, et al: *Discharge Patterns of Single Fibers in Cat's Auditory Nerve.* Cambridge, MIT Press, 1965.)

perceptible auditory sensation. A healthy human ear can register amazingly low energy levels, and some animals do even better. It has been calculated that at the threshold of hearing of the optimum audible frequency, the excursions of the basilar membrane are smaller than the diameter of the hydrogen atom. While such calculations involve questionable extrapolations and may therefore be inaccurate, there is no doubt that we can hear very faint sounds indeed.

In clinical practice the threshold of hearing is rarely measured in absolute physical units. Instead, the hearing of patients is compared to that of the normal average and any deviation is expressed as *hearing loss*. The instrument used is an *audiometer*, a tone generator than can emit tones of adjustable frequency and intensity. Zero intensity is defined as that which is just heard by healthy young adults and is different for different frequencies. This standard has been determined by a committee and is defined in units of absolute sound pressure level (SPL) for certain convenient frequencies. Standard levels have separately been determined for air conduction and for bone conduction. Some people hear slightly better than the standard. The difference (if any) between the threshold of the patient and the standard is plotted for each test frequency on charts printed for the purpose. *Hearing loss* is shown in decibels (i.e. as the logarithm of the ratio of the thresholds of patient and standard: cf. Section 11.2 and Fig. 11.14).

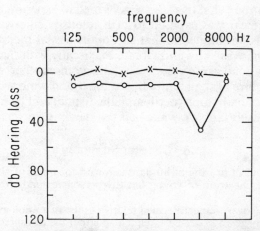

Figure 11.14. Audiograms for the two ears of a (hypothetical) patient. The patient has significant hearing loss at 4000 Hz in one ear only.

Different clinical conditions cause hearing loss characteristically distributed among the various frequency bands. For example, the common partial deafness of elderly people (caused by degeneration of hair cells) is usually worse at higher frequencies. Hearing loss due to otosclerosis is worse for low frequencies, because the middle ear transmission system stiffens.

11.5a. ACOUSTIC TRAUMA

Very loud noise is painful. The pain is caused by stimulation of nociceptive endings in the tympanic membrane. The threshold of pain is given as 140–160 db above 0.0002 dyne·cm^{-1} (see Fig. 11.1). The full operating range of the auditory organ, from minimum perceptible to maximum tolerable is, therefore, a 10^7–10^8-fold variation of auditory pressure.

But loud noises, especially if they are repeated or prolonged, can damage the organ of hearing, even at an intensity which is not strong enough to cause pain. The hearing loss of acoustic trauma is due to damage to the hair cells, primarily to the ciliary mechanism. Unlike taste receptor cells which can regenerate completely (see Section 8.2), hair cells do not heal.

If the damaging sound is dominated by a particular frequency, the hearing loss is limited to that frequency band. The reason is not difficult to surmise. The hair cells that suffer most are the ones exposed to the maximal vibration. That this is so was verified in experiments on guinea pigs. When the ear was exposed to high intensity sine wave tone, the loss of hair cells was limited to that part of the basilar membrane which, from other data, was known to vibrate maximally with that frequency.

Sudden very loud noise can cause damage in another way, namely, by causing rupture of the membrane of the round window, with consequent leakage of perilymph (perilymphatic fistula) and hearing loss. The distinction is important for, while hair cell death is irreversible, a fistula can heal.

11.6. Chapter Summary

1. The threshold of hearing of humans is lowest for tones of about 3000 Hz. The audible spectrum of young healthy persons extends from 20–20,000 Hz.
2. Decibels are logarithmically scaled relative units. In audiology sound intensity is usually given in decibels, relative to either the threshold of hearing of the human ear or some other arbitrarily defined sound pressure level.
3. The tympanic membrane, the middle ear ossicles, and the membrane of

the oval window form a mechanical system by which the acoustic impedance of air is matched to that of the inner ear fluids.

4. When middle ear function in one ear is impaired, sounds transmitted by air are lateralized toward the healthy ear, sounds transmitted by bone conduction toward the deaf ear (Weber's test).
5. Pressure oscillations are imparted to the cochlear fluids by movements of the stapes acting on the membrane of the oval window. These pressure oscillations cause small displacements of fluid, made possible by the "give" of the membrane of the round window. The pressure oscillations cause the basilar membrane to vibrate. These waves travel on the basilar membrane always from the base of the cochlea toward the helicotrema, because the basilar membrane is stiffer at the base than near the apex.
6. As waves travel on the basilar membrane from the base toward the apex of the cochlea, they first increase gradually to a maximum and then they are damped suddenly. The excursions of the vibrating basilar membrane are maximum near the base of the cochlea when the input sound is of high frequency, and near the helicotrema when it is of low frequency.
7. The membrane potential of hair cells is decreased when the ciliae are bent toward the basal body, and increased by their bending in the opposite direction. The cilia are being bent by the tectorial membrane as it shears over the ciliated surface of the hair cells due to vibration of the basilar membrane.
8. Oscillation of the membrane potential of excited hair cells generates the cochlear microphonic potential. These oscillations "ride" on a sustained shift of potential called the summating potential that is generated by sustained depolarization of hair cells.
9. Cochlear microphonic potential, summating potential, and the action potential of the auditory nerve fibers can be recorded clinically (electrocochleography).
10. Endolymph is rich in potassium, poor in sodium, and is at 80 mV positive potential relative to other extracellular fluids, including perilymph.
11. Excitation is transmitted from hair cells to auditory nerve endings probably by the cooperation of a chemical and an electrical mechanism. The former is probably more important for transmission of high-frequency stimuli, the latter for low frequencies. The electric mechanism may be responsible for the phase locking of impulses in auditory nerve fibers to low-frequency auditory stimuli.
12. Most auditory nerve fibers are tuned to a narrower band of frequencies than the resonance curves of points of the basilar membrane would suggest.
13. In audiometry, hearing loss is measured for several frequencies of tones, and it is expressed in decibels of threshold increase relative to the average normal ear.
14. Very loud noises kill hair cells.

Further Reading

See at end of Chapter 12.

Auditory Pathways and Centers

How the neural signals generated by the cochea are processed in the brain stem and cerebral cortex; directional hearing; auditory masking; the consequences of injury to auditory centers.

12.1. The Afferent Neurons of the Cochlea and Their Projections

The bipolar cell bodies of the auditory nerve fibers are in the spiral ganglion, within the cochlea itself. The peripheral process of these cells is, therefore, quite short. The centrally directed axon is much longer and terminates in the cochlear nuclei at the pontomedullary junction of the same side. The auditory centers of the brain are, besides the cochlear nuclei: the superior olivary complex; the trapezoid body and its nucleus; the lateral lemniscus and its nuclei; the inferior colliculi of the midbrain tectum; and the medial geniculate nuclei. These scattered groupings of gray matter are interconnected in intricate ways. Except for the cochlear nuclei which receive input only from the ear on their own side, there are bilateral connections among most other auditory nuclei (see Fig. 12.3). Throughout these multiple interconnections topographic relations are preserved with remarkable precision, so that the spatial representation of frequencies, which originates in the cochlea, is maintained in all nuclei of the auditory pathway. This is termed *tonotopic representation*, and will be discussed shortly (Section 12.3).

The medial geniculate body is the auditory thalamic nucleus. Its input comes from the auditory nuclei of the brain stem, and its relay cells project to the auditory cortex. In man the latter is contained in the superior aspect of temporal lobe, mainly in the transverse gyrus of Heschl (areas 41 and 42) (Fig. 7.5 and Carpenter, Fig. 13.16).

12.2. Descending Auditory Pathways

It has been recognized for several decades that some of the nerve endings in the cochlea, at the base of the hair cells, are not of the fibers of the VIIIth nerve. These have been identified as efferent axonal terminals. Some of these efferents contact hair cells, others the afferent VIIIth nerve terminals. Their function in both cases is inhibitory. Their parent neurons were traced to the superior olives, mostly of the contralateral, a few from the ipsilateral side. These axons form the olivocochlear bundles.

The significance of the olivocochlear fibers for hearing has not exactly been determined. Two suggested roles have advocates among investigators. One of their functions could be the suppression of input, when attention is directed to some sensory modality other than hearing. Another suggested function for olivocochlear efferents is the sharpening of the tuning curves of VIIIth nerve fibers by lateral inhibition. Lateral inhibition has indeed been demonstrated for auditory units in the VIIIth nerve, and for cells in successively higher levels of auditory processing (see Section 12.5 and Fig. 12.2), but the possible specific role of the olivocochlear bundle in such lateral inhibition is not clear. An amended version of this theory proposes that olivocochlear fibers screen background noise by suppressing excitation that is widely and randomly distributed along basilar membrane while interfering little with the transmission of more locally concentrated excitation.

We know the function served by the afferent synapses between hair cells and VIIIth nerve fiber terminals, but the transmitter has not been identified. On the other hand, for the efferent inhibitory terminals of the olivocochlear bundle, we know the transmitter, but are uncertain of the function. Acetylcholine is the likely inhibitory transmitter of the olivocochlear terminals.

The olivocochlear bundle is but one of many efferent fiber systems in the auditory pathways. There seems to be two-way traffic between most, if not all, auditory nuclei of the brain stem. Many of the efferent connections are inhibitory, but some are excitatory. It is reasonable to

conclude that auditory information is analyzed by integrated cooperation among the auditory brain stem nuclei, which precedes the higher
processing that subsequently takes place in the cortex.

12.3. Tonotopic Representation

In the late 1930s Lorente de Nó made the important discovery that
the VIIIth nerve fibers from the basal turn of the cochlea project to a
different part of the cochlear nucleus than do the fibers from the cochlear
apex. This suggested that the positions of the receptors within the cochlea
are mapped in the brain in a manner similar to the retinotopic organization of the visual pathways and to the dermatomal distribution of
input in the somatic sensory pathways. Since different tonal frequencies
excite different parts of the cochlea to different degrees, a "cochleotopic"
representation is the equivalent of a *tonotopic* representation. The latter
term implies that different tone heights cause maximal excitation at
different loci in auditory nuclei.

Tonotopic representation was first clearly demonstrated by recording
evoked potentials from the surface of the auditory cortex and then
confirmed by recording the responses of individual neurons (Fig. 12.1).
Brief tones of high frequency evoke maximal potential responses in the

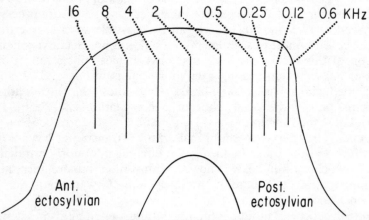

Figure 12.1. Tonotopic map, or the representation of auditory frequency on
the primary auditory receiving area of the cerebral cortex of a dog. *Ant.
ectosylvian*, anterior ectosylvian gyrus. (Modified and redrawn after A. R. Tunturi:
American Journal of Physiology 162:489–502, 1950.)

anterior parts of the cortex, low frequencies in the posterior parts. Between them an orderly representation of the entire auditory spectrum is laid out. Each frequency band excites maximally another strip of cortical tissue, so that the representations of octave intervals fall at approximately equal distances on the cortex, almost like a piano keyboard; a well-tempered cortex indeed.

Tonotopic "maps" have been demonstrated in almost all the subcortical auditory nuclei. In some of these nuclear complexes there are two or more tonotopic sequences. For example, in the cochlear nuclei there are two such representations on each side.

It seems likely that the topographic organization in the visual and in the somatic sensory systems has to do with the decoding of spatial information. For similar reasons it seems an almost inescapable conclusion that tonotopic organization is in some way necessary for the brain's ability to identify tone height and to determine the interrelationships between the pitches of sounds. At the same time it is also clear that, in and of itself, the topographic organization of the gray matter of the brain does not explain all phenomena of psychoacoustics.

12.4. Frequency Theory of Pitch Representation

Toward the end of the 19th century, Rutherford proposed a theory of the neural representation of tone height, which he called the "telephone theory." He suggested that the basilar membrane acts like the membrane of a telephone receiver, and that the vibrations cause electric waves in the VIIIth nerve, synchronized with the motions of the basilar membrane. We have seen already that the basilar membrane does not behave like a microphone membrane (the basilar membrane surface does not vibrate in phase). It also has been known for some time that nerve fibers cannot generate action potentials at the frequencies found in the higher reaches of the audible spectrum.

The idea that the frequency of sound could, somehow, be represented by the frequency of nerve potentials was, however, too attractive to be abandoned, and around 1930 a new version was devised, known as the "volley theory." It was based on the fact that action potentials in the auditory nerve tend to be phase-locked to the stimulating sound (see Section 11.4d and Fig. 11.11). It seemed that, even if individual nerve fibers could not represent auditory frequencies higher than perhaps 500 Hz, the assembly of many VIIIth nerve fibers acting in concert could. Several difficulties prevented general acceptance of the volley theory. First, phase locking is completely lost at frequencies higher than 2000 or 3000 Hz, and it is not very secure even between 1000 and 2000 Hz.

Second, while phase locking is preserved in the action potentials of some of the neurons in the cochlear and superior olivary nuclei, it becomes less pronounced as one ascends in the auditory pathway and it cannot be detected at all in the discharge of cortical neurons. Third, when the auditory stimulus is composed of several frequencies, action potentials tend to be locked to the component waves of the largest amplitudes and not the minor component frequencies. Yet complex sounds of similar dominant frequency but containing different mixtures of lesser frequencies do sound different; therefore, in the brain there must be a neural code representing even minor components of a complex stimulus.

In spite of these theoretical difficulties, there are investigators who hold the opinion that, at least for lower frequencies and in the lower brain stem nuclei, the sequencing of auditory action potentials is significant for the coding of pitch. It is for this reason, that a brief description of the frequency theory has been included in this text.

The question may be asked whether the phase locking of auditory action potentials may have some significance other than representing tone height. The answer is clearly yes. One of them is the auditory system's ability to detect the direction of a sound source (see Section 12.7). Another is the accurate encoding of the temporal sequence of sound patterns, so important in discriminating, for example, human speech.

12.5. Tuning Curves of Central Auditory Neurons

The thresholds for exciting (or inhibiting) the discharge of nerve impulses by auditory stimulation of various tonal frequencies has been determined for many neurons, in many brain stem and cerebral structures, in many animals. While differing in detail, the overall forms of such tuning curves seem similar to those found for fibers in the VIIIth nerve. It has been claimed that in each successively higher center of the auditory pathway, the tuning curves become more and more narrow. While this may be true for some parts of some nuclei, this rule has not proved to be generally valid.

The greatest diversity in the shape of tuning curves was found among neurons of the auditory cortex. While for some cells the customary asymmetrical V-shaped configuration was found (as in Fig. 11.13), others had irregular tuning curves, sometimes with more than one minimal point (more than one "best frequency"). There also were cells that responded poorly to tones of constant height and intensity, but were intensely excited either by tones of rising or by falling pitch; and in other cases by tones of either increasing or decreasing intensity. These were taken to be examples of *feature detection* in the auditory sphere, comparable to contrast detectors, and cells selectively sensitive to moving stimuli in the visual and somatic sense modalities.

Tones and noises emitted by people and other animals are recognizable by their temporal cadence and by the relative changes of pitch. Absolute tone height, while important in music, is not essential for the recognition of such sound patterns. For example, a word remains recognizable whether uttered in a high or in a low voice, by man, woman or child (although changes of pitch may alter the word's emotional coloring). It has been suggested that the main function of the auditory cortex is to detect the features in sound that make the identification of sound patterns possible.

Numerous examples of inhibitory effects of auditory stimulation on central auditory neurons have been found. A relatively simple example is that of lateral inhibition of the form illustrated in Figure 12.2. In this case a limited band of frequencies excites the cell while tones of higher or lower frequencies inhibit it. Other, more intricate response patterns have also been described.

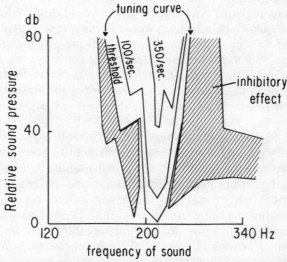

Figure 12.2. Lateral inhibition of a neuron in the auditory pathway. (Reprinted with permission from G. Somjen: *Sensory Coding in the Mammalian Nervous System.* New York, Plenum Press, 1975; after data of D. D. Greenwood and N. Maruyama: *Journal of Neurophysiology* 18:863–892, 1965.)

12.6. The Consequences of Injury to the Auditory Cortex

Injury or disease affecting the cochlea, the auditory portion of the VIIIth nerve, or the cochlear nucleus of the brain stem cause deafness in the ear of the affected side. Loss of hearing can extend over the entire auditory spectrum, or it may be limited to certain frequencies depending on the extent of the lesion.

Injury to the higher auditory centers has more subtle consequences. Experiments have been performed in which all known auditory areas of the cerebral cortex of both hemispheres of a cat have been destroyed surgically. These lesions included not only the primary auditory receiving area (A-I), but all the surrounding cortical areas that are major targets of auditory input. After they recovered from surgery, these animals were not deaf. They could still learn to discriminate between tones of different frequencies. What they did lose was the ability to recognize patterned sequences, consisting of three or more tones sounding in succession, what we might call simple musical phrases. In addition, after lesions of the primary auditory cortex, cats lose the ability to detect the direction of a sound source, a point to which we shall return soon.

Bilateral destruction of the auditory areas of the two hemispheres is rare in human patients. Any injury which would destroy the superior temporal gyri of both hemispheres would in most cases destroy so much of the rest of the brain that the question of auditory function would become moot. When, after bilateral loss of the auditory cortex, auditory testing was nevertheless still possible, there was severe impairment of the patient's hearing. In man, the consequences for auditory function seemed much worse than in animals that sustained lesions of comparable size.

One-sided lesions of the cortical auditory receiving area are more common and cause relatively minor impairment of auditory function. There are two reasons for this. *First,* because sound normally reaches both ears, so that minor hearing loss affecting one side may be compensated to some extent by turning the head. *Second,* because auditory projections within the brain are bilateral (Fig. 12.3). The bilaterality of the anatomical connections does not mean, however, that auditory function is equally divided between the two hemispheres. Careful testing after one-sided brain injury reveals impairment of hearing in the contralateral half of auditory space. Three sets of deficiencies have been described. (1) The auditory threshold is higher in the ear contralateral to the injured brain half than in the ear of the same side. (2) The

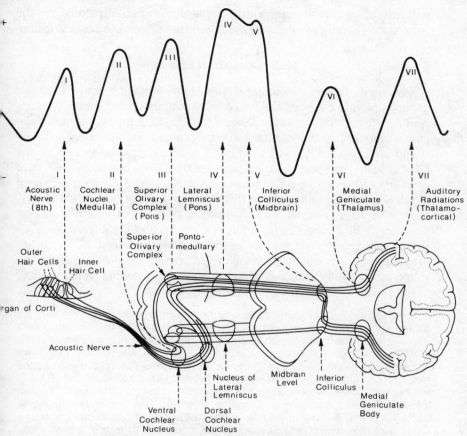

Figure 12.3. Auditory evoked potentials and the central structures responsible for their generation. The *curve* shows the potential waves recorded from the top of the skull (termed point Cz by the convention used in EEG) in response to a brief auditory stimulus (click). The waves labeled *I–VI* are the "far-field" responses, so called because they are generated at a distance from the point of recording. Note the very small amplitude of these potentials, which could not be registered without electronic averaging (cf. Fig. 21.1). The entire sequence of waves *I–VII* lasts about 10 msec. For auditory evoked potentials that occur later, see Figure 21.1. (Reprinted with permission from D. D. DeWeese and W. H. Saunders: *Textbook of Otolaryngology*, 6th ed. St. Louis, C. V. Mosby, 1982.)

direction from which sound comes is less accurately detected by the patient in the contralateral half of his auditory space. (3) Complex patterns of sound are less easily recognized when presented in the contralateral auditory space than on the same side as the cortical lesion.

12.7. Directional Hearing

The ability to detect whether sound comes from the left or the right depends mainly on using the two ears in conjunction. Patients who are deaf in one ear do have some residual directional hearing, but it is quite poor compared to the normal binaural population. To detect whether sound comes from ahead or behind, the head must be turned. If the head is held quite still, and the sound source does not move, left-right determinations can be made within a few degrees of arc, but it is hard to tell whether the sound came from the front or the back. This ability, to be able to determine the left or right position of a sound source, depends on differences in (1) interaural *timing* and (2) interaural *intensity*. Sound reaches the ear turned toward the source just a little earlier than it does in the ear turned away. Furthermore, the near ear hears the sound more loudly than the far ear because the latter lies in the shadow of the head.

From the velocity of sound in air and the distance between the two ears the maximal timing difference between the two ears can easily be calculated for a sound source that is exactly to one side of the subject. For an average adult head, it is around 0.6 msec. The effect of interaural timing differences was demonstrated in psychophysical experiments as follows. A subject was equipped with two earphones. Two accurately timed sound generators delivered clicks to the two ears. If the two clicks were separated by an interval between 0.006 and 0.6 msec, the subject heard it as coming from one side, the side of the ear to which the sound was presented first (illusion of laterality). At shorter intervals a single click was heard in the center of the skull, and at longer intervals two separate clicks, one in each ear. By making the two clicks coincide in time, but one louder than the other, a similar lateralization can be achieved.

When listening to tones, instead of clicks, the direction of the sound source is detected by the phase difference. The phase is advanced in the nearer ear relative to the farther ear. Phase differences can, however, be detected only for low frequencies. With frequencies of 2000 and higher, the successive waves (periods) of the sound vibration follow one another at intervals of 0.5 msec or less. Phase difference then becomes useless as a directional clue because the interval between successive sound waves becomes shorter than the interval between the arrival of the waves in the two ears. Besides, at higher frequencies phase locking of action potentials fails (see Section 11.4d). Fortunately, as phase difference becomes useless, intensity difference becomes the optimal clue. The long waves of low-frequency tones can diffract around the skull, so that the head casts no shadow and so the intensity difference vanishes. The higher the frequency, the more marked the intensity differences between the two ears become.

The superior olives are believed to be the first station in the auditory pathway where directional information is analyzed. Input from the two ears converges upon neurons in the superior olivary complex. The dendrites of these cells are bunched in two arbors, one oriented medially, the other laterally. The medial dendrites receive afferents from the cochlear nucleus of the contralateral side, the lateral dendrites from the ipsilateral side. Input from the one side is excitatory, that from the other inhibitory, for some cells. Sound reaching both ears at equal intensity will not affect these cells, because excitation and inhibition will mutually cancel; but if the sound in the one (excitatory) side is louder, it will win over the competing inhibitory side. Other superior olivary cells are excited by sound reaching either ear, but excitation is preferential for certain specified timing differences between two ears.

Cats are especially good at detecting the direction of a sound source. They use this talent while hunting in darkness. Two types of experimental lesions can impair this faculty. Bilateral lesion of either the superior accessory olives or the primary auditory cortex will deprive them of all but the most rudimentary directional hearing. As we have seen earlier, such lesions do not cause deafness in cats (cf. Section 12.6). While the primary processing of the information required for directional hearing seems to be performed in the superior olivary complex, the decoding of the processed information is in the auditory area of the cerebral cortex.

As may be expected, neurons have also been found in the auditory cerebral cortex, the excitation of which depends on the direction of the sound source. Cells dominated by ipsilateral and by contralateral sound input are arranged in zones. Thus superimposed on the tonotopic map of the auditory cortex is a map of auditory space. While tone height is represented in an anteroposterior sequence, auditory space is represented in a mediolateral sequence. The result is a *columnar organization*, similar to those in somatic and visual cortices. Within any one column of cells in the auditory cortex, cells have a similar best frequency and represent the same zone in auditory space.

12.8. Auditory Masking

Generally speaking, when two different tones or noises sound simultaneously, both are perceived, and both are identified by the subject separately and as coming from different directions. It has been argued that we can thank the topographic method of decoding auditory frequencies for our ability to discern multiple frequency patterns simultaneously. The spatial resolution of sound sources is an additional aid in the process, for if two sound patterns are heard as coming from two different directions, this will help in telling them apart. Conductors of orchestras rely on this faculty more than the average person. The celebrated "cocktail party effect" depends on our ability to attend to the source of a sound occupying a particular position in space, and to screen out all others.

Even though the auditory system's capacity to analyze complex vibration patterns is truly awe-inspiring, it does not always work. Under certain circumstances one sound can prevent another from being heard. This is termed *auditory masking*. Not surprisingly, the louder of two tones is the one that may mask the softer one. Also rather obviously, if both sounds come from the same direction in space, masking is more likely to occur than if the sources are widely separated. If the two sounds have similar frequency ranges, masking is also more probable. Finally, and less obviously, lower tones have a greater power to mask high tones than the other way around.

Attempts to explain all cases of auditory masking by a single simple principle have not been successful. It seems there must be two sets of factors involved. One is the interference of vibration patterns within the resonant structures in the middle and inner ears. The other is synaptic interaction within the central nervous system.

12.9. Auditory Evoked Potentials

Recording of potential waves evoked in the brain by auditory stimulation, along with its visual and somatosensory counterparts, is gradually becoming part of the clinical diagnostic laboratory's repertory. The greatest significance of this procedure lies in the testing of hearing in infants. There have been cases in which young children have been treated as retarded, when in fact they were of normal intelligence but hard of hearing.

In auditory evoked potentials it is possible to resolve the earliest responses which are generated in the brain stem and not in the cortex (Fig. 12.3). It is remarkable that this is possible with electrodes fastened to the scalp. When a potential generated in the brain stem is registered by an electrode on the scalp, it is called a *far-field response*. The recording of far-field responses is made possible by the high degree of synchrony, due to phase locking, when auditory neurons in the brain stem respond to click stimuli.

The clinical diagnostic use of electrocochleography was mentioned in the previous chapter (see Section 11.4c and Figs. 11.9 and 11.10).

12.10. Chapter Summary

1. Efferent fibers innervate cells in most of the nuclei of the auditory pathway. These efferent synapses are for the most part but not exclusively inhibitory in function. The olivocochlear bundle, mediating inhibition from superior olives to the hair cell-VIIIth nerve ending synapse, is the best known of these.
2. Fibers in the auditory nerve originating in different parts of the cochlea terminate in different parts of the cochlear nucleus, thus creating an orderly representation of the basilar membrane and hence of the best frequencies of excitation. Such tonotopic maps are found in all nuclei of the auditory pathway and in the auditory receiving areas of the cerebral cortex.
3. Some neurons in the auditory nuclei exhibit lateral inhibition: tones higher and lower than the exciting frequency band inhibit the firing of the cell.
4. Directional hearing depends on differences in loudness and in phase between the two ears, when sound is coming from one side. Directional hearing requires the integrity of superior olivary nuclei and of the auditory cortices.
5. Damage to the auditory receiving area of the cerebral cortex of one hemisphere causes in the contralateral ear only some impairment in the ability to discriminate tonal patterns and the direction of a sound source, and also some elevation of the threshold of hearing.
6. Of two tones sounding simultaneously, the louder and lower is likely to mask the softer and higher one, especially if the two come from similar directions and are composed of similar frequencies.

Further Reading: Chapters 11 and 12

Books and Reviews

Békésy G: *Experiments in Hearing.* New York, McGraw-Hill, 1960.

Carpenter MB: *Core Text of Neuroanatomy.* Baltimore, Williams & Wilkins, 1978.

Dallos P: *The Auditory Periphery.* New York, Academic Press, 1973.

Davis H, Silverman SR (eds): *Hearing and Deafness,* ed 4. New York, Holt, Rinehart and Winston, 1978.

Keidel WD, Neff WD, (eds): *Auditory System, Handbook of Sensory Physiology,* vol 5. Berlin, Springer, 1975.

Neff WD: Localization and lateralization of sound in space. In DeReuck AVS, Knight J (eds): *Hearing Mechanisms in Vertebrates,* CIBA Foundation Symposium. London, J and A Churchill, 1968, pp 207–231.

Articles

Diamond IT, Goldberg JM, Neff WD: Tonal discrimination after ablation of auditory cortex. *J Neurophysiol* 25:223–235, 1962.

Merzenich MM, Knight PL, Roth GL: Representation of cochlea within primary auditory cortex in the cat. *J Neurophysiol* 38:231–249, 1975.

Robertson D, Johnstone BM: Effects of divalent cations on spontaneous and evoked activity in single mammalian auditory neurones. *Pflueger's Arch* 380:7–12, 1979.

Russel IJ, Sellick PM: Intracellular studies of hair cells in the mammalian cochlea. *J Physiol (Lond)* 284:261–290, 1978.

Wersäll J, Flock A, Lundquist PG: Structural basis for directional selectivity in cochlear and vestibular sensory receptors. *Cold Spring Harbor Symp Quant Biol* 30:115–132, 1965.

chapter 13

The Vestibular System

*How the organism orients in space, and how it senses
displacement of its own body.*

13.1. The Vestibular Sense Organs

The sense organs detecting the position and the movements of the
head are intimately connected with those sensing sound vibration. Not
only are they in close proximity in the temporal bone, but the receptor
cells are nearly identical. The hair cells of the cochlea, the saccule, the
utricle and the semicircular canals are all similar in both structure and
biophysical function. Moreover, the cochlear duct communicates with
the saccule, it in turn with utricle, and the latter with the semicircular
canals. The membranous labyrinth is thus filled with endolymph of the
same composition as the cochlear duct.

The immediate, adequate stimulus of all hair cells is the bending of
cilia. The role of the tectorial membrane of the cochlea is played in the
utricle and saccule by the *otoliths* (literally, "ear stones") and in the
ampullae of the semicircular canals by the *cupulae*. These accessory
structures are in contact with the ciliated surface of the hair cells, and
their displacement provides the force that bends the cilia.

The semicircular canals sense the turning of the head. The otolith
organs detect the direction in which gravity acts and from that determine
the position of the head relative to the horizon. They also measure the

direction and the magnitude of linear acceleration acting on the head. Modern physical theory does not distinguish gravity from acceleration, and neither do the otoliths. Pilots need an artificial horizon when they fly at night, because during turns acceleration acting on their otolith organs confounds their orientation with respect to gravity.

In the past there has been some debate whether the saccule functions as a sense organ for low-frequency vibrations. Whatever its significance may be in some vertebrates as an accessory organ of hearing, in mammals such a function does not seem to be important. Rather, the two saccules and two utricles of the two sides of the head are a foursome of sense organs of shared function.

1.1a. THE SEMICIRCULAR CANALS

If the head—and with it the semicircular canals—are turned, the endolymph in the canals tends to lag behind. Since both ends of each canal open into the utricle, the fluid could flow in a complete circle if it were not prevented from doing so by the cupula (Fig. 13.1). The cupula is an elastic trapdoor that occludes the ampullae. When the

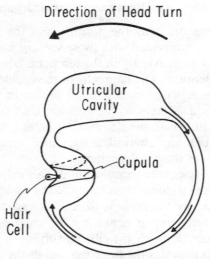

Figure 13.1. The mechanics of a semicircular canal. The *arrows* inside the canal show the direction of the (relative) movement of endolymph when the head is turning as indicated.

endolymph is set into motion it presses on the cupula, and so bends it. The motion of the cupula in turn bends the cilia of the hair cells and therefore excites them.

Bending the stereocilia toward the kinocilium causes depolarization of the hair cells; bending them the other way causes hyperpolarization. All the hair cells of each crista ampullae are lined up one way. In the lateral semicircular canals the kinocilia are on the side that faces the utricle, in the superior and posterior canals they are on the side away from the utricle. When the head is stationary, nerve fibers innervating the hair cells of the crista ampullaris fire impulses at a steady rate. If the endolymph in a lateral canal flows from the canal toward the ampulla, thereby bending the cupula toward the utricle, the firing quickens; fluid streaming in the opposite direction depresses the firing. For example, turning the head to the left (counter-clockwise) will cause fluid to stream to the right (clockwise) in both lateral (horizontal) canals. In the lateral canal on the left side of the head, this will cause increased firing, on the right, decreased firing (Fig. 13.2).

The two lateral semicircular canals lie in the same plane, tilted 30° from the horizontal if the head is erect. Because of this tilt, it is misleading to call them the horizontal canals, as is the widespread custom. The anterior (superior) canal stands at 90° to both the lateral and also to the posterior canals. The anterior canal of the right side stands in a plane parallel with the posterior canal of the left, and the two form a complementary pair, excited in a reciprocal manner, similar to the lateral canals of the two sides (Fig. 13.3). Together the three pairs of semicircular canals represent the coordinates of three-dimensional space. Turning the head in any plane will stimulate at least one and usually two pairs of semicircular canals.

Investigation of semicircular canals originally posed the question, whether excitation of these organs measures the angular velocity or the angular acceleration of the movements of the head. During rotation at a constant velocity, friction between the fluid and the wall of the canal imparts momentum to the fluid and gradually sets it into motion. As the fluid gathers the same velocity at which the head turns, it will no longer press on the cupula. Since the cupula is elastic, it will right itself when it is relieved of the pressure of the endolymph and cease to stimulate the hair cells. During continued rotation at constant angular velocity the rate of discharge of the nerve fibers will, therefore, be the same as with the head motionless. When rotation stops, the fluid in the canal will tend to keep moving because of its inertia. It then will exert

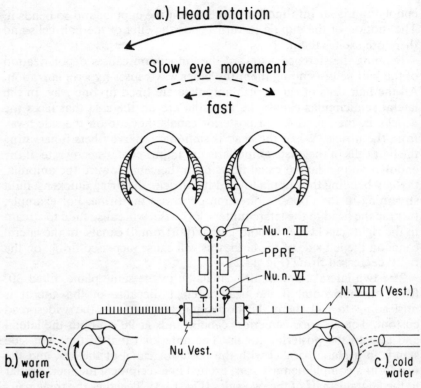

Figure 13.2. Stimulation of the lateral semicircular canals and resulting eye movements (vestibulo-ocular reflex). Note that turning the head to the left (*a*) has the same effect as warming the left lateral canal (*b*), and as cooling the right lateral canal (*c*). *Nu.n.III*, oculomotor nucleus; *PPRF*, parapontine reticular formation; *Nu.n.VI*, abducens nucleus; *N.VIII*,: eighth cranial nerve, vestibular division; *round nerve endings* symbolize excitatory connections, *flat terminals* inhibitory connections.

pressure on the cupula once more, this time in a direction opposite to that taken at the onset of rotation.

Probably all readers have experienced post-rotational stimulation of the semicircular canals and its consequences: post-rotational nystagmus and vertigo. Stepping off a merry-go-round (rotating piano stool, or other instrument of masochistic entertainment), a blurred image of the world is seen whirling around, and one's self is felt spinning in a direction opposite to the original rotation. The illusion of a moving visual world is caused by the nystagmus (see Section 13.3 and Fig. 13.2) and the

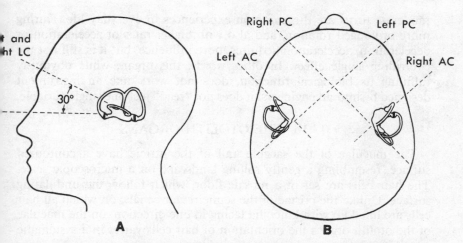

Figure 13.3. The relative positions of the three pairs of semicircular canals. *LC*, lateral canal; *AC*, anterior canal; *PC*, posterior canal. (Reprinted with permission from H. Barber and C. W. Stockwell: *Manual of Electronystagmography*, ed 2. St. Louis, C. V. Mosby, 1980.)

sensation of head and body spinning by the post-rotational stimulation of the canals themselves. The associated unsteady gait and peculiarly never failing merriment stem from the confusion of vestibular, visual and proprioceptive senses sending contradictory signals to the brain.

These simple observations confirm that, first, there is little or no stimulation of the semicircular canals during steady rotation; and second, stimulation caused by deceleration is in a direction opposite to that of acceleration. These two facts suggest that the semicircular canals react to the first derivative of angular velocity, namely, angular acceleration. Actual measurements, however, do not confirm this simple conclusion.

A complete set of equations describing the displacement of the cupulae must take account of at least the following parameters: the viscosity and mass of the endolymph; the friction between the fluid and the wall of the canal; the mass of the cupula as well as its elasticity and friction. The result is not a simple function of either velocity or acceleration. During brief turns of the head as long as acceleration is moderate, the excitation of nerve fibers innervating the semicircular canals reflects the velocity of the head more closely than its acceleration. For most of us, except aviators, acrobats and dancers, such brief, moderate turns are the common experiences in everyday life. During more prolonged rotation, and also with higher rates of acceleration or deceleration, acceleration acquires more influence, but it is still not the overriding single effect. In other words, this organ, while obviously fulfilling its biological function, does not work like an instrument designed by human engineers: it does not "read" just one single variable.

13.1b. THE OTOLITH ORGANS

The maculae of the saccule and of the utricle have a contoured surface, resembling a gently rolling landscape on a microscopic scale. The hair cells are set in a mosaic floor, which follow the undulating surface. Unlike the cristae of the semicircular canals, on which all hair cells are lined up with kinocilia facing in one direction, on the maculae of the otolith organs the orientation of hair cells varies in a systematic way (Fig. 13.4).

The otoliths are denser than the endolymph in which they are submerged, and thus weigh down on the hair cells. They are only loosely attached to the substratum. When the head is tilted this way and that, the otoliths shift about and excite different groups among the hair cells upon which they rest (Fig. 13.5). The macula of the saccule stands in a plane at roughly right angles to that of the utricle (Fig. 13.4). The distribution of excitation among the assemblies of hair cells of the two pairs of otolith organs of the two sides of the head can encode all possible head positions and all possible directions of linear acceleration.

Because the otoliths are only loosely anchored, they can become dislocated by violent acceleration, such as a blow to the head, with consequent loss of function.

13.2. Vestibular Nuclei

Fibers of the vestibular division of the VIIIth nerve are addressed to the vestibular nuclei in the pons and medulla oblongata and to the vestibular (nodulofloccular) portion of the cerebellum (see Section 18.3e). The superior, and to a lesser degree the medial, vestibular nuclei control the vestibulo-ocular reflex (see the next section). Output fibers from the superior vestibular nucleus join the medial longitudinal fasciculus, a collection of axons needed for the coordination of eye movements. The lateral (Deiters') nuclei, descending nuclei, and part of the medial nuclei coordinate the vestibulospinal reflexes. The direct connections of the vestibular nuclei to the spinal cord are, of course, the

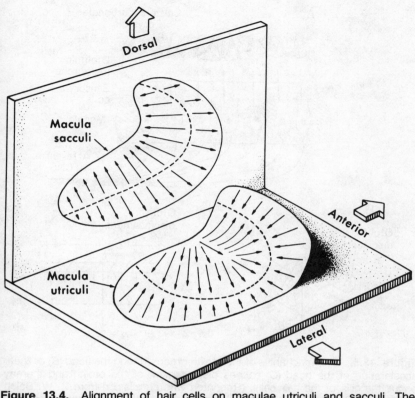

Figure 13.4. Alignment of hair cells on maculae utriculi and sacculi. The directions of the arrows show the direction in which bending of the cilia causes increased excitation. (Reprinted with permission from H. Barber and C. W. Stockwell: *Manual of Electronystagmography*, ed 2. St. Louis, C. V. Mosby, 1980; after data from H. H. Lindemann: *Ergebnisse der Anatomie und Entwicklungslehre* 42:1–113, 1969.)

vestibulospinal tracts, but in addition, there is an indirect path through the vestibuloreticular connections and the reticulospinal tracts. The vestibular nuclei receive input not only from the labyrinths, but also from stretch receptors of the neck muscles and from the cerebellum. The flocculus of the cerebellum is, in particular, involved in coordinating reflex movements of the eyes and neck muscles, and also in performing the computations required for balancing the body (see Section 18.3e).

Individual neurons in the vestibular nuclear complex respond to stimulation of the labyrinths in numerous ways. Separate populations of neurons are

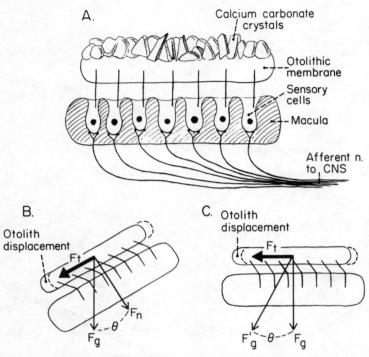

Figure 13.5. The mechanics of the otolith organs. Tilting the head (*B*) or linear acceleration of the head (*C*) causes displacement of the otolith and thereby bends the cilia of the hair cells. (Reprinted with permission from R. W. Baloh and V. Honrubia: Clinical neurophysiology of the vestibular system. In *Contemporary Neurology*, vol. 18. Philadelphia, F. A. Davis, 1979.)

stimulated by fibers from the semicircular canals and from the otolith organs. Thus one population of cells is concerned with turning the head and another group with linear acceleration and tilting of the head. As may be expected from what has been said in the previous paragraph, the cells concerned with rotary movements are concentrated in the superior nucleus and in the rostral portion of the medial nucleus; the cells concerned with otolith input are in the other components of the vestibular nuclear complex.

Within each nucleus there are several classes of neurons that respond differently to various inputs. For example, four different types of behavior occur during turning of the head. Some neurons are excited when the head is turned to the right, and inhibited during turns to the left; others behave in the exact reverse. Yet other cells are excited if the head is turned, no matter in which direction, and others are inhibited by all turning movements. Different response repertoires have also been described for otolith input.

Even though the cell populations concerned with otolith input are segregated anatomically from the populations responding to semicircular canal excitation, their functions are not independent. Intricate synaptic interactions of otolith and semicircular canal excitation have been demonstrated. Since during movements occurring under natural (as opposed to laboratory) conditions, otolith organs and semicircular canals are simultaneously stimulated, interaction in the central processing of their signals is necessary for the coordination of the complex movements the musculature must execute to respond appropriately to vestibular stimulation.

As head and body move under everyday conditions, the vestibular nuclei and the circuits in the nodulofloccular part of the cerebellum continuously keep account of present and past input, to compute position, velocity and acceleration of the head. The resulting compensatory reflex movements enable the eyes to fix on a target, for example as the head is bobbing up and down during walking. Similarly, such computations make it possible to keep the head up during various changes of body posture and also when the floor is moving in a vehicle.

Vestibular input also reaches the cerebral cortex. The cortical projection of the labyrinth lies just behind the face representation of the somatosensory cortex (see Fig. 7.5B) in the interparietal sulcus. Stimulation of this region of conscious human patients evokes the subjective sensation of turning.

13.3. Vestibular Reflexes

The most studied functions of the labyriths are the two complementing sets of reflexes: (1) those that aid keeping the eyes fixed on a target as the head and/or body turns; and (2) those that keep the body balanced upright during movements of the substratum, and during self-produced movements—walking, running and jumping.

People can manage without labyrinths, and sometimes loss of their function goes unnoticed. Streptomycin is an antibiotic which, in overdose, damages hair cells. In the days before its toxic effect was widely known, some patients treated with streptomycin became deaf, others lost labyrinth function, and some lost both. In one case, a young man who had been treated with the drug found out that his labyrinths did not function only when he dove into a swimming pool. Once submerged he could not tell up from down and did not find the way to the surface until he was pulled out, just in time.

This case illustrates that under ordinary conditions loss of labyrinth functions can be compensated for by other sense organs, notably vision, proprioception, and tactile input. Birds and free-living monkeys need their labyrinths more than humans; but humans do need them under special conditions, not just in swimming pools but also walking at night or with eyes closed.

When the head or the body are turned, our eyes normally move in the opposite direction in order to maintain a stable visual world. This compensatory eye movement is partly controlled by input from the retina (see Section 10.4), but even with eyes closed, head turning evokes a compensatory eye movement: this is the *vestibulo-ocular reflex*. If, instead of a brief turn, head and body are spun around for one or more full turns, *vestibular nystagmus* is provoked, which is a special case of the vestibuloocular reflex. As with optokinetic nystagmus (Section 10.4), the eyes move first with a velocity equal to the turning of the head but in the opposite direction (compensatory movement), and then with a quick saccade (corrective, follow-up, or return component) in the same direction as the turn (Fig. 13.6).

Figure 13.2 illustrates schematically the minimal neuronal circuit required for the slow component of vestibular nystagmus. In reality, the synaptic connections are probably considerably more complicated. With

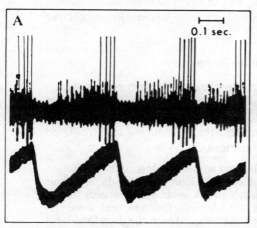
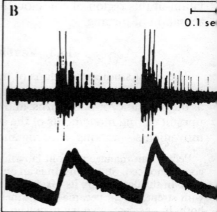

Figure 13.6. Vestibular nystagmus. The *upper tracings* are recordings from a small bundle of motor fibers in the abducens nerve, the *lower tracings* the contractile force of the lateral rectus muscle. *A*, nystagmus with slow component toward the side from which the recordings were taken; *B*, with fast component toward the side of recording. (Reprinted with permission from Y. Yamanaka and P. Bach-y-Rita: *Experimental Neurology* 20:143–155, 1968.)

the head turning to the left, excitation of the left lateral semicircular canal is increased, that of the right canal decreased. The left canal then sends increased excitatory signals that stimulate the motoneurons innervating the lateral rectus muscle of the right eye and to the medial rectus muscle of the left eye; and at the same time inhibits the motoneurons of the right medial and left lateral recti. The result is conjugate movement of the two eyeballs to the right, helping to keep the eyes on a target. Not shown in Figure 13.2 are the reciprocal connections of the right lateral canal. Because excitation of the right canal decreases, it sends *decreasing* excitatory signals to the left lateral and right medial recti, and decreasing inhibitory signals to the right lateral and left medial recti, thus enhancing the effectiveness of the input from the left canal.

When the eyeballs have moved as far to one side as possible during the slow component of the nystagmus, they are reset by the rapid component, or saccade. This quick resetting is believed to be initiated and coordinated by the paramedian pontine reticular formation (PPRF: shown without its synaptic connections in Fig. 13.2).

When a person is spun in a rotating chair with eyes closed, he may make compensatory movements not only with his eyes, but also with his head. This movement of the neck muscles is mediated by vestibulospinal reflexes operating on the upper cervical segments. Vestibulospinal reflexes also act on the innervation of the legs, aiding in the maintenance of the upright position. These balancing reflexes require input from the otolith organs (see also Sections 13.1b and 18.4a).

13.3a. THE TESTING OF VESTIBULAR FUNCTION

Traditional clinical tests of vestibular function depend on observation or measurement of such behaviors evoked by labyrinth stimulation as: (1) nystagmus; (2) the tendency to fall when standing, usually with eyes closed; (3) errors in judging direction, with eyes closed (past-pointing). Two standard methods of stimulating the labyrinths are: (1) the rotating chair; and (2) caloric stimulation. Both were first introduced into clinical practice by Bárány, and both are sometimes referred to by his name.

In a rotating chair, eye movements can be evoked (1) by imposing a sudden acceleration or deceleration; (2) by sinusoidal oscillatory motion; (3) by prolonged accelerating rotation. Before the invention of electric recording of eye movements (see Section 9.4b), the only way to judge vestibular stimulation caused by rotation was to turn the patient around at a predetermined velocity for a predetermined time, then suddenly stop the rotation and then observe the following signs: (1) *post-rotational nystagmus* (slow component in the direction in which the patient had been turning; remember the patient experiences illusory turning in a direction opposite to the original rotation); (2) *past-pointing* (in the direction of the preceding rotation) and (3) *tendency to fall* when attempting to get up from the chair (in the direction of the previous rotation). *Note: past-pointing and falling are always in the direction of the slow component of the nystagmus.*

In specialized clinical laboratories the electro-oculogram is now recorded both during and after spinning the patient in a motor-driven chair. A variety of standardized tests have been designed involving various rotary motions, either unidirectional or oscillatory.

During oscillatory rotation of moderate amplitude and frequency, the eyeballs make compensatory movements which keep them directed very nearly to one and the same point, even if the eyes are kept closed. This means that the vestibulo-ocular reflex generates eye movements that are 180° out of phase with the movements of the chair and have an amplitude exactly matched to the movements imposed on the subject. Using terms borrowed from engineering, the vestibulo-ocular reflex is said to have a "gain" close to −1. The negative sign indicates that the eye movements oppose the rotation.

The gain of the vestibulo-ocular reflex can, however, be changed. An interesting and frequently repeated psychological experiment consists of wearing prismatic eyeglasses that reverse the visual field. If such glasses are mounted in the frame so that left and right seem reversed to the subject, then the reflexes evoked from the retina (optokinetic reflexes) conflict with those evoked from the vestibular organ. The wearing of such glasses is for a while confusing. If, however, they are worn during all waking hours, the subject gradually becomes used to his abnormal visual world. As such adjustment is achieved, the vestibulo-ocular reflex is suppressed (i.e., its "gain" is reduced). In a few such instances, actual reversal of the direction of the vestibulo-ocular reflex has been recorded. When monkeys have been made to wear such prismatic eyeglasses, it could be shown that the modification of the vestibulo-ocular reflex is a function of changes in the neuronal circuits in the cerebellar flocculus (cf. Section 18.3e).

The caloric testing of the labyrinth is especially useful, because with it the semicircular canal function of one side can be examined without involving the other side. The caloric test makes use of convection currents set up in the semicircular canal by warming or by cooling the endolymph. Only the lateral canal is accessible to caloric testing because it is the one close enough to the external auditory meatus to be cooled or warmed.

For this test the head is positioned so that the lateral canal is in an upright position. For this, the head must be tilted 60° back if the patient is seated; if he is lying down, it must be tilted 30° forward (cf. Fig. 13.3A). The external meatus is then irrigated with cool (30°C) or warm (40°C) water or air. If, for example, the lateral canal of the right side is cooled, the endolymph closest to the external auditory meatus will become dense and will stream away from the ampulla (Fig. 13.2c). This will induce the illusion of the head turning toward the left. Thus nystagmus is evoked, and past-pointing and the tendency to fall may be demonstrated. The patient may also feel giddy. The slow compensatory component of the nystagmus will be toward the right, and so will be past-pointing and the tendency to fall.

A note on clinical nomenclature. The convention used to be to name nystagmus after its fast component. "Nystagmus to the right" meant slow component to the left, quick to the right. Naming the nystagmus after the quick components is, however, ambiguous, because the slow component is the compensatory movement and is therefore considered functionally important. For this reason the custom is spreading to specify both the movement and its direction, writing, for example: "Nystagmus with slow component to the right." The popular mnemogram by which generations of medical students learned the rules of caloric nystagmus is however based on the old naming: the "COWS" stand for "*c*old *o*pposite, *w*arm *s*ame" referring, respectively, to the temperature of the caloric stimulus and the direction of the quick component of the nystagmus (relative to the irrigated ear).

13.3b. VERTIGO AND NAUSEA

It is important to distinguish between two complaints, both often described as "dizzyness" in everyday language. *Vertigo* is the giddy illusion of the world turning or of the floor moving and the associated difficulty in maintaining an upright posture. *Nausea* is the ill feeling associated with the need to vomit. The two often go together, but need not do so. If a patient complains of feeling dizzy, the physician must find out what he means.

Both vertigo and nausea are common clinical complaints. Both can be caused by abnormal excitation of the vestibular system, but can have other causes as well (e.g. see Section 5.3a). Vertigo is commonly associated with past-pointing and a tendency to fall.

Ménière's syndrome consists of attacks of vertigo, often with nausea and vomiting, and frequently with auditory symptoms. The pathophysiology of the condition is not completely understood, but it usually is associated with degenerative changes of the labyrinths.

13.3c. UNILATERAL DAMAGE TO THE LABYRINTH

Having just one vestibular organ is worse than having none. While bilateral loss of vestibular function may go unnoticed for a while (see Section 13.3) unilateral damage is immediately apt to cause severe disturbance. The reason is that under normal conditions, at rest, the three complementary pairs of semicircular canals send balanced, opponent signals to the brain stem vestibular nuclei of both sides (see Section 13.1a). If one member of a pair is taken away, the unilateral input evokes the illusion of constant, unilateral turning, and consequently the triad of nystagmus, vertigo and nausea. The illusion is of turning toward the intact side, so that the slow compensatory eye movement of the nystagmus is toward the side of the lesion. There is improvement with time, and if the loss is gradual rather than sudden, the symptoms are much less severe.

13.4. Chapter Summary

1. The semicircular canals sense the turning of the head, but they are not excited during protracted constant velocity rotation.
2. The lateral semicircular canals of the two sides form a reciprocally antagonistic pair. That is, at rest both emit a steady stream of impulses, the effect of which on the vestibular nucleus is balanced; during turning of the head excitation increases in the lateral canal on the side toward which the head turns, and it decreases in the canal of the opposite side. The anterior canal of one side forms a similar reciprocally opposing pair with the posterior canal of the other side.
3. The adequate stimulus of the hair cells of the semicircular canal is the bending of the cilia; the cilia are bent by the bending of the cupula, which is moved by the pressure exerted by endolymph during head turns.
4. Nystagmus elicited by vestibular stimulation normally supplements optokinetic nystagmus. Thus the slow (compensatory) component of the nystagmus is in the direction opposite to the direction of the head turn, and the fast (resetting, saccadic) component is in the same direction as that of the head turn.
5. The utricle and saccule sense linear acceleration of the head and the position of the head relative to gravity.

6. Hair cells of the utricle and of the saccule are excited by the bending of the cilia caused by the sliding of the otoliths over the surface of the hair cells.
7. Caloric testing of semicircular canal function makes use of convection currents set up by warming or cooling of endolymph. Caloric testing has the advantage that the vestibular organ of each side can be tested independently of the other.

Further Reading

Books and Reviews

Nauton RF: *The Vestibular System.* New York, Academic Press, 1975.
Wilson VJ, Jones GM: *Mammalian Vestibular Physiology.* New York, Plenum Press, 1979.

chapter 14

Muscle Contraction

How muscles do their work.

14.1. The Contractile Machine of Skeletal Muscle

It has been known for centuries that bones are moved by the shortening of muscles. How muscles shorten remained a mystery until the electron microscope revealed the structural basis of muscular contraction. Figure 14.1 shows a reconstruction of the fine structure of muscle, and Figures 14.2 and 14.3, diagrams of the moving parts.

The contractile proteins are arranged in two sets of filaments. The thick filaments are composed of myosin, a protein of two parts, a long chain (light meromyosin) and a compact group called heavy meromyosin. The light myosin tails are aligned in bundles to compose the thick filaments, and the heavy myosin head groups protrude from these filaments at regularly staggered intervals. Actin, a globular protein, forms the thin filaments as its molecules are linked in intertwined helical chains (Fig. 14.2). Long tropomyosin molecules are inserted in the grooves of the helix in the thin filaments, and troponin molecules are attached at the end of each tropomyosin filament.

The thick and thin filaments are arranged in regular arrays. Where they overlap, the muscle fiber is optically anisotropic, forming the A band; where only thin filaments are present the fiber is isotropic, the I band (Figs. 14.1 and 14.3). In the center of the A band there is a lighter

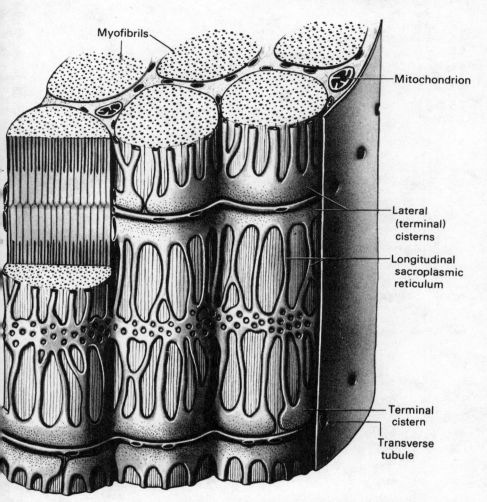

Figure 14.1. The fine structure of the interior of a vertebrate skeletal muscle fiber. (Reprinted with permission from W. M. Copenhaver, D. E. Kelly, and R. L. Wood: *Bailey's Textbook of Histology*, ed. 17. Baltimore, Williams & Wilkins, 1978.)

zone where thin filaments do not reach, the H band. In the middle of the I band is the Z line, a thin line formed by a disk of yet another protein. The regular alignment of the banding of the filaments in skeletal and cardiac muscle fibers gives them the cross-striated appearance well

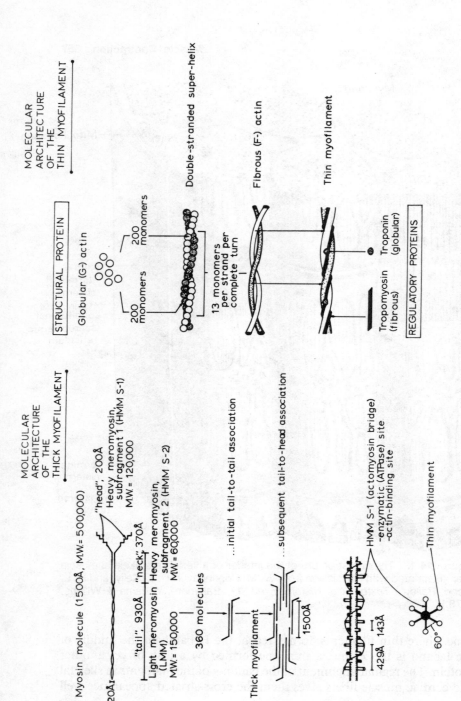

Figure 14.2. The components and the molecular structure of the thick and thin filaments in vertebrate skeletal muscle. (Reprinted with permission from W. M. Copenhaver, D. E. Kelly, and R. L. Wood: *Bailey's Textbook of Histology*, ed. 17. Baltimore, Williams &

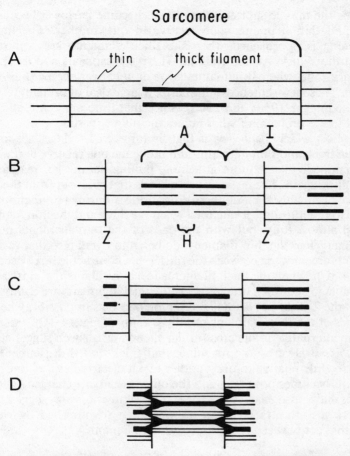

Figure 14.3. Relative positions of the thick and thin filaments in various degrees of stretch and contraction of skeletal muscle. *A*, the fiber is stretched to the point where thick and thin filaments no longer overlap, so that contractile force cannot develop; *B*, thick and thin filaments overlap so that contractile force can effectively develop; *C*, with thin filaments doubly overlapping contractile force diminishes; *D*, the fiber cannot shorten any further than the length at which the free ends of the thin filaments abut the Z lines (compare with Fig. 14.5).

seen even in unstained preparations, but accentuated by various staining methods. Smooth muscle fibers also contain parallel bundles of actin and myosin, but they are not all arranged in a regular geometrical pattern and so do not appear striated.

When the muscle shortens, the I bands become narrower because the thick and thin filaments slide relative to one another. The limit of shortening is approached when the thick filaments are compressed against the Z disk. At that time the H band disappears and is replaced by a dark zone, where thin filaments are doubly overlapping (Fig. 14.3C and D). These few sentences summarize a great deal of brilliant research published in the 1950s and 1960s. Since that time much attention has shifted to the problem of what makes the filaments slide.

The most widely held view is that multiple cross-bridges are formed between thick and thin filaments and move the one relative to the other in a centipede-like motion, attaching, pulling, letting go, reattaching, and pulling again. The heavy myosin heads that stick out from the thick filaments probably become these cross-bridges during contraction (Fig. 14.2). Contractile force is maximal when the thick and the thin filaments overlap almost fully, but with the ends of the thin filaments not yet touching. When the thin filaments do begin to overlap so that two thin filaments are jammed between the thick ones, contractile force decreases (Fig. 14.3C). When the thick filaments reach the Z line the muscle fiber is still able to shorten a little more as the thick filaments are compressed against the Z disk, but further shortening becomes impossible when the free ends of the thin filaments reach the Z lines (Fig. 14.3D).

As an alternative to the cross-bridge theory, it has been suggested that muscle is an electrostatic machine; that thick and thin filaments are forced to slide relative to one another by an electric field, as one set of filaments becomes positively and the other negatively charged. The two theories have also been combined. The synthetic view suggests that cross-bridges are attached, moved, and then relinquished by electric forces that act between the bridge and the filament.

14.1a. THE FUEL OF MUSCLE CONTRACTION

Myosin is not just a moving part, it also serves as the sparkplug of the muscle engine. Myosin is an adenosine triphosphatase (ATPase): it splits ATP into adenosine diphosphate (ADP) and inorganic phosphate, liberating the energy of the phosphate bond that powers contraction and also generates heat.

ATP is not split by myosin when the muscle is at rest because the ATPase activity is inhibited by tropomyosin. This inhibitory effect is lifted—disinhibited, if you like—when calcium binds to troponin. At rest Ca^{2+} activity in the sarcoplasm is only about 3×10^{-7} M. Just before contraction begins it rises to about 10^{-5} M, which is still low compared to that of interstitial fluid (10^{-3} M; see Table 2.1) but high enough for binding to troponin. The result is suppression of ATPase inhibition and the splitting of ATP to fuel cross-bridge formation.

How $[Ca^{2+}]_i$ rises to initiate contraction and then declines again when it is time to relax is the topic of the next section.

14.1b. EXCITATION-CONTRACTION COUPLING

Muscle fibers contain two elaborate intracellular systems of channels (Fig. 14.1). The *transverse* or *T tubules* are open at one end to the interstitial space and contain extracellular fluid. In fact T tubules are narrow invaginations of the surface membrane (the sarcolemma). They are located near the Z lines. The *sarcoplasmic reticulum* is a network of intercommunicating canals and cisterns that is entirely within the muscle fiber and does not communicate with the outside. The wide *terminal cisterns* of this reticulum are near the T tubules but do not touch them; the thinner longitudinal canals interconnect the cisterns (Fig. 14.1). Elements of the sarcoplasmic reticulum have been isolated from muscle fibers. After the fairly drastic treatment needed to isolate them, they re-form into closed vesicles of submicroscopic size. Isolated sarcoplasmic reticulum vesicles accumulate Ca^{2+} from the environment against a steep gradient of concentration. ATP is required for this work. In intact muscle the role of sarcoplasmic reticulum is believed to be the same; namely, the removal of Ca^{2+} from the sarcoplasm and its storage until needed to initiate contraction.

What induces sarcoplasmic reticulum to release some of the sequestered Ca^{2+} at the onset of contraction is not exactly known, but the muscle action potential does initiate the process. Since the membrane of the T tubules is continuous with the surface membrane of the muscle fiber, the impulse propagates into the T tubules. With the action potential Na^+ ions enter the sarcoplasm near the terminal cisterns of the sarcoplasmic reticulum. Ca^{2+} is believed to be released from these cisterns either under the influence of the electric potential change of the nearby T tubular membrane, or of the entering Na^+, or through the mediation of some unidentified intracellular messenger substance.

Once Ca^{2+} is released, some of it is bound to troponin and thus indirectly initiates the splitting of ATP and cross-bridge formation as already explained (see Section 14.1a).

For contracted muscle to relax, Ca^{2+} has to be removed from the sarcoplasm again. This is the job of the longitudinal canals of the sarcoplasmic reticulum. Thus, Ca^{2+} released from the terminal cisterns is taken back by the tubules that are continuous with the cisterns. Once it is recaptured, Ca^{2+} must be redistributed within the reticulum to be stored in the terminal cisterns again, ready for the next contraction.

Uptake of Ca^{2+} is necessary but not sufficient for relaxation. Some ATP must also be present. During contraction some of the available ATP is used up, but normally supply can keep up with demand so that the concentration is only slightly decreased. If for any reason ATP is not regenerated from ADP, so that all ATP is consumed, the cross-bridges are never broken. This state is called *rigor*. ATP is not split while it catalyzes relaxation; the presence of the intact molecule in low concentration suffices. This is called the *plasticizing* action of ATP and is distinct from its role as recyclable fuel. After death the supply of oxygen as well as metabolic substrates ceases and therefore ATP eventually vanishes and *rigor mortis* sets in. In general, if a muscle shortens without firing action potentials, we speak of *contracture*. Rigor is just one form of contracture; certain poisons can cause it too. Myotonia is not contracture, because it is caused by the abnormal firing of action potentials (see Section 3.4d).

14.2. Whole Muscle Function

Under certain conditions entire muscles can be removed from the body and examined *in vitro*, with or without the motor nerve attached. This is easily done in frogs, but in mammals is possible only with certain thin muscles. But much has been learned about mammalian muscles by detaching the tendon from the skeletal insertion and attaching it to some recording device. If such a muscle is stimulated by a single pulse, applied either to the motor nerve or to the muscle itself, it will briefly contract and then relax. This, in technical language, is a *twitch*. In the external ocular muscles it takes less than 0.01 second to contract and about 0.02 second to relax: in a large "slow" muscle (see Section 15.1a) such as soleus it takes about 0.1 second to reach its peak and 0.3 second from onset of contraction to complete relaxation.

If a weight is hung on the tendon of the muscle, then at the onset of contraction its force rises rapidly until it matches the weight; after that the force remains constant while the weight is lifted: this is described as *isotonic contraction*. If the weight stretches the muscle before the contraction starts, we speak of pre-loaded condition. If the weight is initially supported so that the muscle is slack before it contracts and then picks the weight up on its way, we speak of post-loaded condition.

Within limits the maximal velocity of isotonic contractions is an inverse (but non-linear) function of the load (Fig. 14.4). The muscle shortens at the highest velocity if it carries no weight at all. If the load exceeds the maximal force of which the muscle is capable, of course velocity will be zero.

If the ends of a muscle are fixed so that it cannot shorten and the muscle is stimulated, the resulting contraction is said to be *isometric*. Isometric contractions are normally used, for example, to support or to carry a weight without lifting it, or to stiffen a joint in a given position without moving it.

The maximal isometric contractile force developed by a muscle depends on the length at which it is immobilized (Fig. 14.5). When the muscle is attached to its normal origin and insertion, the limits to length change are set by the range of movement allowed by the skeleton. The force a muscle can develop is maximal when it is stretched to its greatest anatomical length. Most muscles attain this length when the bones to which they are attached have least leverage, when they are in the mechanically least advantageous position. Thus they develop maximal force when they need it most. For example, the flexors of the elbow develop maximal force when the arm is fully extended and the extensors when the arm is fully flexed.

If a muscle attains a length greater or smaller than normally allowed by its skeletal stops, it rapidly loses contractile force, for the reasons explained earlier (Figs. 14.3 and 14.5). In practice this occurs when joints are dislocated or bones are broken. In setting a fracture, muscles

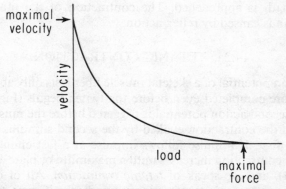

Figure 14.4. Velocity of contraction as a function of load during isotonic contraction of vertebrate skeletal muscle.

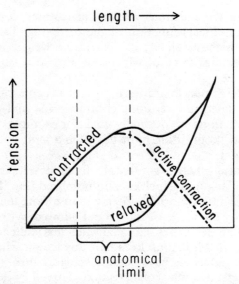

Figure 14.5. The tension measured by a strain gauge attached to the tendon of a vertebrate skeletal muscle (cf. Fig. 14.6*A*) as a function of the length of the muscle, measured under isometric conditions, in the relaxed and in the actively contracting state. *Vertical dashed lines* indicate limits to shortening and lengthening when the muscle is in its normal anatomical position; *dashed curve* shows difference between contracted and relaxed states, i.e. the net contractile force.

may offer little resistance at first, but then resistance mounts as their normal length is approached. The contraction of the muscles of an injured limb is caused by reflex action.

14.2a. TETANIC CONTRACTION

The action potential of a skeletal muscle fiber lasts only about 2 msec. It is therefore completed even before the twitch begins (Figs. 14.6 and 14.7). If a second action potential is triggered before the muscle relaxed, the force of the contraction evoked by the second stimulus is added to that of the first. If impulse follows impulse at a fast enough rate, the force of the contraction increases until a maximum or plateau is reached (Fig. 14.6*A*), and we speak of *tetanic contraction*. All of our normal movements are tetanic contractions; we rarely if ever twitch. The frequency of stimulation at which the contraction becomes smooth

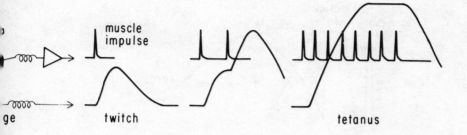

muscle
impulse

twitch

tetanus

ge

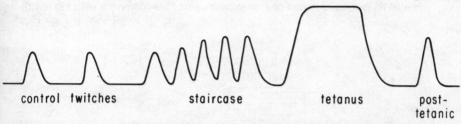

control twitches   staircase   tetanus   post-
tetanic

Figure 14.6. Electric and mechanical responses of a skeletal muscle. *A*, the recording of the muscle action potential and the force of contraction during an isometric twitch, the summation of two twitches, and a smoothly fused tetanic contraction. *B*, illustrating the staircase phenomenon and post-tetanic potentiation of the contractile force in skeletal muscle.

instead of oscillating is the *fusion frequency*. It is different for different types of muscles: the shorter the twitch time, the higher the fusion frequency (see Table 15.1 and Section 15.1a).

The *active state* of muscle fibers, the state in which force is being developed by the contractile machinery, is shorter than the time it takes for a twitch to reach maximum force (Fig. 14.7). The delay is caused by the elastic elements that are in series with the contractile proteins. As a simplified model, imagine that the sliding filaments are coupled to a spring, and that a force-measuring device is attached to the other end of the spring. If the contractile elements suddenly pulled on the spring, it would take some time for the spring to transmit the force (Fig. 14.8). The interposition of elastic elements between contractile components and the insertion of the tendon is also the main reason that the

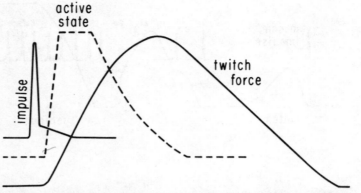

Figure 14.7. The time courses of the action potential, the active state and the force of an isometric twitch of a skeletal muscle fiber (compare with Fig. 14.8).

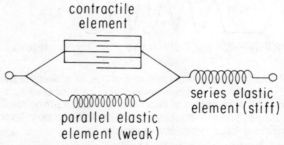

Figure 14.8. Model of the mechanical components of a skeletal muscle fiber to explain the unequal time courses of active state and contractile tension (Fig. 14.7) and the length-tension diagram (Fig. 14.5) of vertebrate skeletal muscle. The contractile element, symbolically represented as an electrostatic force generator, is responsible for the active state. The spring shown as the elastic element in series with the force generator is responsible for the delay in the development of the force at the tendon compared to the development of the active state. When the relaxed muscle is stretched, only the weak parallel elastic element offers resistance, hence the minimal tension of relaxed muscle within its anatomical limits to its length; beyond those limits the series elastic element is stretched.

maximum force of a twitch is less than the maximum force developed during tetanic contraction. When the active state of a twitch ceases, its full force has not yet been transmitted to the load. During tetanic contraction the spring cannot relax, and the full force of the active state is transmitted.

The active state itself is not invariable, as can be demonstrated as follows. If a muscle is stimulated at repeated intervals but not quite frequently enough for a fused tetanus, then the amplitude of subsequent twitches gradually increases at first and then a constant level is reached. The initial increase of repeated twitches is the *staircase* phenomenon, and it is even more marked in cardiac than in skeletal muscle (Fig. 14.6B). Moreover, if the muscle has been stimulated tetanically and then allowed to relax, and then stimulated again with single pulses, the twitches after the tetanus are stronger than those before. This post-tetanic potentiation of contractions is distinct from the post-tetanic potentiation of synaptic transmission discussed in Section 4.3 and is related to an enhancement of active state. Opinions differ concerning the mechanism of these changes, but many investigators attribute the enhanced contractions following previous activation to the lingering of residual calcium, not yet reabsorbed by the sarcoplasmic reticulum following a contraction.

The force and shortening of contracting muscle are normally controlled by the rate of motor nerve impulses and by the recruitment of motor neurons. How such grading is achieved and how several muscles are coordinated in movements will be discussed in Chapter 15.

14.2b. MUSCLE FATIGUE

Being tired has many aspects, and muscle fatigue is just one of them. By muscle fatigue physiologists mean the failure of contraction of normal muscle during prolonged stimulation. A distinction must be made between fatigue during voluntary effort and fatigue during artificial (electric) stimulation. Voluntary contraction could fail because of fatigue of: (1) the central nervous system; (2) the neuromuscular junction; (3) the muscle excitable membrane; (4) excitation-contraction coupling; (5) the energy supply to the contractile mechanism; and (6) the contractile mechanism itself.

Early research was concerned mainly with whether fatigue of voluntary contraction was central or peripheral. In the first experiments it appeared that when a subject's voluntary contraction began to weaken, electrical stimulation could still cause a strong contraction. It thus seemed that voluntary fatigue was mainly central, a failure of "effort" rather than exhaustion of the muscle itself. It was later shown, however, that voluntary effort can in fact mobilize all the contractile power of a muscle, provided that three factors are optimal: motivation, training and feedback. The importance of the first two of these three factors are intuitively obvious; the third needs some explanation. If a subject is just asked to push as hard and as long as he can, he usually will slacken his contraction earlier than if he can see the result of his effort, for example the needle of the meter or some other visible or audible indicator.

It seems, then, that central factors play a part in fatigue but need not do so. What is it that makes some subjects give up their effort before their muscle is exhausted? A feeling of discomfort in the exercised muscle seems to be the obvious immediate cause. The nature of this discomfort is not entirely clear, but nociceptive nerve endings in the muscle itself may play a part. These endings may be stimulated by lactic acid and by H^+ ions. Furthermore, during sustained isometric contraction the circulation is impaired and oxygen tension in the muscle may fall.

As we have seen, a well-trained, well-motivated, well-informed subject can maintain voluntary effort in spite of rising discomfort until his muscle is truly exhausted. To explain the fatigue in these cases we are still left with five alternatives. Research is now focused at distinguishing between electrical and chemical factors, of which the former include nerve-muscle transmission and muscle impulse generation, the latter all the other ingredients of muscle function from excitation-contraction coupling onward. In this respect different types of muscle fibers seem to behave differently. In the next chapter we will learn the differences between fatigue-prone (type FF) and fatigue-resistant (types FR and S) muscle fibers. In the fatigue-prone fibers the biochemical machinery seems to fatigue at a time when impulses are still transmitted to, and generated by, the muscle fibers. In the fatigue-resistant fibers electric and chemical failure appear to go hand in hand. Whether the electric failure is at the nerve-muscle junction, at the muscle membrane, or both, is controversial. The majority of investigators now seem to be of the opinion, however, that the human nerve-muscle junction never fails, except in myasthenic patients (see Section 3.4e) and some other pathological and toxic conditions, leaving the ionic mechanism of the muscle membrane the more likely site of electric fatigue.

A beginning has been made with sorting out the different components that may be responsible for fatigue of the biochemical equipment of muscle. The ATP content of fatigued muscle is only slightly decreased, but the turnover of ATP seems slowed. Whether the diminished energy turnover is cause or effect of fatigue is not yet clear. The factors that are currently much discussed include the possible fatigue of excitation-contraction coupling, in other words of the sarcoplasmic reticulum; the acidification of the sarcoplasm which may adversely affect several enzyme systems; and the accumulation of lactic acid which is mainly responsible for the acidification.

14.3. Cardiac and Smooth Muscles

Properties and functions of cardiac and smooth muscles are described in detail in texts dealing with the cardiovascular and gastrointestinal systems. Only a brief summary will be given here, highlighting the most striking differences between visceral and skeletal muscles. Any such summary must be simplified, neglecting the details concerning, for example, the wide variety of smooth muscles and the properties of cardiac muscle in different regions of the heart.

The contractile mechanism of all muscles is controlled by the intracellular activity of free calcium. The details of the mechanism are different in that free Ca^{2+} in the cytoplasm of smooth muscle interacts with a protein called calmodulin, and the Ca-calmodulin complex initiates a chain of enzymic reactions which result in the splitting of ATP by myosin. A perhaps even more important difference is that while skeletal muscle contains a store of calcium sequestered in the sarcoplasmic reticulum and is therefore independent of calcium in interstitial fluid, many types of smooth muscle need to take in Ca^{2+} from their environment to initiate contraction. This intake occurs with action potentials, which in these cells are generated by inward current of Ca^{2+} instead of Na^+ (see Section 3.11).

Some other smooth muscle cells generate mixed Ca^{2+}-Na^+ spikes. Cardiac muscle is also intermediate in this respect. While it does have a sarcoplasmic reticulum, this is not as well developed in cardiac as in skeletal muscle. The level of $[Ca^{2+}]_o$ does influence cardiac contractility. When $[Ca^{2+}]_o$ is too low, cardiac contractions weaken; when it is high, they become unduly strong; and when $[Ca^{2+}]_o$ is raised to a great excess, the heart stops in a contracted state—systolic arrest. Such extremes of $[Ca^{2+}]_o$ jeopardize other vital functions and are rarely seen in clinical practice.

The dependence on Ca^{2+} is especially marked in the smooth muscles of microvessels. Blocking the entry of calcium with Mg^{2+}, Co^{2+}, Mn^{2+} or the organic calcium channel blockers causes arterioles to relax. Organic calcium channel blocking drugs are prescribed to achieve vasodilatation. These drugs also weaken cardiac contraction, but less so than vascular smooth muscle contractions.

Cardiac muscle is rhythmically active without being driven by the nervous system. So are many but not all smooth muscles. The smooth muscle of the intestines and of the microcirculatory vessels are, for example, autorhythmic. Both cardiac and intestinal muscle cells are linked by gap junctions that are freely permeable to ions (see Section 2.5c) so that action potentials of one cell are conducted without hindrance to its neighbors. Such electrotonically continuous nets of cells are often described as functional syncytia. Neuroglial cells also form such electrotonic nets, but their function is quite different (see Section 5.9b).

The pacemaker potentials of cardiac muscle are relaxation oscillations of the membrane potential (see Section 4.6; see also Smith and Kampine, Figs. 5.4 and 5.6). The action potentials of cardiac muscle are much longer than those of any other muscle cell. As a consequence the cardiac cells have prolonged refractory periods so that tetanic fusion of cardiac contractions is not possible. Each cardiac systole can be considered a twitch; a slow one to be sure, but a twitch nonetheless (see also Smith and Kampine, Fig. 5.5).

The pacemaker activity of smooth muscle is manifested in more or less sinusoidal oscillations of the membrane potential. Trains of action potentials are triggered by the depolarization phase of these oscillations, and cease during the repolarization phase. The muscle contracts while action potentials are fired and relaxes during repolarization. Blocking the impulses, for example by calcium channel blockers, suppresses contraction even though the slow oscillations continue.

The heart can contract in a coordinated and effective manner without any assistance from nerves. The intestines are too long, and the conduction velocity in their smooth muscle too slow, to achieve coordination of the organ by muscular conduction alone. The movements by which food is propelled and mixed are coordinated by the intramural nerve plexus of Meissner and Auerbach. The neuron circuits either inhibit or enhance the autorhythmicity of the smooth muscle and coordinate the muscular action over long distances of gut (see Section 17.3c).

Not all smooth muscles are autorhythmic and not all are syncytial. The vas deferens and the piloerector muscles are entirely under nervous control, and each muscle cell acts independently of the others. These are described as *multi-unit* or motor-unit type muscles, in contrast to the syncytial, or *single-unit*, or unitary type such as is found in the intestines. Some organs, such as the urinary bladder, are intermediate between these extremes. Under normal conditions the bladder is under neural control but if its innervation is destroyed, after some weeks it acquires automaticity (see Section 17.3d).

The excitability of smooth muscles is also influenced by circulating hormones. Adrenaline affects most of them, inhibiting bronchial and intestinal, but stimulating vascular muscles. Gonadal hormones and oxytocin have strong effects on uterine smooth muscle.

14.4. Malignant Hyperthermia

Malignant hyperthermia is a fortunately rare but unfortunately occasionally fatal complication of general anesthesia, especially if halothane is used. The excessive rise of body temperature is caused by activation of contractile mechanism and oxidative metabolism of muscles, skeletal and cardiac. The muscles are activated by entry of Ca^{2+} through the sarcolemma, initiating the splitting of ATP and all that it entails. The consequence may be circulatory collapse.

14.5. Chapter Summary

1. Skeletal muscle contracts when the thick filaments, composed of myosin, and the thin filaments, composed of actin with troponin and tropomyosin attached, slide upon one another.
2. According to the most commonly held theory, the sliding motion is caused by the action of cross-bridges between the thick and the thin filaments. The cross-bridges are formed by the heavy "heads" of the myosin molecules.
3. The excitation represented by the action potential triggers the contraction by releasing Ca^{2+} from the terminal cisternae of the sarcoplasmic reticulum into the sarcoplasm. The action potential gains access to the interior of the muscle fiber through the T tubules.
4. In the relaxed state of the muscle, in the absence of free Ca^{2+}, tropomyosin inhibits the ATPase effect of myosin. The Ca^{2+} released from the sarcoplasmic reticulum binds to troponin and inhibits tropomyosin. As the Ca-troponin complex inhibits tropomyosin, myosin is allowed to split ATP and initiates, as well as provides fuel for, contraction.
5. Muscle relaxes when Ca^{2+} is retrieved by the longitudinal canals of the sarcoplasmic reticulum. Some ATP must also be present to provide plasticizing action for relaxation. If all ATP has been split, rigor ensues.
6. During an isotonic twitch, the velocity of shortening is an inverse nonlinear function of the load.
7. The maximum isometric contractile force developed by striated muscles is a bell-shaped function of the muscle's length. For most skeletal muscles the maximum force is developed when the muscle in its normal anatomical position attains the maximum length its skeletal stops allow.
8. Tetanic contraction of skeletal muscle is possible because the duration of the twitch is much longer than the duration of the refractory period of the action potential.
9. True muscle fatigue is mainly caused by an exhaustion of the contractile mechanism itself. The occurrence of transmission failure at the endplate of fatigued but otherwise healthy muscle is the subject of controversy. Discomfort due to exercise may occur before true muscle fatigue (as just defined).
10. Cardiac muscle, and most smooth muscles, must derive part or all the Ca^{2+} required for excitation-contraction coupling from their environment. Ca^{2+} ions enter the cytoplasm of these cells with the action potential.
11. In cardiac muscle and in so-called single-unit type smooth muscle, action potentials are conducted freely from any one muscle fiber to all of its neighbors.

Further Reading

Books and Reviews

Bülbring E, Brading AF, Jones AW, et al: *Smooth Muscle.* Austin, University of Texas Press, 1981.

Ebashi S: Regulation of muscle contraction. *Proc R Soc Lond (Biol)* 207:286, 1980.

Huxley AF: Muscle structure and theories of contraction. *Prog Biophysics Biophys Chem* 7:257–318, 1959.

Huxley HE: The mechanism of muscle contraction. *Science* 164:1356–1365, 1969.

Porter R, Whelan J (eds): *Human Muscle Fatigue: Physiological Mechanisms:* CIBA Foundation Symposium No. 82. London, Pitman Medical, 1981.

Smith, JJ, Kampine, JP: *Circulatory Physiology: The Essentials.* Baltimore, Williams & Wilkins, 1980.

Treagear RT, Marston SB: The crossbridge theory. *Annu Rev Physiol* 41:723–736, 1979.

Vanhoutte PM, Bohr DF (eds): Calcium entry blockers and the cardiovascular system. *Fed Proc* 40:2851–2888, 1981.

Articles

Hill AV: The development of the active state of muscle during the latent period. *Proc R Soc Lond (Biol)* 137:320–329, 1950.

chapter 15

Organization of Muscle and Spinal Reflexes

How the specific properties of various types of muscle fibers are matched to the tasks they are called to perform; the properties of stretch receptors in muscle and their central connections; reflexes of normal and injured spinal cords; hypertonias of muscle.

15.1. Motor Units

A motor unit consists of an alpha motor neuron, its axon with all its terminal branches, and all the muscle fibers that axon innervates. No smaller movement is possible than that caused by the contraction of one motor unit, because if one alpha motor neuron discharges one action potential, that action potential will invade all the terminal branches of the axon and be transmitted to all muscle fibers of the unit. Less than one whole motor unit moves at the command of a nerve impulse only in certain diseases of the neuromuscular junction and under the influence of certain poisons, and perhaps in extreme muscle fatigue (see Section 14.2b).

The use of the term "unit" in this context needs a qualification. Motor units are not all of equal size. In the muscles of the middle ear one motor axon innervates 10–20 muscle fibers; in gastrocnemius muscle of humans the average is 1700 muscle fibers. Not only does the average size of motor units differ from muscle to muscle, but even within a single muscle, the size of motor units varies over a wide range.

The muscle fibers belonging to one motor unit are not packed compactly, but mingle with those of its neighbor. This was strikingly demonstrated in the following experiment. A single spinal motor neuron of an animal was stimulated until the muscle fibers it innervated became fatigued. At that time nearly all the glycogen in those fibers was exhausted. The muscle was then prepared for histochemical examination, and the sections were stained for glycogen. The glycogen-depleted fibers did not form a continuous field in these sections, but were scattered among glycogen-rich fibers of the surrounding, rested units. The need for interdigitation and overlap in the architecture of motor units will become obvious shortly (see Section 15.1c).

15.1a. MOTOR UNIT TYPES

Motor units vary not only in size, but also according to physiological and biochemical properties. In many animals, including cats and rabbits, certain of the differences are obvious from simple inspection of some muscles. Soleus, for example, has a conspicuously deep red color, while tibialis anterior muscle is much paler. It has been found years ago that red muscles contract more slowly and fatigue less readily than do pale ("white") muscles. The difference in color is due to variation in myoglobin content, red muscle fibers having much more of this material than pale ones.

The majority of skeletal muscles is neither purely red nor purely pale but of mixed composition. Microscopic examination shows that individual muscle fibers have a distinctive character, but red and pale fibers lie side by side within the same muscle. In man, no muscle is as pure in composition as the just-quoted example of the soleus muscle of cats and rabbits, but even in people some muscles are redder than others.

More recently it has been shown that there are more than two distinct classes of muscle fibers. All red muscle fibers have in common that they are more resistant to fatigue than pale fibers, but by other criteria they fall into separate groups. One classification is based on cytochemical characteristics, another on physiological criteria. The physiological classes were defined in experiments in which single motor neurons (or their axons) were stimulated, and the resulting contraction of individual motor units was recorded. The three cytochemical types were designated by the letters A, B and C; the motor unit types by the following abbreviations: FF, meaning "fast-contracting fatigue-prone"; FR standing for "fast but fatigue-resistant", FI for "fast-intermediate"; and S for "slow." A summary of chemical and physiological characteristics may be found in Table 15.1, but the smaller subgroup FI has been deleted for the sake of simplification.

Since most muscles contain different types of muscle fibers, it was natural to

Table 15.1.
Muscle Fiber Chemical and Physiological Characteristics

Muscle Fiber Type*	A	B	C
Appearance	Pale	Intermediate to red	Red
Myoglobin	Poor	Rich	Rich
Glycogen	Intermediate	Poor	Rich
Glycolytic activity	High	Variable	Low
Mitochondria	Few	Intermediate	Many
Mitochondrial ATPase	Poor	Intermediate	Rich
Myofibrillar ATPase	Rich	Intermediate	Poor
Fiber diameter	Large	Small to intermediate	Small
Adjacent capillaries	Few	Many	Many
Motor Unit Type	**FF**	**FR**	**S**
Twitch time	Short (~20 msec)	Short	Long (>50 msec)
Fusion frequency	High	High	Low
Fatigue†	1–2 min	5–10 min	30–90 min
Size (number of muscle fibers)	Large	Small to intermediate	Small
Power	Powerful	Medium	Weak
Parent Motor Neuron	**Large**	**Intermediate**	**Small**
Recruitment	Late	Intermediate	Early
Maximum firing frequency	High	Intermediate	Low
After-hyperpolarization	Minimal	Intermediate	Marked

* Note that some authors designate the intermediate group as C, and the red group as B. Note also that "white" and "pale" are synonyms in this context. Furthermore, the A group is sometimes classified as type I and sometimes as type II. A unified nomenclature is badly needed.

† The time taken for contraction to fail during prolonged tetanic stimulation of the motor axon.

Note also that certain parameters, e.g. myofibrillar ATPase, are reported differently by different authors. This table was compiled by selecting data that seemed consistent one with another from reviews by R. I. Close: *Physiological Reviews* 52:129–197, 1972; and R. E. Burke: Motor units: anatomy, physiology and functional organization. In *Motor Control, Handbook of Physiology*, vol. 2, edited by V. B. Brooks. Bethesda, American Physiological Society, 1981, pp. 345–422.

ask whether different fiber types could mingle in the same motor unit. The answer is "no": each motor unit is made up of just one type of muscle fiber. The next question then is: what safeguards this homogeneity of motor units during embryonic development? Motor axons grow from the central nervous system (CNS), and their numerous branches must find their target cells among the many making up a muscle. In theory, there could be two ways for axons to make the right connections. Either each axonal branch would seek out the appropriate type of muscle fiber. Or, the germinal muscle cells could be undifferentiated, and each motor axon could impose specific properties on the developing muscle fibers with which it forms a junction. There are reasons to believe that the latter is the true explanation. The differentiation of muscle fibers is not yet completed at birth, but continues into the first weeks or months of postnatal life. If in a young rabbit two motor nerves are surgically crossed, so that a nerve originally innervating a pale muscle is forced to regenerate into a red one, and *vice versa*, after a few months the properties of the two muscles will be altered. The muscle that should have been pale will, under the influence of its new nerve, be significantly redder than normal and acquire physiological properties resembling normal red muscle. A similar change, but in the reverse direction, occurs in cross-innervated red muscle.

15.1b. MOTOR UNIT TYPE AND MUSCLE FUNCTION

If we reflect for a moment on what people and animals do all day, it is obvious that the demands made on muscles vary greatly. As we stand still, we contract some muscle fibers tonically, others intermittently as the body sways and its weight shifts. Carrying an object requires steady force; playing the piano, speed and finesse. A watch is repaired by finely graded but sustained contractions. A long jump places loads on the musculature in a way that is very different from the exertion needed to move furniture. Yet the same muscles often participate in such very different acts. Having muscles built of motor units with varying functional specifications undoubtedly aids in carrying out each of these tasks the right way.

When a single axon innervating red muscle fibers is stimulated, the resulting contraction is slow and feeble compared to that evoked by stimulating an axon innervating pale fibers of the same muscle (see Table 15.1). The red, S motor units are weaker than the FF units, because the red muscle fibers are thinner and because fewer muscle fibers belong to one motor axon (*lower innervation ratio*). These two factors, innervation ratio and average thickness of muscle fibers, determine the total cross-sectional area and hence the number of myofilaments available for activation in one motor unit, and so the maximal force it is capable of exerting.

We know from electromyographic recordings and from other observations that our muscles, especially those responsible for maintaining body postures, are rarely completely inactive. Some motor units fire almost always, even in most stages of sleep (see Chapter 19). Not surprisingly, the units that are most engaged throughout our lifetimes are the S units. Feeble and slow, but indefatigable, red muscle fibers are suited for carrying sustained but smaller loads. The FR units are available when both speed and precision are important, but only moderate forces are needed. FF units are in reserve for the occasions when a long leap, a hard blow, or a sudden push is called for.

The key to the fatigue resistance of red muscle fibers is that (1) they are much better supplied with capillaries; and (2) they are better equipped for oxidative respiration (Table 15.1), and hence do not build up lactate and so do not run up an oxygen debt. Pale muscle fibers, on the other hand, are less dependent on oxygen because of high glycolytic activity. But while pale muscle fibers are better off on the short haul, they become energy-depleted and run up an oxygen debt on the long run.

15.1c. THE GRADING OF MUSCULAR STRENGTH

As with the intensity coding of sensory signals, contractile force is controlled by the combined use of two principles: (1) by varying the numbers of motor units *recruited*; and (2) by modulating the *frequency* of impulses fired by motor axons. In principle any number of combinations of mean frequency multiplied by number of units recruited could produce a certain force. In fact, however, a given force is always produced by the same fixed number of motor units and firing frequency. This seemingly arbitrary limitation presumably simplifies the programming of the central control mechanisms.

When the force of contraction of a muscle is gradually increased, first the smallest motor neurons innervating the smallest motor units are called into action, and then gradually the larger and larger ones. This is Henneman's *size principle of recruitment*. With very few exceptions the size principle was found valid for normal reflex and voluntary movements, and also for pathological reflex contractions and for convulsive movements. It is this principle which insures that weak but sustained postural contractions are carried out by the small S units (see Section 15.1b). Another consequence of recruiting small units first is that weak contractions can be graded with greater finesse than strong contractions. Recruiting one small motor unit adds but a few muscle fibers to those already contracting; recruiting a large unit throws in several hundred

more. Fig. 15.1 shows how various types of motor units are recruited as
a cat is using a leg muscle of mixed composition for different movements. During quiet standing the cat uses 25% of the motor unit pool
of the gastrocnemius muscle, but this fraction of the population brings
forth only 5% of the total force of which this muscle is capable. Insofar
as data collected by observing cats are applicable to humans, it would
appear that people who sit all day never use the largest part of their
muscle mass. The physiological and biochemical consequences of keeping so much tissue idle do not belong in this text, but should be borne
in mind when advising patients.

It will be recalled that when nerves are stimulated by electric pulses, the axons

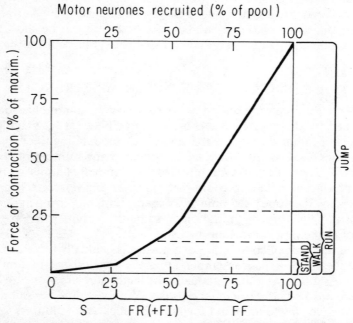

Figure 15.1. Recruitment of motor units in a hindlimb extensor muscle of a
cat. Note that recruiting 50% of the motor units develops less than 25% of the
total force of the muscle. The figure has been constructed with the assumption
that recruitment proceeds strictly by FR units being called into action after S
units, and FF units after FRs. In reality there may be some overlap in the
recruiting order, which would, however, not change the main idea conveyed by
this diagram. (Modified and redrawn after B. Walmsly, J. A. Hodgson, and R. E.
Burke: *Journal of Neurophysiology* 41:1203–1216, 1978.)

of largest caliber are excited by the weakest stimulus. The size principle of recruitment seems to run counter to this rule of electrical excitability. It will also be remembered, however, that the apparent threshold to extracellularly applied electrical stimulation is determined by the manner in which axons in an electric field admit current (see Section 3.1d and Fig. 3.7). Motor neurons in the central nervous system are, however, not normally excited by electric fields, but by chemically transmitting synapses, where the rules of electrical excitation do not apply. It has been observed that small neurons receive disproportionately large excitatory postsynaptic potentials (EPSPs) compared to larger neurons, and this probably explains their early recruitment. The reasons for the large EPSPs are, however, not clear.

That small motor neurons are more excitable through synapses than large ones enables calling small cells into action without activating large ones. It is clear enough that this is an advantage for performing slow, sustained contractions. The question is, would it not be an advantage also to be able to recruit the faster large motor units without simultaneously activating small ones in order to perform fast movements? To do this, the recruitment order would have to be reversed, in other words, the size principle overruled perhaps by selective inhibition of small neurones. Unfortunately, it is difficult to record the discharge of motor units while a muscle is rapidly shortening, and for this reason data are scarce. Examples of reversed recruitment order have been reported, but mostly in rather artifical conditions involving electrical stimulation of nerves. Actually, on further reflection, the need to recruit large, fast units at the exclusion of small, slow ones may arise only rarely. Most rapid, phasic movements require a tonic, postural underpinning. Small S type motor units may have to contract before, during and after FR and FF units do their job to provide stable start and finish positions of the skeleton.

It should be clear that muscles with two or more heads and dual or triple action must have more than one motor neuron pool, so that each head can be controlled independently of the other. Muscles having wide origins and/or insertions such as the deltoid and the masseter are special cases. Strands of fibers in these muscles contract in various proportions to move their joints in different directions. It may be assumed that their motor neuron populations are topographically organized and can be called into action in groups, as the intended movement requires.

Red muscle fibers are slow to contract and to relax, and therefore their fusion frequency (see Section 14.2a) is lower than that of pale muscle fibers (Table 15.1). Electromyography has revealed that during weak or moderately strong contractions motor units of any type often fire impulses at a rate below that required for a smoothly fused tetanic contraction. The shortening of normal muscle is nevertheless neither jerky nor tremulous. This is because motor units do not all fire at the same time. Since the fibers of neighboring motor units mingle and since units take turns tugging at their common tendon, their contraction, which would be intermittent if acting singly, is combined and smoothed.

15.2. Muscle Receptors

Charles Bell is remembered especially for two ideas. One was the insight that dorsal roots contain afferent fibers and ventral roots only efferents. Bell and Magendie discovered this independently at about the same time. The Bell-Magendie law seemed valid without exception until aberrant afferent C fibers were recently discovered in ventral roots.

Bell's other major contribution was his proposal that skeletal muscle contains sense organs and that muscle nerves are therefore not purely motor but also contain sensory fibers. When Bell wrote his paper on muscle sense, he had no idea what the sensory receptors in muscle might look like.

15.2a. MUSCLE SPINDLES

Muscle spindles were described toward the end of the 19th century, but at first were taken to be "germinal sites" from which muscle fibers grew during development and perhaps regenerated after injury. Decades passed before the afferent innervation and sensory function of these organs was discovered. Then, in the early 1920s, Bryan Matthews recorded impulses of afferent fibers of spindles in frog muscle and established the relationship between stimulus intensity and frequency of firing. His was, in fact, the first demonstration of the impulse discharge of a single sensory fiber. In the more than half century since Matthews' experiment, generations of researchers have studied these marvelous little organs, and there seems to be no end yet to the new detail still being discovered.

What seemed like germinal muscle cells to the histologists of the 19th century turned out to be complete, if miniature, striated muscle fibers (See Fig. 15.2). The motor fibers controlling them were discovered in the 1930s, and christened *fusimotor* or *gamma motor* fibers. The tiny muscle inside the capsule of spindles became known as *intrafusal*, to distinguish it from the regular or *extrafusal* muscle that does all the work. Intrafusal muscle is so feeble that its contraction cannot be recorded at the tendon of the muscle. Its function is to regulate the sensitivity of the sensory nerve terminals.

The sensory endings of muscle spindles are mechanoreceptors. Their adequate stimulus, as is that of other mechanoreceptors (see Section 6.4), is the deformation of the sensitive nerve terminal. Such deformation is achieved in one of two ways: (1) by stretching the muscle (and with it, its spindles); and (2) by the contraction of the intrafusal muscle (see Fig. 15.3). Contraction of the extrafusal fibers relieves the tension that stretches the sensory nerve terminals of the spindle, and so *diminishes* their excitation (Fig. 15.3). This happens during both isotonic and isometric contraction.

There are two types of each, intrafusal muscle fibers, fusimotor nerve fibers, and sensory terminals in each spindle (Figs. 15.2 and 15.4) and there are further subdivisions in some of these categories. By appearance, intrafusal muscle fibers are classified as *nuclear bag* and *nuclear chain* fibers, depending on whether nuclei are collected in a cluster in the middle of the fiber (the "equator"), or spread along its length. Nuclear bag fibers are further subdivided into bag 1, or dynamic bag, and bag 2 or static bag fibers. The two categories of gamma motor fibers are the *dynamic* and the *static* fusimotor fibers. Dynamic fusimotor fibers form

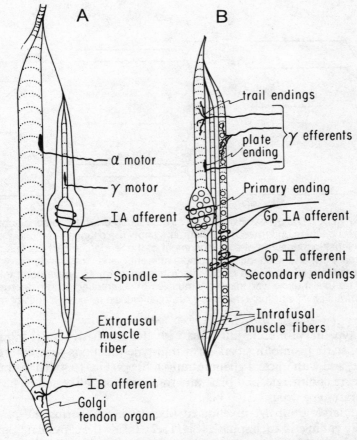

A

B

trail endings

plate ending
$\rangle \gamma$ efferents

α motor

γ motor

IA afferent

Primary ending

Gp IA afferent

Gp II afferent
Secondary endings

Spindle

Extrafusal
muscle
fiber

Intrafusal
muscle fibers

IB afferent
Golgi
tendon organ

Figure 15.2. The structure and innervation of muscle spindles. *A*, a spindle alongside the extrafusal muscle fibers; *B*, the main components of the spindle.

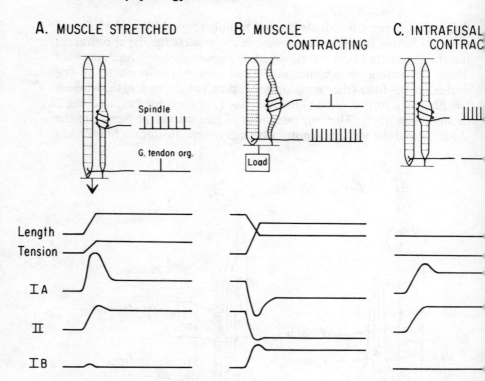

Figure 15.3. The behavior of muscle stretch receptors in three conditions. The idealized tracings underneath the diagrams show the changes of muscle length, of the tension measured at the attachment of the tendon, and of the firing rates of primary (*IA*) and secondary (*II*) spindle afferents, and Golgi tendon organ (*IB*). *A,* passive stretching of the muscle (length increasing); *B,* active contraction of the extrafusal muscle with intrafusal muscle not contracting (length decreasing); *C,* contraction of intrafusal muscle, extrafusal muscle relaxed, length of muscle fixed.

plate-type nerve-muscle junctions with the bag 1 (dynamic) intrafusal fibers; static fusimotor fibers form trail-type junctions with both bag 2 (static) and with nuclear chain intrafusal fibers (Fig. 15.4). All fusimotor fibers are cholinergic, and plate and trail junctions alike can be blocked by curare-type drugs.

One large group IA myelinated fiber (Fig. 6.4) forms the *primary* sensory endings in each spindle (Fig. 15.2). Inside the capsule it branches and forms coiled sensory terminals wrapped around the middle or "equatorial" portion of each intrafusal muscle fiber. Usually there are

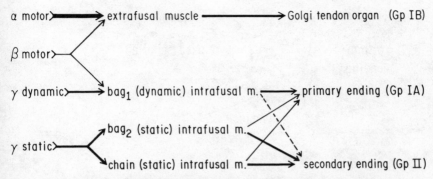

Figure 15.4. Actions of nerve and muscle fibers in skeletal muscle. The *arrows* indicate which component influences which; the thickness of the arrows shows the strength of the influence. Note that beta motor fibers, branches of which innervate both extrafusal and intrafusal muscle fibers, were known since many years to exist in amphibian muscles but have only recently been discovered in mammalian muscles. They are included here to complete the diagram but their significance is uncertain for the present. (Modified and redrawn after R. B. Stein: *Nerve and Muscle: Membranes, Cells and Systems.* New York, Plenum Press, 1980.)

more than one of the thinner, group II fibers which form *secondary* sensory terminals. The secondary endings lie outside the equatorial region, adjacent to the primary endings, mainly on chain muscle fibers, to a lesser degree on bag 2, and rarely on bag 1 fibers (Fig. 15.4). Primary and secondary endings used to be called annulospiral and flower-spray endings, but these names became obsolete when it turned out that both types of terminals form coils wrapped around intrafusal muscle fibers.

With so many components interacting, the functioning of muscle spindles had to be first analyzed in a simplified state. In acute experiments it is possible to interrupt all efferent connections of a muscle by cutting the appropriate ventral roots, and examine the afferent fiber discharge of muscle spindles while neither intra- nor extrafusal muscle contracts. Controlled stimuli can then be applied to selected efferent fibers and their influence examined one by one. If a relaxed muscle is stretched, both primary and secondary endings give both static and dynamic responses (Figs. 15.3 and 15.5), in other words, they adapt partially (see Sections 4.5 and 6.1). The dynamic sensitivity of primary endings is, however, much greater than that of secondary endings, and it is further enhanced if dynamic gamma motor fibers are stimulated to cause the contraction of bag 1 intrafusal fibers (Figs. 15.4 and 15.5).

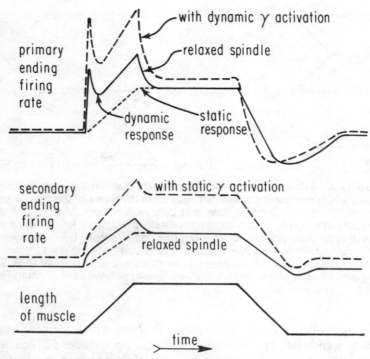

Figure 15.5.   Responses (firing rates) of primary and secondary spindle endings before, during and after stretching the muscle, without concurrent intrafusal contraction (*solid lines*) and with intrafusal muscle activated (*dashed lines*). The *dotted lines* show the static component in the responses of the afferent endings in a spindle (in the absence of intrafusal contraction).

The static sensitivity of primary endings is only moderately enhanced by contraction of the bag 1 fibers, and the responses of secondary endings are barely influenced by it.

The static (adapted) firing rate of the spindle sensory endings depends on the length of the muscle. While a muscle is in its anatomical position, attached to intact skeletal parts, the range of lengths it can take is limited by the range of motion of the joints. In a relaxed muscle the static discharge rate of both primary and secondary endings is a linear function of the length of the muscle, at least within the operating range of that particular sensory ending; that is from the threshold of firing to the upper anatomical limit of elongation of the muscle. In the absence of intrafusal contraction the static responses of primary and secondary endings are approximately parallel functions of muscle length (Fig. 15.6).

When the static fusimotor fibers are stimulated, the static responses of the secondary endings are greatly enhanced, those of the primary endings somewhat less (Figs. 15.5 and 15.6). Primary endings are distinguished by several features. When the muscle is being stretched, they show an onset-transient response consisting of a brief high frequency response which seems to signal the transition from the stationary to the moving state (Fig. 15.5). Furthermore, their dynamic sensitivity is non-linear, in that they respond disproportionately to small movements of relatively low velocity. And finally, when the muscle shortens, whether by the active contraction of extrafusal fibers, or passively by just being allowed to retract, the firing of primary endings decreases, sometimes to zero (Fig. 15.3). This highlights the significance of the resting discharge of the primary spindle afferents: it is the decrease of the firing rate below the resting level which signals "negative stretching," i.e. the shortening of the muscle.

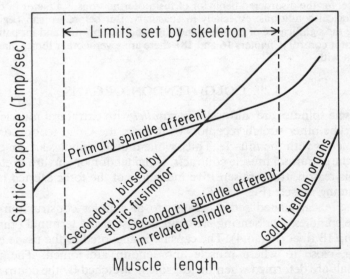

Figure 15.6. The static (adapted) firing rates of muscle stretch receptors at varying muscle length. There is a wide range of variation in the absolute firing frequency of both primary and secondary endings in different spindles that is not indicated in this diagram. More importantly, the static sensitivity (Δ firing rate/Δ length) of primary and secondary endings in a relaxed spindle is very similar, but static fusimotor activity influences secondary endings more strongly than primary endings.

In summary: the response of secondary spindle endings is dominated by the length of the muscle; the response of primary endings is more strongly influenced by rate of change than by actual length. The sensitivity of secondary endings is influenced by the excitation of static but not of dynamic fusimotor fibers; that of primary endings is influenced by both static and dynamic fusimotor fibers, but more by the latter. The primary endings are further distinguished by onset-transient responses; by excessive sensitivity to small stretches; and by strong suppression of the response during shortening of the muscle.

Complicated as it may seem at first reading, the foregoing is a simplified summary of the abundant detail known about muscle spindles. Thus the behavior of these organs under the controlled conditions of the laboratory is now rather well understood. The use to which they are put during normal movements is more controversial. In the last several years researchers did, however, succeed in recording the discharge of spindle afferents under relatively normal conditions as well, and so the analysis of their physiological function began in earnest. Understanding their function is also important for medical practice, for the disordered behavior of fusimotor neurons is a factor in certain neurological conditions, especially in spasticity. But before we can begin discussing the significance of muscle spindle function for normal and for pathological motor control (Chapters 16 and 18), there are several other topics that must be dealt with.

15.2b. GOLGI TENDON ORGANS

Muscle spindles are said to lie *in parallel* with extrafusal muscle (Fig. 15.2). The other stretch receptors of muscle, the Golgi tendon organs, are *in series* with the muscle. Thus, while muscle spindles are unloaded when the extrafusal muscle contracts, Golgi tendon organs are stretched. For this reason, they are sensitive indicators of the force exerted by the contracting muscle (Fig. 15.3*B*).

These encapsulated sense organs are of simpler construction than muscle spindles. The sensing elements consist of the terminal branches of group IB fiber (Fig. 6.4). The capsule is anchored to the tissue of the tendon, close to where muscle and tendon are joined. The nerve terminals are deformed when the capsule is stretched by the contraction of the muscle. A small number of muscle fibers contribute to the stretching of any one Golgi tendon organ. Because of the way in which muscle fibers belonging to adjacent motor units mingle (see Section 15.1), the muscle fibers acting on one Golgi tendon organ always belong to several motor units. Each tendon organ thus "samples" and averages the contractile force exerted by several motor units.

In the laboratory, with the tendon surgically detached from its skeletal insertion, Golgi tendon organs can also be stimulated by stretching a relaxed muscle, but the threshold of excitation is reached only when the muscle is stretched near to or beyond its physiological limit (Fig. 15.6). Under normal conditions, in an intact organism, Golgi tendon organs discharge only weakly and transiently when a relaxed muscle elongates because its antagonists shorten. This is because within the physiological range of lengths, a relaxed muscle offers little resistance to stretching (Fig. 14.5). The fibers of the tendon in which the Golgi tendon organ is embedded are stiffer than the muscle is in the relaxed state; therefore the Golgi tendon organ is protected and not deformed. But when the muscle contracts, the force applied to the tendon stretches the elastic fibers of the tendon and so deforms the Golgi tendon organs.

15.3. Spinal Connection of Stretch Receptors

15.3a. MUSCLE SPINDLES

In 1940 Renshaw noticed that when he stimulated a spinal dorsal root by an electric pulse, motor axons in the ventral root discharged so quickly that in the interval between stimulus and response not more than one synapse could have been traversed. Shortly thereafter, Lloyd established that the afferent limb of the *spinal monosynaptic reflex* arc is formed by the primary afferent fibers of muscle spindles. At that time it also became clear that the so-called *tendon reflexes* are in fact special examples of *stretch reflexes* of skeletal muscle, mediated by the mono-synaptic connections of the primary afferents in muscle spindles (see also Section 4.2a).

Some years later it became apparent that not only the primary, but also the secondary, afferent fibers of muscle spindles excite synaptically the alpha motor neurons of their own muscle. Both monosynaptic and polysynaptic excitatory connections exist from both primary and secondary endings to their own alpha motor neurons. Under conditions where both types of spindle endings are excited, their synaptic effects reinforce one another.

What is the effect of the stretch reflex of skeletal muscle? Since stretching the muscle excites spindle afferent fibers, which in turn excite alpha motor neurons and cause contraction of the extrafusal muscle, a stretched muscle will resist elongation. Now it should be quite obvious that such a stretch reflex cannot be active under all circumstances. By deliberately relaxing one's muscles, it is easy to make a limb quite limp, so that it does not resist manipulation by another person. In medical terminology, a muscle's resistance to passive stretching is its *tonus*, or *tone*. To a large degree, though not entirely, a muscle's tone is determined by the stretch reflex. It has been suggested but not proven that in order to relax a muscle, the stretch reflex must be inhibited. The condition in which muscles cannot be relaxed, so that they offer abnormal resistance to passive manipulation, is called muscle *hypertonia*. This is a neurological sign of considerable importance (see Section 15.7).

What then can turn the stretch reflex of skeletal muscles on and off, and thereby regulate muscle tone? There are two ways to do this: either by varying the activity of the afferent endings of muscle spindles via

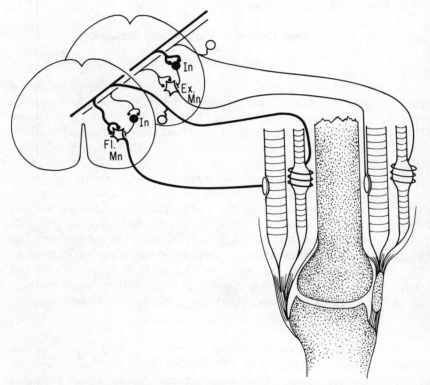

Figure 15.7. Reciprocal innervation between a flexor and an extensor muscle. A single spindle with a primary afferent fiber, and a single extrafusal muscle fiber with its alpha motor neuron were drawn for both muscles to represent all spindles and muscle fibers of those two muscles. Nerve fibers innervating the flexor muscle were drawn in *heavy lines*, those of the extensor muscle in *thin lines* to aid the eye. *In*, inhibitory interneuron; *Fl. Mn*, flexor motor neuron; *Ex. Mn*, extensor motor neuron.

changing intrafusal contraction by changing gamma (fusimotor) firing, or by varying the excitability of motor neurons via direct input to alpha motor neurons. The responsiveness of afferent terminals of the muscle spindles is controlled, or biased, as we have seen, by the intrafusal muscle, and the activity of fusimotor neurons is an important factor in the control of muscle tone. As far as the excitability of motor neuron pools is concerned, there are many inputs that could influence it (cf. Fig. 15.10), and so also influence the stretch reflex. Clinicians make use of this fact to bring out sluggish tendon reflexes in the so-called Jendrassik's maneuver (see Section 15.5b). Conversely, inhibition of either alpha or gamma motor neurons or both decreases stretch reflexes and diminishes muscle tone.

Stiffness is properly defined as the ratio of the change of elastic force and the length change causing the force. At least one of the functions of the stretch reflex of skeletal muscle is to regulate the stiffness of muscle (see Section 16.3b).

The afferent fibers of muscle spindles send branches to many motor neurons. In fact, in a muscle such as the cat's soleus or gastrocnemius, any primary spindle afferent is connected with up to 90% of the motor neurons innervating that same muscle. Whether the distribution is equally widespread in the much larger limb muscles of humans is not known. It seems likely, although it is not proven, that in muscles such as, for example, the deltoideus or latissimus dorsi, where one part of the muscle can be contracted independently from the other parts, the distribution of spindle input among motor neurons is regionally restricted.

In addition to the connections with motor neurons of their own muscle, spindle afferents also send monosynaptic excitatory connections to motor neurons of synergist muscles. The connections to synergists are, however, sparser and weaker than those made with motor cells of their own muscle. There also are connections from muscle spindles to the motor neurons controlling muscles of opposing action. Such connections to *antagonist* muscles are, however, *inhibitory*. The inhibitory connection between primary afferent nerve and antagonist motor neuron is made through an inhibitory interneuron (Fig. 15.7). The arrangement of connections through which a muscle spindle excites its own muscle and inhibits its antagonist, while the spindles of the antagonist muscle excite the antagonist and inhibit the agonist, are an example of *reciprocal innervation*, so called by Sherrington. When a muscle shortens it often is an advantage if its antagonist relaxes, but this need not always be the case. We will discuss this matter in a little more detail later (Sections 15.4 and 16.3a).

Information from the spindles of skeletal muscles reaches not only spinal neurons but also the cerebellum and the forebrain. Connections to the cerebellum are made from the lower half of the body by way of Clarke's column neurons and the spinocerebellar tract, from the more rostral segments by way of the cuneocerebellar tract (see Sections 7.2c and 18.3a). The pathway to the forebrain runs by way of the sensory thalamus and reaches not only the primary sensory cortex but also the motor cortex (see Sections 7.2, 7.7, and 18.1c).

15.3b. CENTRAL CONNECTIONS OF GOLGI TENDON ORGANS

Like muscle spindles, Golgi tendon organs also are connected to neuron circuits in the spinal cord, in the cerebellum and in the forebrain. At the spinal level the action of Golgi tendon organs opposes that of spindle afferents. Afferent nerve fibers of Golgi tendon organs inhibit the motor neurons of their own muscles, and excite those of their antagonist muscles. Both excitatory and inhibitory effects of the IB afferents are disynaptic, mediated by short-axon interneurons (Fig. 15.10).

Since Golgi tendon organs are excited by the force exerted by the contracting muscle, and since they inhibit the motor neurons of their own muscle, they seem to limit the force of contraction. They appear to function as negative force feedback elements (Fig. 16.4). Common sense suggests that there must be a way in which motor neurons can temporarily be exempted from Golgi tendon organ inhibition or else no muscle could ever develop the maximum punch it was designed to deliver. Golgi tendon organs have, however, no built-in controller similar to the intrafusal muscle of spindles. Presynaptic inhibition (see Section 3.2c) would, in principle, be a mechanism well suited for either admitting, or excluding, Golgi tendon organ input to a pool of motor neurons, as the circumstances demand it. While there is some evidence that group IB presynaptic terminals in the spinal cord receive presynaptic inhibitory input, we do not yet know in what way these are used in the normal course of events.

The combination of spinal reflex effects of muscle spindles, namely excitation of their own muscle, weaker excitation of their synergists, and inhibition of their antagonists, has been termed the *myotatic reflex*; that of Golgi tendon organs, the *inverse myotatic reflex*.

15.3c. THE RENSHAW CIRCUIT

In Chapter 4, the principle of recurrent inhibition was described, and the Renshaw circuit was mentioned (see Section 4.7). To recapitulate:

collateral branches of alpha motor axons curve medially to re-enter the ventral horn, where they form excitatory synapses with small inhibitory interneurons known as Renshaw cells. Branches of the axons of Renshaw cells form inhibitory synapses with the same motor neurons whose collaterals innervate them, their synergist motor neurons, and also certain interneurons. Some of these interneurons are inhibitory cells in the pathways acting on antagonist motor neurons. By inhibiting these inhibitory interneurons, Renshaw cells disinhibit the antagonist motor cells (cf. Section 4.10). Thus Renshaw cells can put the brakes on the very cells which excite them, while they unfetter their opponents (Fig. 15.8).

The transmitter substance of the recurrent collateral of the motor axons is acetylcholine, just as it is at the nerve-muscle junction. This has often been quoted as the prime example of Dale's principle (see Section 2.5e), because the recurrent collateral and the motor terminal belong to the same neuron. The acetylcholine released by the recurrent collateral terminals excites the Renshaw cells. Renshaw cells use glycine

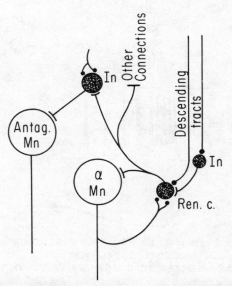

Figure 15.8. Some connections of Renshaw cells. Renshaw cells inhibit motor neurons of their own motor nucleus and disinhibit motor neurons of the antagonist muscles. *In,* inhibitory interneurons (other than Renshaw cells); *Antag. Mn,* antagonist motor neurons; *Ren. c.,* Renshaw cell.

as the inhibitory transmitter. Glycine is also the transmitter of the inhibitory interneurons in the myotatic and inverse myotatic reflex pathways (Figs. 15.9 and 15.10).

Renshaw cells receive synaptic connections from other sources besides recurrent motor axon collaterals (Fig. 15.8). This suggests that the Renshaw circuit can be turned on and off by input from other parts of the CNS. Exactly how this circuit is used is not clear. One of its possible roles may be the stabilization of the output of motor neurons. The idea of stabilization may be understood from the self-limitation imposed by the recurrent inhibition. As long as motor axons fire at a low rate, recurrent inhibition is weak. But, as their firing rate increases, so does recurrent inhibition, making it harder and harder to increase the firing rate any further.

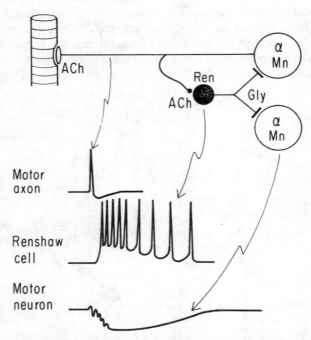

Figure 15.9.   Intracellular potential recordings and transmitters substances of the Renshaw circuit. An impulse conducted in an alpha motor axon propagates into the recurrent collateral branch of that motor axon and liberates acetylcholine at the terminals innervating the Renshaw cells. This depolarizes the Renshaw cell and causes its firing a burst of impulses. This burst releases glycine at the terminals of the Renshaw cell's axon causing the hyperpolarization (inhibitory postsynaptic potential) of the alpha motor neurons and of other cells innervated by Renshaw cells. *ACh,* acetylcholine; Gly, glycine; Ren, Renshaw cell.

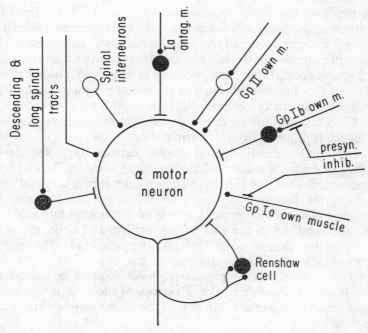

Figure 15.10. Some of the synapses acting on alpha motor neurons. *Ia antag. m.*, primary spindle afferent from antagonistic muscle; *own m.*, the muscle innervated by the alpha motor neuron. Round terminals indicate excitatory synapse, flat terminals inhibitory synapse.

Another theory of the the significance of Renshaw cells emphasizes the importance of the input received from sources other than the recurrent collateral. This theory suggests that the Reshaw circuit serves as a variable gain control of the output of motor neurons. The more the Renshaw cells are facilitated by descending pathways, the more they limit the output of their motor neurons (low gain). The more Renshaw cells are inhibited, the freer the reigns on the motor cells (high gain). Several other hypotheses have been proposed, but none yet backed by solid factual evidence.

15.4. Motor Programs of the Spinal Cord

A headless frog can jump. Mammals, however, are more dependent on brain function. The increased reliance on the rostral end of the neuraxis in higher vertebrates is attributed to the evolutionary process of encephalization (see Section 1.1). Thus, decapitated mammals could never duplicate the motor coordination of a spinal (i.e. headless) frog. Nevertheless, the programs for certain simple movement patterns are "wired in" the gray matter of our spinal segments as well. Among these movement patterns are flexion and extension of the limbs and simple stepping sequences. In an intact nervous system, spinal motor mechanisms are subordinate subroutines of the motor programs controlled in the brain and in the cerebellum. When severed from the higher levels of the CNS, the gray matter in the spinal segments acquires a life of its own, which is different from its normal state.

A spinal reflex described and studied extensively is the flexion-withdrawal of a limb, usually referred to as the *flexor* (or *flexion*) *reflex*. To understand what this entails, imagine a cat stepping on a hot ember and lifting the foot out of harm's way. This movement consists of contraction of the flexor muscles acting on the several joints of a leg: ankle, knee and hip in the case of the hindleg, and wrist, elbow and shoulder in the case of a forelimb. At the same time, the extensor muscles, which otherwise would oppose the withdrawal of the limb, relax. This is another example of *reciprocal innervation* (see Section 15.3a). It can be shown that the relaxation of the extensor muscles is brought about by synaptic inhibition of the motor neurons innervating those muscles.

Pain is not felt in the skin innervated by spinal segments which had been disconnected from the brain. Nevertheless, a limb innervated by such detached segments is withdrawn when a noxious stimulus is applied to it.

A note is in order here concerning the designation of flexion and extension movements. Following Sherrington, physiologists include among the extensor muscles all of those which oppose gravity. For example, the muscle group which anatomists call the flexors of the ankle and of the toes (e.g. flexor hallucis longus) belong to the physiological extensors; and conversely, their antagonists (e.g. tibialis, extensor digitorum longus, etc.) are physiological flexors. When it comes to the muscles acting on the knee or elbow, anatomical and physiological nomenclatures fortunately do agree.

Flexor withdrawal thus involves the simultaneous contraction of numerous muscles and the relaxation of several others. To achieve this combination, an extensive network of interneurons must be activated in the proper pattern. To evoke the flexor reflex in an intact animal, noxious stimulation is required. The flexor reflex jerks away a hurt finger even before pain is felt. In a paraplegic individual, however, stimuli that are not truly noxious, such as moderate squeezing of a limb, can also evoke reflex withdrawal. It generally is assumed that after spinal transection, the spinal flexor reflex mechanism is *released* from inhibitory control (see Section 4.10). The afferent fibers, stimulation of which is capable of evoking the flexor reflex, are sometimes collectively referred to as "flexor reflex afferents," sometimes abbreviated FRAs. What type of sense organs do and which do not belong into this group cannot accurately be defined, since the ability to evoke the flexor reflex changes according to the state of the nervous system.

When the cat that stepped on a hot coal lifts a paw, it must adjust its posture, or it will topple. In doing so, it shifts more weight onto the leg opposite to the one lifted, and therefore it must increasingly engage the antigravity muscles of that leg. This compensatory action is the *crossed extensor reflex*. A flexor reflex may occur without a crossed extensor response, but the crossed extensor reflex is rarely if ever seen without a flexor reflex. If, after transection of the upper cervical spinal cord (quadriplegia), an animal is kept alive by artifical respiration, stimulation of one limb may, under favorable conditions, evoke a combined response in all four limbs. Sherrington called such coordinated four-legged responses *reflex figures*. If, for instance, the left hindlimb is stimulated, the typical response is flexion (the flexor reflex) of the stimulated hindleg, plus flexion of the right foreleg, accompanied by extension of the right hindleg (crossed extension) and also of the left foreleg (Fig. 15.11). Such a diagonally symmetrical reflex figure can be evoked by stimulating any one of the four limbs. Such diagonally symmetrical movements occur also during four-legged stepping. Quadruped mammals walk by lifting and then swinging forward two diagonally opposite limbs simultaneously, while the other two legs support the body. It is a reasonable guess that the interneuron circuits that provide for the withdrawal of a limb in a flexor reflex are, in part or whole, identical with those that control the lifting of the leg during walking. The "program" for flexion is then also a "subroutine" of the more complex program of walking. Such a multi-purpose arrangement seems more economical than employing separate and independent populations of interneurons for two movements which have much in common.

A variety of other spinal reflex responses have been described, but need not be catalogued here. The interested reader should consult the works mentioned at the end of this chapter.

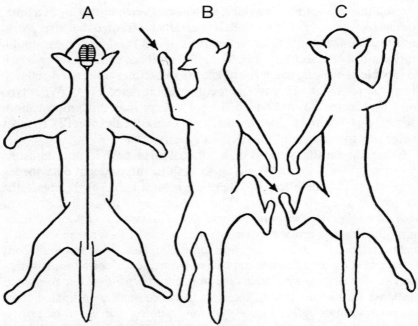

Figure 15.11. Four-limb coordination (reflex figures) in a decerebrate cat. *A,* position of the unstimulated decerebrate animal; *B,* reflexive movements evoked by stimulating the left forelimb; *C,* stimulating left hindlimb. (Reprinted with permission from C. Sherrington: *The Integrative Action of the Nervous System.* New Haven, Yale University Press, 1947.)

15.5. The Consequences of Spinal Transection

15.5a. SPINAL SHOCK

When the victim of an accident in which the spinal cord is severed or crushed is brought to the emergency room, the muscles innervated by the segments below the transection offer little resistance to passive manipulation, and no reflex response can be evoked in them. This state of areflexia is called *spinal shock.* Apart from its name, spinal shock has nothing in common with acute failure of the circulation. There can be spinal shock with or without concomitant circulatory shock. In human victims of spinal transection, the areflexic state may last for days or a few weeks. In lower mammals spinal shock is of shorter duration, in cats only an hour or so.

As the spinal cord recovers from shock, reflex responses reappear, and eventually a state of increased reflexes replaces the areflexic state. The detached segments are characterized by three groups of motor signs: (1) *hyperreflexia*, or increased liveliness of reflexes that are qualitatively normal; (2) moderately increased muscle tone, or *hypertonia* (1 and 2 together constitute *spasticity*); and (3) the appearance of *abnormal reflexes* that cannot be produced by normal spinal cords.

Neither the reason for the initial loss of all reflex movements, nor for their return and eventual abnormal state, are altogether clear. With the cord transected, all connections descending from and ascending to the brain and the higher spinal segments are irreversibly broken (paraplegia or quadriplegia, see Section 7.4). The lost descending fibers include both excitatory and inhibitory connections. Loss of background facilitation of motor neurons may in part account for their diminished responsiveness. While spinal shock lasts, ventral horn cells are relatively hyperpolarized, and this has been attributed to the absence of tonic excitatory (depolarizing) input from the transected descending tracts.

As reflexes return, and then become hyperactive, EPSPs evoked by afferent stimulation acquire an excessively large amplitude. Different explanations have been offered for the phenomenon of enhanced synaptic transmission, but none has been proven at this time. Both muscle hypertonia and hyperreflexia are, in part, related to abnormal continuous activity of fusimotor neurons. This causes contraction of intrafusal muscles, which sensitizes the afferent fibers of muscle spindles and so enhances the stretch reflex. We do not know, however, what drives the fusimotor neurons in paraplegic spinal cords.

If a paraplegic cat is placed on a treadmill, initially it will walk only with its front legs, and drag its hindquarters. If the exercise is repeated daily, the hindquarters will eventually develop stepping movements on their own, but the rhythm of the stepping of the hindlegs will not be coordinated with that of the forelegs. With time and exercise such an animal will be able to walk in a straight path, though it will topple when trying to turn. In human paraplegics, even though muscle tone is abnormally strong, the extensor reflexes never acquire enough power to support the body weight. Nor has effective stepping ever been achieved after total transection of the human cord.

15.5b. REMARKS ON THE TESTING OF REFLEXES

The reflexes commonly examined by physicians are classified as *cutaneous* and *tendon* reflexes; or, sometimes, as *superficial* and *deep* reflexes. The former are evoked by stroking the skin, the latter by tapping with the reflex hammer a tendon, or a bone to which a muscle is attached.

Of cutaneous reflexes, the abdominal and the cremaster reflex are the two most frequently tested. The former is evoked by stroking the skin of the abdomen; the response is contraction of the abdominal muscles. The latter is evoked by stroking the inside of the thigh; the cremaster muscle responds by lifting the scrotum. These cutaneous reflexes disappear after lesions that interrupt the corticospinal tracts. Sometimes, however, they are difficult or impossible to elicit even in persons who have no neurological deficit, and therefore they are not considered very reliable diagnostic signs. Although the circuits which mediate these reflexes are presumably contained within the spinal cord, they seem to require the support of impulses arriving through descending fibers.

The so-called tendon reflexes are examples of muscle stretch reflexes. The brief, small amplitude stretch imposed on a muscle by tapping its tendon preferentially excites primary spindle endings (see Section 15.2a) and so activation of the monosynaptic reflex. The masseter reflex, evoked by tapping the chin, is also a stretch reflex of the jaw-closing muscles. The ease with which these reflexes are elicited varies greatly even among perfectly healthy individuals. In some patients the knee will not jerk no matter how skilfully the patellar tendon is tapped. The physician then asks the patient to link hands and forcefully try to pull them apart without letting go (i.e. isometrically). While straining, the patient automatically tenses all muscles. As muscle tone is increased, stretch reflexes are facilitated. This diagnostic trick is called *Jendrassik's maneuver*.

Rarely, there are cases where nothing will bring out a stretch reflex. On the other hand, there are also people whose muscles will jerk at the slightest touch of the reflex hammer. Neither variant need be a sign of disease. The student may well ask why a procedure whose outcome is so unpredictable be part of routine examination. There are in fact good reasons for this. Absent or excessive tendon reflexes, even if inconclusive by themselves, are a red flag that suggests a thorough neurological examination. If other neurological signs are found, abnormal tendon reflexes do acquire diagnostic meaning. For example, hyperreflexia combined with clonus is a reliable sign of "upper motor neuron" disorder (see Section 18.1f). Furthermore, if there is a marked asymmetry between the tendon reflexes of left and right sides, that definitely should cause concern.

The spinal monosynaptic reflex can also be recorded with electronic equipment. Figure 15.12 shows how this is done. Only muscles with innervation accessible to electric stimulation through the skin are suitable for this test. An electromyographic (EMG) electrode (cf. Section 3.3a) is used to record the compound action potential of the muscle.

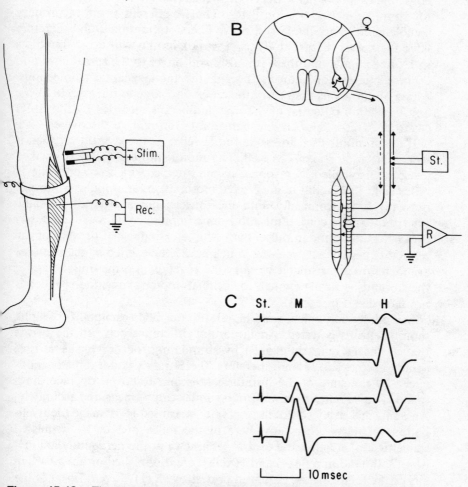

Figure 15.12.   The recording of the H reflex in the calf muscles of a human subject. A, schema of recording and stimulating equipment; B, the principal nerve connections involved; C, four tracings obtained with the arrangements shown in A and B; St., stimulus artefact; M, M response; H, H reflex; the stimulus strength was increased for the tracings from the top down.

The stimulating electrode pair is placed on the skin over a nerve containing the fibers destined for the muscle. A strong electric pulse will then stimulate both motor and sensory fibers but the intention is to stimulate only the latter. We can now put to good use the fact that the larger the caliber of nerve fibers, the weaker the electric current required for stimulation (see Section 3.1d). The IA afferent fibers of primary spindle endings are the largest nerve fibers of mammals, and therefore have the lowest threshold. Thus, a weak stimulus will evoke impulses in IA fibers only, and these impulses will travel to the spinal cord and excite alpha motor neurons through the monosynaptic connections. Alpha motor axons then carry the reflex discharge to the muscle fibers, and the action potential of the muscle fibers is recorded by the EMG electrode. This is the *H reflex*, named for Hoffman, its discoverer.

If the stimulus used to evoke the H reflex is made stronger, then it will excite motor axons as well. The motor impulse volley so evoked causes the so-called M response in the muscle, which precedes the H reflex (Fig. 15.12). But in the excited motor axons an impulse will travel not only orthodromically, into the muscle, but also antidromically, toward the spinal cord. If the antidromic impulse collides with a reflexly evoked orthodromic impulse, both will be extinguished because of the refractory period. Motor axons which have been excited by the stimulus are therefore not available to carry the H reflex into the muscle, and if the stimulus is strong enough to excite all motor axons, the H reflex is not recorded (Fig. 15.12).

By both tendon reflexes and H reflexes, the reflex excitability of alpha motor neurons is tested. An important difference between the two is that as the H reflex is evoked by stimulating the nerve, the muscle spindles are bypassed and, therefore, the H reflex is not directly influenced by the state of the intrafusal muscle. Moreover, on recordings made of the H reflex the timing of the reflex can be measured accurately. An abnormal delay could, in principle, be caused by damage (demyelination) of nerve fibers anywhere in the reflex arc, or by depressed transmission, either at the central synapse or at the nerve-muscle junction. Both tendon reflexes and H reflex are diminished or absent when any of the following are damaged or destroyed: (1) afferent fibers of the muscle spindle; (2) spinal dorsal roots; (3) alpha motor neurons; (4) ventral roots; (5) alpha motor fibers of the muscle; (6) neuromuscular junctions. More advanced techniques are now developed that should enable a distinction among these six alternatives. Both tendon reflexes and H reflex are unusually lively when motor neurons are excessively excited, or when inhibitory restraint is lacking.

15.5c. ABNORMAL REFLEXES OF THE PARAPLEGIC SPINAL CORD

Interruption of the corticospinal pathway, whether in the spinal cord, the brain stem, or within the forebrain itself, is recognized by *Babinski's sign*. To evoke it, the sole of the foot is stroked with a blunt instrument moving from heel toward the toes in a shallow arc. Ordinarily, the only response is a slight to moderate bending of the big toe towards the sole of the foot—plantar flexion (physiologically extension; see Section 15.4). In young infants or at any age after a lesion that interrupted the corticospinal tract, the response consists of dorsiflexion of the big toe and fanning (abduction) of the other toes. This is Babinski's sign.

With time, the character of the response tends to change. Some months or years after complete transection of the spinal cord blunt stimulation of the sole may evoke not just Babinski's sign, but flexor withdrawal of the leg. This is an example of the release of the flexor reflex from control by higher levels of the CNS. Since Babinski's response is the precursor of this hyperexcitable flexor reflex, some neurologists regard Babinski's sign itself as an incomplete flexor reflex.

It should be noted that in clinical parlance Babinski's sign is often described as an "extensor" response. "Plantar response: flexor" is the way the normal response is conventionally reported; "plantar response: extensor" designates the pathological condition. This terminology follows anatomical nomenclature, as explained in Section 15.4.

In some, but not all, paraplegics a so-called *mass reflex* develops eventually. This consists of flexion-withdrawal of both legs, sometimes followed by after-contractions of cramp-like, or almost seizure-like, quality, and sometimes accompanied by emptying of the bladder and/ or rectum. In severe cases, such storms of mass movement can be touched off by quite innocuous stimuli, such as attempts to dress the patient. It has been claimed that physical therapy and proper care, which includes the avoidance of bladder infection, help to prevent the development of violent mass reflexes.

The repertory of reflex movements of the spinal cords of two patients who have suffered similar accidents and lived with their paraplegic condition for a similar number of years need not be identical. Detached segments of the spinal cord seem to go through a series of "plastic" changes (cf. Sections 20.3 and 20.5), and this evolution may not be the same in all. It is almost as if each cord acquired a "character" of its own, some easier to live with than others.

The problems of bladder function in paraplegics will be discussed in Chapter 17 (Section 17.3d).

15.6. The Decerebrate State

Occasionally a patient brought in after a street accident may be breathing without assistance, have normal or near normal heart beat and blood pressure, but show little or no evidence of forebrain function. His limbs may be stiffly extended, arms internally rotated, jaw clenched, and neck retracted. The chillingly apt diagnosis in these cases is *decerebration*. In animals the condition can be produced either by removing or by causing ischemic necrosis of all brain structures rostral to the plane between superior and inferior colliculi of the midbrain. This is the mid-collicullar decerebrate preparation of Sherrington.

In cats and dogs the most conspicuous manifestation of the decerebrate state is stiffness of extensor muscles of all four limbs, known as *decerebrate rigidity* (Fig. 15.11A). In the fully developed case not only are all extensor muscles contracted, but also the jaw is clenched, and the tail curves upward: all antigravity muscles are contracted, and antagonists of antigravity muscles are relaxed. In the human, the decerebrate posture includes plantar flexion of the foot and bending of the fingers at the interphalangeal joints, once more illustrating that the anatomical flexor muscles acting on these joints are "physiological extensors" (cf. Section 15.4). A decerebrate cat can be propped up so that its stiff legs support its body weight.

The extensor muscles of decerebrate organisms are kept contracted by hyperactive stretch reflexes. This can be demonstrated by cutting the dorsal roots of several segments of the spinal cord on one side. The decerebrate rigidity then disappears from the limb or limbs innervated by the segments now deprived of afferent input. Extensor movements can still be evoked in the deafferented limb, by stimulating the other side where dorsal roots have been spared (that is, the crossed extensor reflex is active in the deafferented limb). Being a hypertonia of reflex origin, decerebrate rigidity is properly classified as a spastic state.

A number of reflexes have been described which occur in decerebrate animals. Some can also be evoked in human victims and are, therefore, of clinical importance. The flexor and crossed extensor reflexes are present in the decerebrate state. Usually stronger stimuli are required to evoke the flexor reflex in decerebrates than after spinal transection. This is because in the decerebrate state, motor neurons of flexor muscles are under continuous inhibition, while extensor motor neurons are excessively excited.

The extensor spasm can be modified by reflex influences. The extensor tone is maximal when the animal is prone and minimal when it is supine. This difference is attributed to input from the vestibular nuclei; it does not occur if the vestibular organ or its pathways have been destroyed.

Of the specific decerebrate responses, perhaps most important are the *tonic neck reflexes.* Passive bending or twisting of the neck causes a characteristic combination of postural adjustments. The input for these reflexes is from the proprioceptors of the joints of the cervical vertebrae. If the experimenter raises a decerebrate cat's head, this causes front legs to straighten and the hindlegs to bend as though the cat were looking up. Lowering the head causes front legs to bend and hindlegs to straighten, as though looking under a sofa. Turning the head to the left causes the left front leg to extend and right front leg to flex, as though the cat were looking up on a shelf; turning the head to the right evokes a movement that is the mirror image of that to the left.

Tonic neck reflexes can also be evoked in decerebrate humans. If, for example, the examiner turns the patient's head to one side, the arm on the side toward which the head is turned is extended, abducted and supinated.

Recovery from the decerebrate state is possible only insofar as brain tissue has not been killed, but only temporarily put out of commission by trauma or poison. In today's practice the prognosis is usually made by electroencephalograph (EEG) examinations repeated several times over a two- or three-day period. If the brain produces detectable EEG activity, then there is some hope, although recovery from temporary decerebration is rarely complete. If the patient's breathing becomes irregular, apneustic, or atactic, it is a bad sign, for it indicates encroachment by the lesion into the lower brain stem (cf. West, pp. 115–116).

15.6a. CHRONIC DECEREBRATES

A few experimenters have succeeded in keeping decerebrate animals alive for weeks or months. If the lesion is confined to the rostral midbrain, breathing and circulation remain normal. Decerebrates do not spontaneously feed, however. Nor do they regulate body temperature, since they lack a functioning hypothalamus. A number of other autonomic functions are disturbed, but these do not threaten survival.

The experimenter's task, then, is to artifically feed the decerebrate animal, to control the temperature of its environment, and to prevent infection.

After some weeks, decerebrate rigidity lessens and posture becomes more nearly normal. Almost immediately after decerebration liquids dropped in the mouth are swallowed. Chewing and eating solid food that has been placed in the mouth return later. Decerebrate cats eventually resume coordinated, though aimless, walking movements. Humans who are in decerebrate coma for long periods remain, however, permanently unable to stand or walk.

15.7. Spasticity

Muscle hypertonia is a frequent disorder in many neurological conditions besides paraplegia and decerebration. Not all hypertonic conditions depend on afferent input. Those that do are sometimes described as *gamma-driven*. In these cases hyperactive stretch reflexes are blamed for the stiffness. Hypertonias that do not depend on afferent input are said to be *alpha-driven*. In these it is assumed that alpha motor neurons are facilitated by input from other parts of the CNS.

The term *spasticity* is reserved for reflexly driven muscle hypertonia, characterized by *excessive tendon reflexes*, the *clasp knife phenomenon* and *clonus*. "Clasp knife" is turn-of-the-century English for a pocket knife, and it aptly describes the effect. If a spastic muscle is forcibly stretched, it first resists the stretching, then it suddenly yields just like a jacknife. The mounting resistance offered by the muscle is the consequence of the hyperactive stretch reflex. The muscle then yields when inhibition supersedes the stretch reflex. The inhibition used to be attributed to the recruitment of Golgi tendon organs, but this explanation has been called into question as a result of recent experiments. Possible remaining candidates for the inhibition that results in the clasp knife effect are nociceptive endings in the tendons and in the muscle.

Clonus is the rhythmically repeated contraction of a stretched muscle, with a regular rhythm between 3 and 7 times per second. Clonus is elicited, for example, by the examiner pushing the patient's foot so as to dorsiflex the ankle, and then keeping it in that position. The stretched gastrocnemius and soleus muscles are then seen and felt to contract rhythmically. In spastic animals clonus is abolished when dorsal roots innervating the muscle are cut. Recordings have been obtained from individual IA spindle afferent fibers in muscles undergoing clonus in both animals and human patients. Spindles were discharging when the muscle was elongating, and were silenced while the muscle was contracting. These observations indicate that clonus is the manifestation of a hyperactive stretch reflex, acting as follows. When the muscle is stretched, sensitized primary spindle afferents send a volley of impulses into the spinal cord, which evokes the synchronous discharge of a large number of motor neurons. The sudden synchronized contraction of extrafusal muscle unloads the spindles, which therefore fall silent, removing the excitatory input from the motor neurons. The extrafusal muscle consequently relaxes, the spindles are re-stretched and re-excited, and the cycle repeats itself. The mechanism of clonus is quite distinct from that of parkinsonian tremor (see Section 18.2c), which is paced by the rhythmic discharge of central neurons, requires no input from sense organs, and is therefore not abolished by interrupting the stretch reflex arc.

Some patients whose main handicap is spasticity and whose muscle strength is nearly normal can be helped by surgical section of alternating dorsal roots or of parts of dorsal roots. Because part of the overlap in dermatomal innervation, if alternating roots are spared, these patients do not lose all sensibility in the affected area. But since part of the excitatory input driving their stretch reflexes is interrupted, in favorable cases the spasticity is significantly diminished.

15.8. Chapter Summary

1. Most skeletal muscles are composed of red and pale fibers in various proportions, but any one motor unit has only one type of muscle fiber. Pale muscle is of the fast fatigue-prone (FF) type; motor units of red muscle may be either fast but fatigue-resistant (FR) or slow (S).
2. When the strength of contraction of a muscle is gradually increased, whether by reflex or by voluntary action, the first to be recruited are the small, weak, slow, fatigue-resistant motor units; last the large, fast units.
3. When a muscle is being stretched, the response of primary muscle spindle endings shows an onset transient and a prominent dynamic response followed by a lesser static response. Secondary endings show mainly a static response with no onset transient and only a small dynamic response.
4. The excitation of dynamic fusimotor nerve fibers causes the contraction of dynamic (bag 1) intrafusal muscle fibers, which enhance the dynamic response of primary spindle afferents, with little or no effect on secondary spindle afferents. Static fusimotor nerve fibers cause the contraction of static (bag 2 and chain) intrafusal muscle fibers which enhance the static responses of secondary spindle afferents and have a lesser effect on primary spindle afferents.
5. Contraction of extrafusal muscle, whether isotonic or isometric, unloads muscle spindles and causes a decrease of their firing. While the muscle shortens, primary but not secondary spindle endings may show a "negative"

dynamic response: a decrease of firing below the static level of firing that would obtain if the muscle were held stationary at a corresponding length.

6. Golgi tendon organs respond to contraction of (extrafusal) muscle. Stretching of a relaxed muscle excites Golgi tendon organs weakly or not at all.

7. Primary and secondary spindle afferents have excitatory synaptic connections with alpha motor neurons of their own muscle, and weaker excitatory connections to synergist motor neurons. They have inhibitory connections, through short-axon interneurons, with alpha motor neurons of antagonist muscles.

8. Golgi tendon organs make disynaptic inhibitory synaptic connections with alpha motor neurons of their own muscle, and excitatory connections with their antagonist muscles.

9. Recurrent collaterals of alpha motor axons excite Renshaw cells, which inhibit motor neurons of their own muscle and disinhibit motor neurons of antagonist muscles. The excitability of Renshaw cells is influenced by fibers descending from brain stem and forebrain.

10. Flexor reflex, crossed extensor reflex, and "long" spinal reflex connections operating between motor nuclei of forelimb and hindlimb muscles provide for coordinated reflex figures which seem to provide the basic programming for stepping movements. In paraplegic cats (but not paraplegic humans) the spinal circuits for stepping can be trained to perform effective locomotion.

11. Spinal shock is associated with hyperpolarization of motor neurons; the hyperreflexia of chronic spinal transection with excessively large EPSPs and excessive fusimotor firing.

12. Tendon jerks are stretch reflexes mediated in the first place by spinal segmental monosynaptic connections of spindle afferent fibers.

13. The H reflex is a clinically useful electrophysiological method of testing spinal segmental monosynaptic reflexes.

14. Babinski's response has been interpreted as a partial release of the flexor reflex from forebrain control. It is a reliable sign of pyramidal tract injury.

15. Spasticity is hypertonia of skeletal muscle, of reflex origin, characterized by excessive tendon reflexes, the clasp knife phenomenon and clonus.

16. Decerebrate rigidity is spastic state affecting extensor muscles. Readily elicited tonic neck reflexes are a sign of decerebration.

Further Reading

See at end of Chapter 16.

chapter 16

Principles of Control Systems

This chapter contains a brief introduction to the elements of control theory. It then discusses the applicability of these principles to the control of the contractions of skeletal muscles.

16.1. Maintaining a Steady State

Equilibrium is a special case of a steady state. A system at equilibrium neither consumes nor produces energy. To maintain a steady, but not equilibrium, condition requires an external source of energy and/or matter.

When we heat our house, we try to keep the flow of heat into the living room equal to the loss of heat through walls, windowpanes and cracks. Thermostats are devices designed to achieve such a steady state. The simplest thermostats are controlled by a thermometer, a relay and a heater (Fig. 16.1). If the temperature of the room is less than the *set point*, the relay activates the heater; when the room has warmed above the set point, the heater is automatically switched off. Such a simple system, however, in which the source of input (the heater, in the illustrated case) is either fully on or fully off, cannot produce a truly steady state. In such a simple system, the *controlled variable* (tempera-

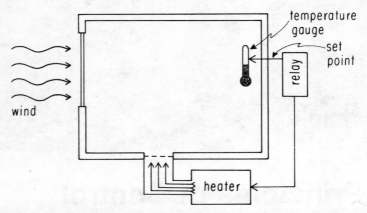

Figure 16.1. Diagram of a simple thermostat regulating room temperature. The relay turns the heater on whenever the temperature falls below the set point, and turns it off when the temperature rises above the set point. See also Figures 16.2*A* and 16.3*B*.

ture) inevitably must *oscillate* (Fig. 16.2*A*) as most of us living in thermostatically controlled homes know well enough.

A more sophisticated system than one controlled by an on-off thermostat is one in which the input is under *proportional control*. In such a system the input need not be fully turned on, but is kept proportional to the deviation of the controlled variable from the desired level. The difference between actual and desired levels is called the *error signal*. If temperature is under proportional control then the colder it gets the more the heater is turned on (Fig. 16.2*B*).

In *negative feedback systems* a perturbation of the output is countered by an opposing change of input. Thermostats provide negative feedback so that increased cooling, i.e. increased heat drain, is opposed by increased heating by the furnace. Watch out here for the meaning of "input" and "output." The output of one component may be the input of the other: the output of the furnace provides input of heat to the room. Output of the system is the heat lost to the outside.

When all goes well, proportional negative feedback can maintain a variable constant. In the case of a thermostat, if heat flow from the furnace is to equal heat loss to the environment, the temperature must settle at a level somewhat below the set point (Fig. 16.2*B*). It could not stay at exactly the set point, because if the difference between actual and desired temperature would be zero, the output of the heater would

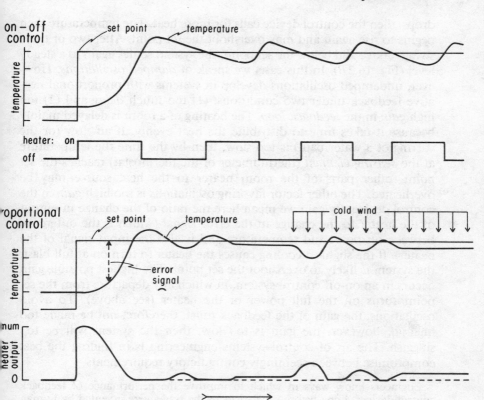

Figure 16.2.   The operations of simple negative feedback devices in regulating temperature. *A*, thermostat with on-off control, such as the one illustrated in Figure 16.1. In such a system the temperature must, by necessity, oscillate. *B*, thermostat with proportional control. The intensity of heating is proportional to the error signal. The error signal is the difference between the measured temperature and the set point. Such a system can, if properly designed, settle to a steady state. Note that while heat loss to the environment is increased (*cold wind*), the output from the heater must be increased; this is achieved at the expense of maintaining a greater error signal (lower steady temperature).

also come to zero and then, as long as heat is lost to the environment, the system would begin to cool down until the furnace is once more activated.

If a system with proportional negative feedback is perturbed, for example by a cold wind blowing at the window, and the temperature drops, then the control device calls for more heat. The temperature then begins to rise again and may overshoot the set point. After two or three swings above and below the set point, the system settles again to a steady level (Fig. 16.2*B*). In this case, we speak of *damped oscillations.* However, undamped oscillations develop in systems with proportional negative feedback under two conditions: (1) too much *delay* and (2) too high *gain* in the *feedback loop.* The heating of a room is delayed mainly because it takes time to distribute the heat evenly. If air flow (or the stirring of a water bath) is too slow, then by the time the temperature at the *sensing element* (thermometer of the thermostat) reaches the set point, other parts of the room nearer to the heat source may be overheated. The other factor favoring oscillations is too high *gain* in the control device. By gain we mean here the ratio of the change in output of the heater to the change in the error signal (which is the difference between set point and temperature and is also the input signal of the heater). If the slightest cooling causes the heater to turn on at full blast, the system is likely to overshoot the set point. The highest possible gain occurs in an on-off control system, in which any departure from the set point turns on the full power of the heater (see above). To avoid oscillations, the gain of the feedback must, therefore, not be made too high. If, however, the gain is too low, then the system will be too sluggish. The art of control-systems engineering is in finding the best compromise between seemingly contradictory requirements.

Engineers know ways in which to improve the performance of feedback control devices. Long before such tricks of the trade were invented by human engineers, they had been incorporated in the physiological systems that govern the functioning of animal organisms. The performance of a negative feedback control device can be improved, for example, if feedback is made to depend not only on the error signal, but also on its rate of change (i.e. first derivative with respect to time, or velocity). To come back to our example, such a device would call for more heating at any given temperature when the temperature is dropping rapidly than when it is cooling down more slowly. Then, when the temperature of the room would start to warm up, the velocity signal in the feedback would become negative and so put the brakes on, therefore as the desired temperature is approached, heating would slow down and the set point would not be overstepped.

Animal organisms make use of velocity-dependent feedback signals in the sense organs that adapt (see Section 6.1). Dynamic responses of sense organs depend on the rate of change of the stimulus. We have already met with examples of this in temperature receptors (see Section 6.6), primary afferent endings in muscle spindles (see Section 15.2a) and in others.

Control systems can further be improved if a way is found to anticipate perturbations before they occurred. In the example of heating a room, such a warning device could be attached to the outside of the building to call for more heat when a cold wind begins to blow against a window, even before the room starts to cool down. Conversely, such a device could turn the heater off when the sun began to shine, before there was a chance to overheat the room. As a matter of fact cutaneous temperature receptors fill precisely this role in the maintenance of body temperature (see Section 17.5a). Regulators which anticipate perturbations may be called feed-forward systems, to distinguish them from feedback systems (Fig. 16.3*A*).

The ideal way of regulating temperature would, however, not rely on thermometers at all. Instead of adjusting heating to the prevailing temperature, the rate of heat production would be matched to the rate of heat loss. To do this, the number of calories flowing from the system to the environment would have to be metered. As we shall see in Chapter 17, the physiological temperature regulation of the body behaves *as if* this information would be available to the central nervous controller. Similarly, respiration and circulation are, under ordinary conditions, adjusted to supply oxygen at the rate at which it is consumed. Whether the nervous system is indeed, in the literal sense, "metering" total heat flow between body and environment and total oxygen consumption is not clear at this time.

While oscillations must be avoided in some systems, they are necessary for the functioning of others. Perhaps the oldest example of a *stable oscillator* is the grandfather clock. In it the energy of the slow, controlled fall of a weight is converted into the swinging of the pendulum. Most electronic oscillators are based on phase delay (or phase advance) in resistance-capacitance (or resistance-inductance) circuits. In mammalian organisms, oscillators control functions too numerous to list, from the *circa diem* (or *circadian*) rhythms coupled to the day-night cycle to the beat of the heart; from the menstrual cycle to the oscillatory potentials of brain cell assemblies.

Oscillations in living systems can, however, also be the expression of a control apparatus that is out of order. The examples include intermittent fevers; periodic breathing; and a variety of motor disorders such as clonus, tremor, and the like (see Sections 15.7, 18.2c, and 18.3c).

16.2. Controlled Change

A number of variables in living organisms are regulated to remain within narrow limits. Others, however, must change widely to enable

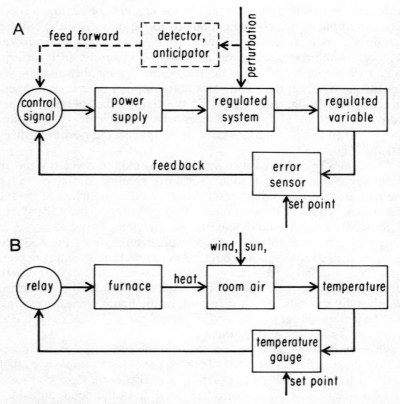

Figure 16.3. Conceptual diagram of the flow of signals in simple regulating systems. *A*, in general; *B*, illustrated on a simple thermostat. (Modified and redrawn after J. C. Houk: Systems and models. In *Medical Physiology*, 14th ed., edited by V. B. Mountcastle. St. Louis, C. V. Mosby, 1980, pp. 227–267.)

the organism to act and to adapt. Change can be guided by feedback in ways similar in principle to those maintaining steady states. The difference is that instead of adjusting the controlled variable to a constant set point, it is forced to move along a prescribed trajectory, as if there were a "moving set point." Some authors reserve the expression "to regulate" to describe the maintenance of a steady state, and use "control" to denote the guidance of a change. This distinction is not strictly adhered to by all. It should be clear that when a variable changes with zero velocity, it remains constant. In other words, to remain steady is the lower limit to change, the upper limit being a step-function, meaning instantaneous change. Control systems in which a variable is forced to follow a command signal are called *servo-controlled systems*, the word having been derived from *servus*, which means slave or servant.

Variables subject to controlled change are more numerous than those that are kept constant. Even the temperature of homoiotherms is not truly constant: in diurnal species it is higher during waking hours than during sleep. The arterial blood pressure certainly rises every time we get out of bed, and again whenever we start physical exercise. But foremost among guided changes are the length and the contractile force of skeletal muscles.

From the realm of weaponry we have borrowed words to describe the two fundamentally different classes of control that can be exerted over moving parts. A ballistic missile is thrown along a trajectory calculated in advance. Once launched, its course cannot be corrected. A guided missile differs from a ballistic missile in that its path can be adjusted in flight. It is believed that certain rapid movements, such as throwing a ball, hitting a nail with a hammer, throwing a punch in a fight, are *ballistic* or *pre-programmed*. Others, which are not so rapid, are guided by *servo-control* throughout their course.

The essence of servo-control is negative feedback that keeps the controlled variable on a prescribed path. A driver adjusts the steering wheel whenever his car does not follow the curvature of the road. In this example, the driver provides the servo-control to the car; his brain is the servo-controller of his hands.

A good part of our central nervous system seems to be devoted to the control of movement. In theory, we can separate the two aspects of motor control: (1) the programming of movement; and (2) its guidance.

In ballistic movements (to be distinguished from "ballismus": see Section 18.2c) only the former is used, for servo-controlled movements both are. Whether programming and servo-control are indeed provided by separate neuron circuits or whether such separation exists only in theoretical analyses is not clear. It is at least thinkable that the same circuits that "chart" the trajectory of a movement before it begins are also the ones that control its path as it is executed. In Chapter 18, we will describe what is known about the roles of the cerebellum, brain stem, basal ganglia and motor cortex in motor control. The exact role of these structures is by no means clear, except that all participate either in the command or in the guidance of skilled movements, or in both.

One thing is, however, quite obvious. In order to guide movements, results must constantly be compared to intentions. All the senses can contribute to this goal. Complex movements may be guided by input from proprioceptive, cutaneous, visual, vestibular, and even by auditory cues. Moreover, movements are guided not only by present performance, but also by past mistakes and successes: skills require learning.

The more skilled an act, the less we need think of it. Yet even when not consciously "thinking" about a particular movement, the brain utilizes all the input, and all the relevant memory traces, as it guides a motor act. How much we depend on our senses for our movements becomes manifest when, if by accident or disease, someone loses a sensory channel. After being blinded, or blindfolded, well-practiced skilled acts become hesitant and deliberate. Then, however, a new strategy, a new program, may be devised in which information through the now-lost sensory channel (sight, in this example) is substituted by those still remaining.

16.3. Control Mechanisms of Skeletal Muscles

The nervous system regulates and controls visceral, respiratory and cardiovascular functions, as well as the movements of skeletal muscles, while internal secretions are governed in part by the central nervous system (CNS) and in part by chemical feedback in endocrine organs. Autonomic functions and certain complex integrated response patterns will be discussed in Chapter 17. The remaining pages of this chapter are devoted to the control of skeletal muscle.

16.3a. POSTURE AND MOVEMENT

To maintain posture, muscles must steady the skeletal parts to which they are attached. To give stability, opposing muscle groups must contract simultaneously: posture is maintained by *co-contraction of antagonists*. In doing so, muscles need not change length: postural contractions are, in the ideal case, *isometric*. Furthermore, postural attitudes may be held for prolonged periods; contraction is then *tonic*.

As we move, certain muscle groups shorten, while opposing muscles lengthen. The relaxation of antagonists may be achieved by an inhibitory effect programmed by *reciprocal innervation* (see Section 15.4). If the load lifted in the performance of a movement is constant, we speak of *isotonic* contraction. Contractions which accomplish movement are generally brief (*phasic*).

Of course in real life most actions require a blend of both tonic-postural and phasic contractions. Even when standing on a parade ground, the bodies of the soldiers make small swaying motions. Incidentally, the stiffer the stance, the greater the danger of fainting. Thus perfectly isometric contraction is rarely achieved, nor is it very often desirable. Similarly, reciprocal inhibition is not an absolute requirement of all movement. Instead of completely relaxing the antagonist muscle group while we move, we sometimes use the braking action of antagonists to smooth and to steady the shortening of the agonists.

It has been suggested that in the CNS separate programs exist for the control of postural and of phasic contractions. These programs would not operate independently, but would be activated in harmoniously combined patterns. Corroborating these expectations are neurological syndromes in which posture is more disturbed than movement and others in which movements are more disturbed and posture is relatively normal. Often, however, these differences are quantitative, not qualitative.

16.3b. MUSCLE STRETCH RECEPTORS AS REGULATORS OF STEADY CONTRACTIONS

Imagine yourself carrying a tray. To do so, you keep your arms bent, and for that purpose the flexor muscles must remain at a prescribed length. If a glass is taken off the tray, or an empty one put on it, the load changes. Nevertheless the arms must retain the same attitude without jerking up when the load is lightened, and without dropping toward the ground when the burden on it is increased. What is it that keeps the position steady?

The regulation of muscle length has been compared to the regulation of temperature by a thermostat. The role played by the temperature sensor of the thermostat could be taken by the muscle spindle which signals the length of the muscle. Instead of a heater, we have the extrafusal muscle. The thermostat relay becomes the excitatory reflex connection of spindle afferent fibers to alpha motor neurons. The set point would be determined by the fusimotor nerve fibers which regulate the responsiveness of the spindle. An extra load placed on the tray is a perturbation, like a cold wind on the windows of a thermostatically controlled room. If an extra load stretches the muscle including its spindles, the stretch reflex activates the motor neurons, which then call on the extrafusal muscle to contract. The latter lifts the weight and unloads the muscle spindles so that the system once more comes to a steady state. When and where the contraction of the extrafusal muscle stops is controlled by the degree of the contraction of the intrafusal muscle (compare Figs. 16.3 and 16.4).

According to this hypothesis, the segmental stretch reflex would serve to regulate the length of the muscle and to maintain it in the face of changes of load. In fact, however, the mechanism which enables one to maintain muscles

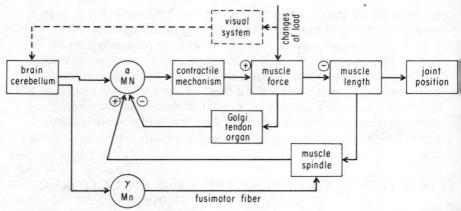

Figure 16.4. Components of the regulator of muscle force and length. Compare this with Figures 15.7, 15.10 and 16.3A. Note that increasing contraction increases the force exerted by the muscle, but decreases its length (shown by *minus sign in circle*). Remember that increasing length (stretch) increases spindle excitation, decreasing length (shortening) decreases spindle excitation. Also, spindle afferents excite, Golgi tendon organs inhibit their own motor neurons. The visual system can sometimes anticipate changes of load and hence serve as a feed-forward signal. (Modified and redrawn after J. C. Houk: Feedback control of muscle. In *Medical Physiology*, ed. 13, edited by V. B. Mountcastle. St. Louis, C. V. Mosby, 1974, pp. 668–677.)

at constant length (and thus limbs at a constant position) is more complex. Experiments on human subjects and on trained monkeys suggest that the short-latency segmental reflexes play but a minor part in the maintenance of posture. In such experiments the subject may be required to hold a handle in a certain position. The experimenter may change the load on the subject's muscles by applying a force which would move the handle, if the subject would not resist it. Electromyographic (EMG) recordings made as the subject resists the perturbation reveal at least three separate bursts of impulses in the muscle. The *first*, beginning after a very short latency, is a manifestation of the segmental stretch reflex. The *second* burst, added on top on the first after a brief delay, is also a spinal reflex but involves more complex interneuron circuits. The *third* burst of EMG potentials superimposed on the preceding two is probably a cortical reflex. It still comes too fast to be voluntary but slowly enough to have been routed through the brain (see also Section 18.1c).

A strong case has recently been made for the proposition that the segmental connections of muscle spindles are not involved in regulating the length of muscles at all, but that they, together with those of Golgi tendon organs, regulate the stiffness of the muscle. Stiffness is the ratio of changes of tensile force over elongation (see Section 15.2a). Since spindles sense muscle length, and Golgi organs the force acting on the tendon, their combined signals may well be used to regulate stiffness. Thus, according to this scheme, the spinal segmental connections of stretch receptors would serve to regulate the stiffness and the supraspinal connections of muscle spindles to regulate the length of the muscle, and the one could be set independently from the other.

16.3c. STRETCH RECEPTORS AND THE GUIDANCE OF MOVEMENTS

Muscle spindles also play a part during the shortening of muscles, but their role here is even less clear than in the maintenance of constant length. Shortly after the discovery of the fusimotor fibers it has been suggested that muscle spindles guide movements in a *follow-up length-servo-system*. The idea was that command signals generated in the brain would activate gamma motor neurons which cause shortening of intrafusal muscle and thus excitation of spindle sensory endings. The spindle afferent fibers would then excite alpha motor neurons through their monosynaptic reflex connections. Shortening of the intrafusal muscle would thus indirectly control the shortening of the extrafusal muscle. If this were the whole story, then all deliberate movement would cease if dorsal roots were torn or cut, because destroying the spindle afferent fibers would interrupt the feedback loop. Loss of dorsal root fibers indeed disturbs movement, but does not stop it (see Section 18.3c).

To accommodate these and other facts, several newer theories have been proposed. I shall briefly describe two, but for an adequate discussion the reader should consult one of the sources listed at the end of the chapter.

1. Muscle spindles may be devices that measure the length of the muscle as it changes. As we have seen (Section 15.2a and Fig. 15.3) the firing rate of spindle afferents indeed reflects muscle length, provided that the excitation of fusimotor fibers is constant. To verify this theory, it must be shown first that gamma motor fiber firing remains constant during the execution of a movement; and second that in normal deliberate movements the firing rate of spindle afferents decreases when the muscle shortens and increases when it lengthens. In some muscles, during some types of movements, some of the spindle afferents behaved as predicted.

2. Muscle spindles may be elements in a *servo-assisted* (but not servo-controlled) system. This means that fusimotor neurons would influence, but not fully control, the excitation of alpha motor neurons, exerting this influence through the *"gamma loop."* This theory suggests that both

alpha and gamma motor neurons are excited by signals received through fiber tracts descending into the spinal cord from the brain (*alpha-gamma coactivation*). It also predicts that the rate of firing of spindle afferents should either remain constant or it should actually increase during shortening of the muscle because the contraction of the intrafusal muscle would keep them excited. It has been reported that this happens in certain types of movements in certain muscles. It has also been suggested that primary endings provide the error signal that enables the CNS to control the velocity of shortening, while secondary endings furnish the error signal that controls its length.

Clearly, muscle length, the velocity at which length changes, as well as the force of contraction are simultaneously controlled during all but the fastest active movements. Current research is concerned not with whether such control exists, but how it is exerted. It is likely that several subsystems of the CNS extract specific aspects ("features") of the information supplied by the various muscle stretch receptors and that parallel and simultaneous computation of different aspects of the movement enables its control.

While the contraction of intrafusal muscle is changing, the firing rate of the spindle afferent fibers is not proportional to the muscle's length. But if the CNS was informed of both the state of contraction of the intrafusal muscle and the degree of excitation of spindle afferents, then muscle length as well as the velocity of its change could always be computed. It has been suspected for many years and for a variety of reasons that the CNS is constantly being informed not only of the state of the sense organs, but also of the output leaving the CNS by way of its efferent fibers. This postulated information has variously been termed "sense of effort," "*corollary discharge*" and "reafferent signal."

In conclusion, if recent experiments seem now to support one and then the other hypothesis concerning the role of muscle spindles, perhaps this is because these signals are utilized by different parts of the CNS in different ways and possibly also because their function may vary according to the type of movement performed. If all this seems obscure and complicated at present, it may become simple and straightforward once the operation of the system is better understood. With the research work currently underway in many laboratories, this may happen in the foreseeable future. For the understanding of neurological disorders, this will be an important breakthrough.

16.4. Chapter Summary

1. Systems regulated by feedback with on-off control always oscillate.
2. Systems regulated by feedback with proportional control can, if properly adjusted, maintain a steady state. They will oscillate, however, if delay and gain in the feedback loop are too high. Their performance can be improved by incorporating feedback proportional to the first derivative of the error signal.
3. The regulation in a system incorporating feed-forward is often superior to that in systems employing negative feedback only.

4. An ideal thermostat would not depend on measuring temperature, but on metering heat flow between the regulated system and its environment. The regulation of temperature (and of certain other variables) in a healthy mammal appears to approach this ideal.
5. The control of movements can, in principle, be analyzed into two parts: programming beforehand and guidance during performance. Fast, ballistic movements must be pre-programmed and cannot be controlled by feedback during their execution. Slower, servo-controlled movements are subject to both programming in advance and guidance by feedback during their performance. The acquisition of skills requires the comparison of the plan (program) to the result of actions and is therefore dependent on memory. This is true of both ballistic and servo-controlled movements.
6. Postural contractions require near-isometric co-contraction of antagonistic muscle groups; phasic movements usually require relaxation of antagonists during shortening of the agonists (reciprocal innervation).
7. Signals of muscle stretch receptors are required for the maintenance of constant muscle length during postural contraction. This involves connections of stretch receptors not only within the spinal cord but also projecting to motor circuits in brain stem and forebrain.
8. The role played by muscle spindles in the control of phasic movements is controversial. Among the proposed theories are the following: (a) that muscle spindles are devices that measure the length of muscles; (b) that muscle spindles are guidance elements in servo-assisted control of movements (also known as the theory of alpha-gamma coactivation); (c) that muscle spindles, in conjunction with Golgi tendon organs, regulate the stiffness of muscle.

Further Reading: Chapters 15 and 16

Books and Reviews

Baldissera F, Hultborn H, Illert M: Integration in spinal neuronal systems. In Brooks BV (ed): *Motor System, Handbook of Physiology*: Section 1, vol II, part 1. Bethesda, American Physiological Society, 1981, pp. 509–596.
Barnes CD, Schadt JC: Release of function in the spinal cord. *Prog Neurobiol* 12:1–13, 1979.
Buchthal F, Schmalbruch H: Motor units of mammalian muscle. *Physiol Rev* 60:90–142, 1980.
Granit R, Pompeiano O (eds): Reflex control of posture and movement. In *Progress in Brain Research*, volume 50. Amsterdam, Elsevier, 1979.
Houk JC: Regulation of stiffness by skeletomotor reflexes. *Annu Rev Physiol* 41:99–114, 1979.
Matthews PBC: *Mammalian Muscle Receptors and Their Central Actions*. Baltimore, Williams & Wilkins, 1972.
Prochazka A: Muscle spindle function during normal movement. In Porter R (ed): *International Review of Physiology*, vol 25. Neurophysiology IV. Baltimore, University Park Press, 1981.
Taylor A, Prochazka A (eds): *Muscle Receptors and Movement*. London, Macmillan, 1981.

West JB: *Respiratory Physiology: The Essentials*, ed 2. Baltimore, Williams & Wilkens, 1979.

Articles

Forsberg H, Grillner S, Halbertsma J: The locomotion of the low spinal cat. *Acta Physiol Scand* 108:269–295, 1980.

Henneman E, Somjen G, Carpenter DO: Functional significance of cell size in spinal motoneurons. *J Neurophysiol* 28:560–580, 1965.

Lloyd DPC: Conduction and synaptic transmission of reflex responses to stretch in spinal cats. *J Neurophysiol* 6:317–326, 1943.

Renshaw B: Central effects of centripetal impulses in axons of spinal ventral root. *J Neurophysiol* 9:191–204, 1946.

chapter 17

Neural Control of Autonomic Functions

How the internal environment and the vital functions of the organism are controlled; functions of the hypothalamus.

17.1. Divisions of the Autonomic Nervous System

Many years before the term "feedback" was adopted in physiology, Walter Cannon used the term *homeostasis* to describe the functions that maintain chemical composition and physical variables of animal organisms within the limits compatible with good health. And many years before Cannon wrote the *Wisdom of the Body*, Claude Bernard pronounced the constancy of the internal environment to be the key to the free life of complex organisms. The maintenance of this constancy, or homeostasis, is mainly the function of the endocrine system and that part of the nervous system which we call autonomic.

Defined in other words, the autonomic nervous system controls the viscera and the organs of circulation, but the boundary between the *somatic* and the *autonomic* functions is not sharp. In the swallowing of food, for example, somatic and autonomic neurons interact. Ventilation of the lungs is one of the functions guarding the constancy of the internal environment, but it is carried out by skeletal muscles controlled by (somatic) alpha motor neurons, and yet it is integrated by autonomic centers in the brain stem (for a definition and criticism of the concept of "centers," see Section 1.3). Many other examples of intimate inter-action between somatic and autonomic systems may be found. The distinction between the two has nonetheless proven useful.

Many authors insist that only efferent nerves should be called auto-nomic. The afferent fibers of sense organs in viscera and blood vessels that are contained in the nerves that also contain the autonomic efferent axons should, strictly speaking, be designated "visceral afferent" and not "autonomic afferent" fibers. This distinction is not adhered to by all.

The autonomic nervous system is divided into the *sympathetic* (for-merly orthosympathetic) and *parasympathetic* divisions. Sympathetic are all the autonomic fibers originating in the thoracic and lumbar spinal segments and the neurons of the paravertebral and prevertebral ganglia. Parasympathetic (meaning "besides the sympathetic") are all the other autonomic nerves: those in cranial nerves and those originating in the sacral spinal segments.

There have been numerous attempts to attach some physiological meaning to this basically anatomical separation of the two divisions of the autonomic system. It has been said, for example, that the sympa-thetic division serves catabolic functions and the parasympathetic ana-bolic functions. Under the influence of generalized sympathetic activa-tion and of adrenaline in the bloodstream, metabolism increases, blood pressure and cardiac output rise and more blood flows through the vessels of skeletal muscles. Such a generalized reaction readies the body for physical effort, in Cannon's words for *fight or flight*, and therefore for greater expenditure of energy. By contrast, the parasympathetic nerves get the digestive juices flowing, ensure the assimilation of food, and inhibit the heart. In short, they slow down the organism and restore its metabolic reserves.

From another point of view, it seems that the sympathetic system usually acts in concert, as a coordinated whole, activating many organs at once. Parasympathetic nerves usually act separately on individual organs. The sympathetic system has been likened to the pedals of a piano, the parasympathetic to its keys. For example, both autonomic divisions influence the size of pupils of the eyes, but the parasympathetic constrictor fibers of the IIIrd cranial nerve are the ones adjusting pupil size according to the amount of incident light (see Section 9.1b). The dilator fibers of the pupils which originate in the cervical sympathetic ganglia are called into action during excitement, be it fright or delight, when the pupillary response is one of the manifestations of the global activation of the sympathetic system.

Such general pronouncements concerning the function of the sympathetic and parasympathetic nerves are attractive to teachers of introductory classes because they allow the organization of otherwise disconnected facts under a few general principles. Still, to avoid misleading one's audience, the limitations of such general rules must be pointed out. Not all sympathetic actions can be termed "catabolic" or "activating," nor all those of the parasympathetic "anabolic" or "conservative." Dilatation and constriction of the pupils, for example, are neutral: they neither enhance nor diminish metabolic activity. Examples are easily found in which sympathetic reactions are limited and not generalized. Blood vessels may be constricted in one limb, for example, without involving vessels elsewhere. Sweating is another example. Sweat glands may be excited as part of a generalized emotional response, but more often their activity serves to cool the body. Moreover, sweating may be limited to a small part of the skin. There are also complex response patterns in which sympathetic and parasympathetic nerves are activated at the same time. For example, the so-called diving response of ducks and marine mammals that is also produced in attenuated form by people submerging in water consists of vasoconstriction (a sympathetic response) combined with bradycardia (parasympathetic). Thus while it is true that sympathetic and parasympathetic nerve endings often have antagonistic effects on specific organs it is *not* correct to say that the two *systems* as a whole are mutually antagonistic.

17.2. Visceral Afferent Nerve Fibers

Viscera are supplied with mechanoreceptors, thermoreceptors, chemoreceptors and nociceptors, though not all viscera have all four. The cell bodies of the visceral afferent neurons may be in the dorsal root ganglia, together with those of somatic afferents. In other cases, the cell bodies are in specialized visceral sensory ganglia, such as those of the vagus and glossopharyngeal nerves at the base of the skull.

Stretch-sensitive mechanoreceptor nerve endings are found, for example, in the airways, especially the small bronchioli. Some of these are the sense organs mediating the classical Hering-Breuer reflexes (West, p. 119). Others give rise to the feeling of respiratory distress (dyspnea) associated with hyperpnea, whether related to vigorous exercise or to suffocation (see Section 17.5b).

Most hollow viscera of the abdomen contain contact-sensitive mechanoreceptors on both their mucosal and the serosal surfaces. In addition, there are stretch- or distension-sensitive mechanoreceptors within the walls of stomach, intestines, bladder and rectum. The signals generated by these afferent fibers serve the complex reflexes that regulate the movements of these organs. We also owe the sensations of fullness of the stomach, and of urgency of the bladder (see Fig. 17.2) and rectum, to the stimulation of mechanoreceptors in the walls of these organs.

Sensory units stimulated by acid or alkali have been found in the stomach and duodenum. Some of these may be nociceptors and are involved in the pain of ulcers. Others respond to more moderate deviations of pH and may be important in regulating the propulsion of the food mass and secretion of digestive juices.

Subjective visceral temperature sense seems to be limited to the pharynx and esophagus. The existence of temperature-sensitive afferents has however been demonstrated for organs of the abdominal cavity as well. These are believed to be linked to thermoregulatory reflexes.

Visceral nociceptors probably all belong to the C fiber, slow nociceptor category (see Section 6.7). Clinical experience speaks of numerous distinct qualities of pain that can arise from different organs under the influence of different pathological conditions. The stimuli that can give rise to these sensations may be chemical or mechanical or a combination of the two. In the case of ulcers, acid and digestive enzymes gain access to nociceptive nerve endings. As with skeletal muscle, hypoxia is a powerful noxious stimulus in the heart and in the viscera and is believed to cause the pain in cases of infarction. Mechanical stimuli are the dominant ones in colic and visceral cramp. Chemical and mechanical stimuli may act in combination in inflammatory conditions. Beyond these generalities, little is known for certain of the neurophysiological substrates of visceral pain. The bradykinin theory has been mentioned earlier (Section 6.7). Referred pain has also been discussed (see Section 7.9d).

17.2a. SPECIALIZED SENSE ORGANS OF THE INTERNAL ENVIRONMENT

Besides the nerve endings in viscera that have much in common with the sensory nerve terminals of the skin and connective tissues, there also are more complex and specialized internal sense organs. Their strategic location in the walls of the blood vessels is related to their function as sensors of intravascular pressure and samplers of the chemical composition of blood plasma. Best known among the former are the baroreceptors of the carotid sinus and the aortic arch, of the latter the carotid and aortic bodies.

Mechanoreceptors are also scattered in the large veins, the walls of the atria, and in several of the large arteries. The best studied, however, are the afferent nerve endings of the carotid sinus. These *baroreceptors* (pressure receptors) fire as a function of the arterial pressure. The branched nerve terminals lie in elastic connective tissues in the wall of the artery. They do not measure pressure in the literal sense, but their adequate stimulus is the deformation of the nerve terminals caused by the stretching of the elastic fibers of the vessel wall. These endings, then, are one more example of a stretch receptor. The baroreceptors of the large arteries are more sensitive to pulsatile pressure than to steady pressure: they are incompletely adapting (see Section 6.1; see Smith and Kampine, pp. 168–172).

The *carotid body* or *glomus caroticum* has, per unit weight, the highest rate of blood flow of all organs. There are two characteristic cell types, the chief or type I cells, and the sustentacular or type II cells. The tissue is richly supplied with nerve endings that are excited by lowering the P_{O_2}, or the pH, and by raising P_{CO_2} and are influenced by the rate of flow of the blood in the capillaries as well. The effects of pH and P_{CO_2} may be interdependent, but P_{O_2} and blood flow is believed to act on the nerve terminals by a separate, pH-independent mechanism. The nerve fibers are nonetheless not specialized for P_{O_2} and P_{CO_2}; each fiber responds to both, changes of P_{O_2} and of P_{CO_2}.

It has been suggested that the chief cells of the glomus are the chemically sensitive elements and that they excite the nerve endings through a synaptic mechanism. Synapse-like junctions between these cells and adjacent nerve endings do appear on electron micrographs. Moreover, the nerve endings are sensitive to acetylcholine and to several other candidate transmitter substances. Some investigators believe, however, that the nerve endings themselves are the sensory transducers, and that the chief cells serve some other unknown function.

Fibers of efferent function are also present in the glomus. In rodents so-called reciprocal terminals have also been found, the same fiber appearing to be the postsynaptic element at some junctions and the presynaptic element at others. The function of these dual-purpose fibers is at present unknown.

17.3. Organization of the Peripheral Autonomic Nervous System

Figure 17.1 is a diagram of the main components of the sympathetic division of the autonomic system and of their connections. *Preganglionic neurons* connect the spinal cord to the sympathetic ganglia. The cell bodies of these neurons are in the lateral part of the intermediate zone of the spinal gray matter, usually referred to as the *lateral horn.*

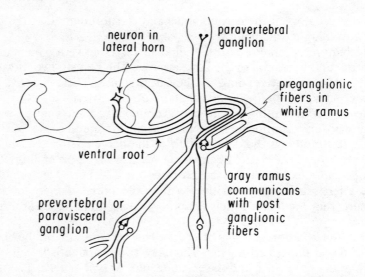

Figure 17.1. The locations of sympathetic preganglionic and postganglionic neurons.

Their axons are in most cases small, B myelinated fibers (see Fig. 6.4), less commonly unmyelinated C axons. These preganglionic fibers exit the spinal cord through the ventral root and then enter the paravertebral sympathetic chain by way of the white communicating branch (*ramus communicans albus*). The cell bodies of the sympathetic *postganglionic neurons* are either in the paravertebral or prevertebral ganglia. The majority of the postganglionic axons are unmyelinated C fibers, although some are myelinated. Those postganglionic fibers which are addressed to the glands and vessels of the skin, skeletal muscles and connective tissues of the limbs and trunk, must join the somatic nerves. This they do by way of the gray communicating branches (*ramus communicans griseus*). The difference in color is due to the predominance of myelinated fibers in the white branch, and of unmyelinated fibers in the gray branch.

Transmission from preganglionic to postganglionic sympathetic neurons is mediated by acetylcholine. Thus, all efferent neurons the axons of which leave the central nervous system (CNS) to join peripheral nerves, including preganglionic sympathetic neurons as well as alpha and gamma motor neurons, are *cholinergic*. The synaptic receptor of the postganglionic neurons is classified as *nicotinic* since it is activated, and in excess it is blocked, by nicotine. It differs, however, from the also nicotinic receptor of skeletal muscle in that the ganglionic junction is more readily blocked by hexamethonium and related drugs than by curare; whereas the muscle endplates are blocked preferentially by curare and its numerous pharmacological relatives.

In the parasympathetic division we also find preganglionic and post-ganglionic neurons. As in the sympathetic division, the preganglionic parasympathetic axons are predominantly B fibers, and their terminals form nicotinic cholinergic synapses with the postganglionic neurons. Unlike most of the sympathetic division, the postganglionic neurons of the parasympathetic are not collected in ganglia, but are scattered within the walls of the organs they innervate. The preganglionic fibers contained in the vagus nerve, for example, find their postganglionic targets in the intramural ganglion cells scattered among the muscle fibers of the heart, airways, esophagus and stomach. The axons of most postganglionic parasympathetic neurons are thus quite short. There are exceptions: the parasympathetic postganglionic neurons innervating the ciliary muscle and the pupils are in the ciliary ganglia, and not within the muscle tissue they innervate.

It should also be remembered that the vagus nerve contains some alpha motor axons that innervate striated (not smooth) muscle fibers in the upper third of the esophagus. In this special case parts of a viscus are moved by skeletal muscle controlled by involuntary reflexes. Although the initiation of swallowing is voluntary, the forwarding of the food is not.

While all the junctions between pre- and postganglionic neurons in both sympathetic and parasympathetic divisions are nicotinic cholinergic, there is more variety among the transmitters and the receptors of postganglionic neuron-effector cell junctions. Postganglionic parasympathetic junctions are all *muscarinic cholinergic*. In these the effects of acetylcholine can be mimicked by low concentrations of muscarine. In some of these the effect of acetylcholine is excitatory, as in the smooth muscle of the intestines and of the airways, in others inhibitory, as in the cardiac pacemaker. All muscarinic junctions, whether excitatory or inhibitory, are blocked by *atropine*.

The majority of the postganglionic sympathetic junctions are noradrenergic. The receptors at noradrenergic junctions have been divided into two types, α and β. This division is based on the relative effectiveness of various chemical relatives of the noradrenaline molecule, either in imitating its action or in blocking it. Some target organs have the one, others the other, and a few have both receptors. α-Receptors and β-receptors similar to those of the peripheral autonomic junctions are believed to be present at central adrenergic synapses as well. Not all the postganglionic sympathetic junctions are, however, noradrenergic. Fibers belonging to the sympathetic division that are muscarinic cholinergic include those innervating sweat glands and the vasodilator fibers of some skeletal muscles and certain regions of the skin.

In summary: in organs that have a parasympathetic innervation (as the heart and most viscera), cholinergic fibers are parasympathetic. In body parts which do not have a parasympathetic innervation (as the skin and skeletal muscle), the cholinergic fibers, if there are any, are sympathetic. Noradrenergic fibers are always sympathetic. In Table 17.1, the transmitters and receptors of the autonomic innervation of major organs are listed.

Adenyl cyclase and cyclic nucleotides may play the role of internal, or "second" (internal) messengers at noradrenergic junctions and also for the effects of circulating adrenaline. Where a catecholamine controls a metabolic function, the cyclic nucleotide is believed to transmit the effect from the membrane receptor to the cell interior. In other cases where noradrenaline influences the permeability of the membrane itself, the second messenger is believed to spread the effect from the synaptic region to the surrounding cell membrane. It should be said, however, that the role of cyclic nucleotides in synaptic transmission is controversial.

17.3a. SYNAPTIC FUNCTIONS IN SYMPATHETIC GANGLIA

Far more postganglionic axons issue from sympathetic ganglia than there are preganglionic fibers entering it. One of the reasons for the existence of peripheral autonomic ganglia is, then, to distribute excitation from a relatively few preganglionic units to a much larger postganglionic population. The terminals of one preganglionic axon often are distributed to more than one ganglion of the paravertebral sympathetic chain. Preganglionic axons thus branch quite profusely. Besides this divergence of synaptic effects, there also is convergence. Each postsynaptic neuron receives terminals from numerous preganglionic units which enables the grading of excitatory postsynaptic potentials (EPSPs) just as in the CNS. If a sufficient number of presynaptic units fire, the summed EPSPs reach threshold and one, sometimes two, postsynaptic impulses are generated.

In recent years it has become clear that the organization of sympa-

Organ	Innervation	Transmitter	Receptor	Effect
Autonomic ganglia	Preganglionic fiber Preganglionic fiber SIF* cell	Acetylcholine Acetylcholine Dopamine?	Nicotinic Muscarinic ?	Fast EPSP† Slow EPSP Slow IPSP
Iris	IIIrd cranial nerve, parasympathetic fibers Sympathetic fibers	Acetylcholine Noradrenaline	Muscarinic α	Constriction of pupil Dilatation of pupil
Ciliary muscle	IIIrd cranial parasympathetic	Acetylcholine	Muscarinic	Accommodation to near vision
Cardiac pacemaker	Vagal parasympathetic Sympathetic	Acetylcholine Noradrenaline	Muscarinic β	Increased gK, slowing of pace Increased gNa, increased rate
Ventricular muscle	Sympathetic	Noradrenaline	β	Increased contractile strength
Vascular smooth muscle, generally	Sympathetic	Noradrenaline	α	Vasoconstriction
Arteriolar smooth muscle, in skeletal muscle	Sympathetic Sympathetic	Acetylcholine Noradrenaline	Muscarinic β	Vasodilatation‡ Vasodilatation‡
Gastrointestinal tract and bronchioles	Vagus or sacral parasympathetic Sympathetic	Acetylcholine Noradrenaline	Muscarinic β	Stimulation of motility Inhibition of motility
Urinary bladder	Sacral parasympathetic Sympathetic	Acetylcholine and ATP? Noradrenaline	Muscarinic β	Detrusor muscle contraction Detrusor muscle relaxation
Sweat glands	Sympathetic	Acetylcholine	Muscarinic	Increased secretion

* SIF, small intensively fluorescing.
† EPSP, excitatory postsynaptic potential.
‡ Vasodilatation is achieved in some muscles in some species by cholinergic, in others by β-adrenergic, sympathetic fibers. In man the adrenergic dilators are said to be more common, perhaps the only ones.

Nicotinic junctions in ganglia are blocked selectively by hexamethonium; muscarinic junctions by atropine; α-receptors by, for example, phentolamine; β-receptors by propranolol.

Metabolic and other effects of circulating adrenaline are mediated mainly by β-receptors, for which the hormone has higher affinity.

thetic ganglia is more complicated than hitherto suspected, and that presumably they have more intricate functions besides routing and distributing the signals of presynaptic fibers. Small cells have been found in these ganglia that do not resemble ordinary postganglionic neurons. Because of their staining characteristics, some have been termed small intensively fluorescing (SIF) cells. The existence of short-axon interneurons indicates that signals issuing from the spinal cord are processed and integrated in some manner within the sympathetic ganglia. While the nature and meaning of this integrative function is not clear, some of its electrophysiological signs have been discovered. Besides the just described nicotinic cholinergic EPSPs, other synaptic potentials have been recorded from ganglion cells. These so-called "slow EPSPs" and "slow inhibitory postsynaptic potentials (IPSPs)" have protracted rise and decay times. The slow EPSPs are cholinergic, but they are mediated by a muscarinic receptor. The slow IPSPs are transmitted either by noradrenaline or by dopamine, probably from SIF cells.

17.3b. AXON REFLEX

In the 1920s, Bayliss demonstrated that intense, prolonged repetitive stimulation of the peripheral stump of a transected dorsal root causes vasodilatation in the skin innervated by the root. At first he concluded that dorsal roots contain efferent vasomotor fibers, but it later turned out that the vasodilatation was caused by impulses traveling antidromically in afferent fibers, specifically in nociceptive C fibers.

Antidromic vasodilatation is related to another phenomenon also discovered in the 1920s, the *triple response of Lewis*. If a small amount of histamine is injected into the skin, there are three distinct responses. First, the injected area reddens by the action of the histamine on vascular smooth muscle. Then the area swells (the *wheal* formation) by local edema, caused by the action of histamine on capillary walls. Finally the skin becomes flushed in an area much wider than where histamine could have spread by diffusion. This is known as the *flare*, and it is mediated by nerve fibers, but without involvement of the CNS. This is called an *axon reflex*. The triple response can also be caused by scratching the skin without drawing blood; and it looks and feels rather like the place of an insect bite.

The following series of observations proved that the third component, the flare, was mediated by an axon reflex. If a cutaneous nerve is cut, the area innervated by it can at first still produce the entire triple response. Later, once the fibers supplying the skin have degenerated, the local redness and wheal can still be evoked but the flare cannot. Moreover, if the dorsal root fibers of two or more segments are cut peripherally from the dorsal root ganglion and the fibers they contain allowed to degenerate, the flare cannot be provoked in the area normally innervated by the roots. Yet if dorsal roots are cut centrally from the dorsal root ganglion so that the fibers in the peripheral stump remain connected to the ganglion cells and therefore do not degenerate, the ability to flare is preserved. Interrupting the autonomic fibers supplying a skin area, removing sympathetic ganglia, or cutting ventral roots never interferes with the ability to produce a flare. The conclusion: in order to produce the flare there must be cutaneous innervation by somatic afferent fibers, but these fibers need not be connected to the CNS. The histamine, or the scratch, irritate sensory nerve endings and other terminals belonging to branches of the irritated fibers release a chemical substance that causes the vasodilatation.

The flare of the triple response and the antidromic vasodilatation described by Bayliss are believed to be produced by the same vasodilator substance released by similar nerve fibers. A variety of substances have been suggested, including histamine itself, but perhaps the most plausible candidate is substance P. This polypeptide may be the transmitter at the central terminals of nociceptive, and perhaps also some of the other, afferent C fibers (see Section 2.5e). Substance P is present not only at the central terminals, but throughout these neurons, including the sensory terminals. There may also be interaction between substance P, released from sensory nerve terminals, and bradykinin, released from damaged tissue cells (see Section 6.7). Release of substance P from sensory terminals into tissue spaces could thus explain some manifestations of inflammations in general.

17.3c. THE INTRAMURAL NERVE PLEXUS OF THE INTESTINES

An isolated piece of gut suspended in a suitable nutrient solution, properly oxygenated and warmed, moves rhythmically. The intestinal tract as a whole, left *in situ*, will perform its digestive and absorptive functions and propel the food mass in a more or less normal way even if deprived of all extrinsic nerves connecting it to the CNS. The functions of such a disconnected intestinal tract will, of course, not be integrated with the activities of the other organs of the body. For example, there will be no inhibition of motility during exercise, and no splanchnic vasoconstriction when vessels in skeletal muscles dilate. But the neurally disconnected intestinal tract will continue to do its main job of providing the body with nutrients.

Rhythmic self-excitation of the intestinal smooth muscle is a property of its cell membrane (see Section 14.3). The proper coordination of peristalsis, segmentation, the opening and closing of sphincters, and the like (see Sernka and Jacobson, Chapter 7), all depend on the integrative action of the system of neurons built into the wall of the intestine. It probably is fair to say that the gut disconnected from the CNS is about as smart as an earthworm with its head ganglion removed. The extrinsic autonomic nerves of the intestines serve to modulate the activity generated within the intestine's own nervous system.

Anatomists distinguish two separate plexuses of nerves in the intestinal wall: the *submucous* plexus of *Meissner*, and the *myenteric* plexus of *Auerbach*. The plexus of Meissner contains predominantly, or exclusively, neurons with a receptor function. Neurons in the plexus of Auerbach process the information gathered by the sensory cells of the Meissner plexus and generate the command signals which coordinate peristaltic and other patterned movements of the muscles. This plexus also contains the terminals of preganglionic parasympathetic nerves and some of its cells play the role of postganglionic parasympathetic neurons.

The simplest scheme that could explain peristalsis in the intestines involves the following local reflex actions. Food mass in the intestine distends it, and therefore stimulates the stretch-sensitive mechanoreceptors, the cell bodies of which lie in the submucous plexus. Axon terminals of these neurons excite inhibitory neurons lying aborally ("downstream") in the myenteric plexus; these inhibitory neurons cause the relaxation of the circular muscle. At the same time other branches of the axons of the sensory neurons of the submucosa excite excitatory neurons of the myenteric plexus at the site of the food mass, and just adorally ("upstream") of it, causing contraction of the circular muscle fibers. This contraction squeezes the food mass into the already dilated aboral segment of the intestine. Experiments show that such local reflexes are indeed operating within the walls of the gut, but in reality the circuit mediating them is more complex than the scheme just presented.

Acetylcholine and noradrenaline are not the only transmitters in the synaptic network of the intestinal plexuses. Purinergic neurons transmit inhibitory effects utilizing a purine nucleotide, perhaps adenosine triphosphate (ATP). Serotonin, dopamine and several peptides are also suspected to have neural function here, but the exact status of these substances is uncertain at present. Enkephalin is one of them, and the presence of enkephalin receptors in the membrane of intestinal smooth muscle explains the well-known inhibitory effect of opium alkaloids on intestinal motility (cf. Section 7.9c).

17.3d. NEURAL CONTROL OF THE URINARY BLADDER

Although there are neurons within the wall of the bladder, it normally is controlled by extrinsic nerves. The detrusor muscle is activated by cholinergic and probably also purinergic (ATP) innervation. Preganglionic fibers derive from the sacral parasympathetic nerves; the postganglionic neurons are located in the pelvic ganglia and also in the bladder wall. Inhibitory noradrenergic postganglionic fibers from the lumbar sympathetic segments act not only on the smooth muscle but also form inhibitory synapses with the postganglionic parasympathetic neurons.

The human bladder does not have an internal smooth muscle sphincter comparable, for example, to the pylorus or the anus. Instead, continence is maintained by a valve-like action of the urethral opening and reinforced by the external sphincter formed by skeletal muscle. The bladder wall is folded over the initial part of the urethra where it leaves the bladder. Pressure inside the bladder keeps this initial segment of the urethra compressed, and this prevents the escape of urine. This valve action is effective as long as the bladder is not too full and the detrusor muscle is relaxed. Beyond a certain level of filling, continence requires the contraction of the external sphincter composed of striated muscle and under combined reflex and voluntary control.

The bladder does not behave like an elastic balloon: the pressure inside is not proportional to the volume it contains. As it fills with urine from the ureters, the tone of the detrusor muscle is progressively inhibited by a reflex, mediated by the sympathetic nerves. This *receptive relaxation* of the bladder is similar to that of the stomach. Because of this relaxation, pressure remains low and relatively constant. When, however, a certain critical volume has been reached, around 400–450 ml in most people, inhibition ceases and the detrusor muscle is activated by parasympathetic fibers (Fig. 17.2). Intravesical pressure then begins to rise, and with it a sense of urgency. The voluntary muscles of the perineum must now be called upon to prevent the escape of urine.

To empty the bladder, the external sphincter is relaxed, and the voiding reflex permitted to take its course. The detrusor contracts and pulls the infundibular portion of the bladder neck, which had been folded before, into a funnel. This change in shape opens the exit port and allows urine to flow into the urethra. Voiding may, but need not be, assisted by pressure exerted on the bladder by the muscles of the abdominal wall.

Coordination of the various reflexes controlling the bladder occurs at several levels of the CNS. Involved are the autonomic neurons in the

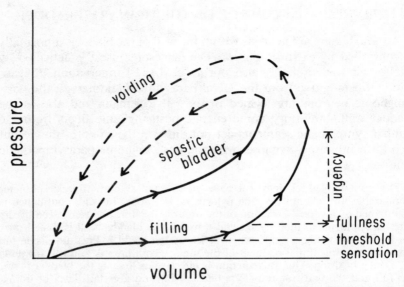

Figure 17.2. Pressure-volume loops of the urinary bladder. The *outer curve* shows the normal condition, the *inner curve* the behavior of a spastic bladder.

tail end of the spinal cord (the conus medullaris) and in the lower lumbar segments, as are neuron circuits in the brain stem and in unspecified "higher centers."

Bladder function in paraplegic patients. What happens to bladder control when the caudal segments of the spinal cord are disconnected from the brain is of great importance for the management of paraplegic patients. During the period of spinal shock (see Section 15.5a) all bladder reflexes are suspended, and the detrusor muscle is *atonic.* Urine is retained until the bladder overfills and urine begins to escape in a trickle. Patients in spinal shock must be relieved by catheter, for the retention of urine has life-threatening consequences.

With the passing of spinal shock, reflex control of the bladder is resumed so that the bladder is emptied at intervals by the contraction of the detrusor muscle. This spinal reflex is initiated by vesical mechanoreceptors. A bladder under reflex control is usually referred to as a *neurogenic bladder.* In many neurogenic bladders neither receptive relaxation nor emptying are complete. This can sometimes lead to a progressive condition known as a *spastic bladder*, in which intravesical pressure is abnormally high, voiding too frequent, and a residual volume of urine always remains (Fig. 17.2). Avoiding bladder spasticity is one of the keys to the successful management of paraplegic patients.

To assist paraplegics in emptying the bladder, neuroprosthetic procedures have recently been devised consisting of permanently implanted stimulating electrodes with which the patient controls the contraction of his detrusor muscle. The electrodes are either fixed in contact with the parasympathetic sacral nerves or are inserted into the lateral horns of the conus medullaris of the spinal cord. As may be imagined, these procedures are fraught with technical difficulties, not all of which have as yet been solved. For this reason they are considered at this time to be experimental.

Patients whose sacral spinal segments have been destroyed and those whose pelvic autonomic nerves have been severed are considerably worse off than paraplegics with neurogenic bladders. Deprived of all central nervous control, the bladder is atonic, but eventually may regain some function governed by the intramural neurons and the intrinsic contractility of its smooth muscle. This condition is referred to as an *automatic bladder* or, sometimes, a *myogenic bladder*. Its function is rarely satisfactory, however, and in these cases the regular use of a catheter for life can seldom be avoided.

17.4. The Central Control of Homeostatic Functions

The controls of respiration, circulation and digestive functions are usually described in detail in the texts dealing with these special organ systems. In the pages that follow the discussion will concentrate on general principles of central autonomic control, and these will be illustrated in the example of temperature control. First, however, we must pay some attention to the part of the brain most essential in the integration of many diverse vital functions, the hypothalamus.

17.5. Functions of the Hypothalamus

The hypothalamus has been described as the "head ganglion of the autonomic nervous system." A catchy phrase, and an acceptable one, as long as it is remembered that autonomic and somatic functions are not independent but interdependent aspects of the integrated responses an organism makes. The vital functions of the hypothalamic area are carried out through a combination of both autonomic and somatic nerves. And, besides, the hypothalamic region is the most important interface between neural and endocrine regulation. *Neuroendocrine cells* are neurons which secrete "transmitter" substances not at a synapse but into capillary blood so that their influence is not limited to a number of target neurons, but is broadcast throughout the circulation. In mammals such neuroendocrine cells are concentrated in some of the nuclei of the hypothalamus.

The hypothalamus is, then, the most comprehensive regulator of numerous vital functions. That this is so had first been suspected on the grounds of clinical observation about a hundred years ago. Modern investigation of this area began in the mid-1930s by the Swiss physiologist Hess. He was one of the first to implant electrodes into deep-lying points in the brain (see Sections 1.2 and 1.4b). With these electrodes he could stimulate nuclei in the hypothalamus while the animal was awake and able to move with relative freedom. Moreover, the same stimulation could be repeated day after day, and the consistency of the response determined.

Hess showed, as did many others after him, that electrical stimulation of certain points evoked reproducible responses. Some of these reactions were relatively simple, such as a rise of blood pressure, but others involved complex integrated activities. For example, when the appropriate stimulation was given to the appropriate point in the hypothalamus, the animal would behave as though enraged. Or, when stimulated at another point and with a different frequency of electric pulses, he would fall asleep. From the observations of Hess and others elaborate maps have been constructed showing the anatomical location of the various stimulated sites, and the effects that stimulation at those sites evoked. Observations of the effects of stimulation were complemented by investigations of the deficiencies caused by destroying specific nuclei, or clusters of nuclei. The disease states caused by these experimental lesions in animals could then also be related to the syndromes of hypothalamic pathology in human patients.

Obesity with hypogenitalism and sexual malfunction is, for example, a well-known hypothalamic developmental disorder known as Froehlich's syndrome. Experimentation on animals enabled the analysis of this complex into its components. It became apparent that destruction of different cells were responsible for the sexual disorder and for the disturbed control of body weight. Sexual development and function are influenced by the hypophysiotropic neurosecretory cells that release their chemical messengers into the portal circulation flowing from the median eminence region of the hypothalamus to the pars distalis of the adenohypophysis. The control of body weight depends on cell groups in the ventromedial and the lateral hypothalamic areas.

Experimental lesions and stimulation experiments have led to the important concept of hypothalamic cell groupings of mutually antagonistic function, examples of reciprocal innervation. For example, in the next section we will learn that the cells coordinating the dissipation of heat and those responsible for heat conservation and production reciprocally inhibit one another. A balancing of similar, reciprocally antagonistic neuron populations controls food intake. If the ventromedial

(VM) region of the hypothalamus is destroyed by an experimental lesion, the animal will eat too much too frequently, and gain a large excess of weight. Electrical stimulation in the same region of an intact brain can evoke an opposite effect: the animal will stop eating, even if it was hungry because of previous food deprivation. The lateral hypothalamus is the reciprocal antagonistic region of the ventromedial area. Bilateral destruction of the lateral hypothalamus causes loss of appetite and weight loss and stimulation there evokes voracious eating. Because of this combination of observations the VM region of the hypothalamus is sometimes referred to as the *satiety center*, and the lateral area, the feeding center or *appetite center*.

A major advance toward understanding the significance of the hypothalamus was made when it became clear that not only electrical stimulation but also certain natural changes excite the neurons of this region. For example, warming the blood that perfuses the hypothalamic region evokes responses that increase the dissipation of body heat (see next section). Another example is that raising the osmotic pressure of the interstitial fluid in the supraoptic nucleus, or in its vicinity, evokes the release of antidiuretic hormone (ADH) by neurosecretory cells, the cell bodies of which are located in the supraoptic nucleus, but their axon terminals releasing the ADH are in the neurohypophysis. Stimulation close to this region also impels animals to seek and drink water, behaving exactly as if they were thirsty. *Thirst* is a complex sensation which can also be caused by dryness of the mouth, tongue and pharynx, as well as by loss of blood and of body fluids, even if the osmotic pressure remains normal. It has long been recognized, however, that a chief factor in thirst is a rise of extracellular osmotic pressure. The experiments just quoted located the sensor of osmotic pressure within the hypothalamus. Excitation of these very sensor cells evokes both conservation of water by the ADH mechanism and its replacement by inducing the animal to drink. A search for the particular cells in the hypothalamuc that act as sense organs of the internal environment has been continued since the early 1950s. Many neurons have been found that change discharge rate as a function of either the osmotic pressure or of the temperature of their environment. Some of these cells may indeed be primary receptor cells, transducing chemical or physical changes of interstitial fluid. In such experiments it is not always possible to distinguish primary receptors from neurons driven synaptically by other nearby cells.

The nervous system interfaces with the glands of internal secretion in two ways. First, neurosecretory cells produce substances which either stimulate or inhibit other cells of endocrine function and neurosecretory cells are integrated into the circuitry of the CNS by synaptic connections with other nerve cells. Second, the influence of the nervous system on the endocrine system is reciprocated by the influence exerted by hormones on neuronal function. Binding sites for circulating hormones have been identified by histochemical and immunofluorescence methods and are especially profuse in the hypothalamic region. Reproductive behavior in particular requires coordination of the endocrine and nervous systems. For further details textbooks of endocrinology should be consulted.

While regional specialization of the hypothalamus is well demonstrated, it would be a mistake to liken this (or any other) part of the brain to an electronic circuit neatly laid out with labeled components and color-coded wire connections. Cell populations of different function occupy overlapping areas, and the fibers connecting these cell groups crisscross various nuclei in a network the finer details of which are hard to trace. Consequently, even the most carefully placed experimental lesions do not necessarily produce a pure defect of just one body function. This is also the reason that functional maps drawn of the same regions by two investigators are not always identical. The more recent practice of using selective poisons, which destroy one kind of cell only, instead of indiscriminate electrolytic lesions, resolved only some of these difficulties in certain special situations. Moreover, the borders that demarcate physiological functions do not always coincide with the boundaries of anatomically recognizable nuclei of the hypothalamus (see also Section 1.3).

The difficulty of analyzing complex functions of the brain by lesion experiments is illustrated by the controversy surrounding the regulation of food intake. It has been claimed that lesion of the ventromedial nucleus of the hypothalamus causes overeating, not because the lesion destroys the cells in this region, but because it interrupts the fibers of the ventral noradrenergic bundle that pass through this area. Based on these results the concept of a satiety center was called a "myth." Similarly, the adipsia (insufficient drinking) and hypophagia (insufficient eating) after lesions of the lateral hypothalamus were attributed to coincidental interruption of the dopaminergic nigrostriate fiber bundle and to the consequently suppressed exploratory behavior and general lack of initiative typical of nigrostriate lesion (see also Section 18.2c). There is, however, considerable evidence, some of it quite recent, confirming a role of hypothalamic neurons in feeding. Neurons were found in these areas that change their firing rate in response to changes in glucose concentration in their environment. Low and high glucose levels are believed to be among the several factors that evoke the feelings of appetite and satiety. Moreover, the administration of gold-thioglucose in appropriate toxic amounts caused death of neurons specifically in those nuclei of the hypothalamus thought to be involved in sensing and signaling glucose concentrations. Loss of these cells was associated with overeating and thus resulted in obesity, similar to the consequence of electrolytic lesions made in the VM nucleus, even though the gold-thioglucose poisoning did not destroy the fibers that pass through the area.

These diverse observations have led investigators to different conclusions, but in reality they are not incompatible. Raw hunger and thirst are not the only motivations influencing eating and drinking. A wide variety of neuronal processes interact in producing, and in inhibiting, such complex behaviors. The monoamine systems probably have much to do with governing those states of the nervous system relating to reward or leading to defensive and aggressive behaviors; in a word, with feelings that in common parlance are called fear, anger, desire, contentment, placidity and the like. It may be true that one of the functions of hypothalamic mechanisms is to keep glucose or other nutrients (e.g. lipids) at an optimum level in the bloodstream. At the same time it may also be correct that a function of the monoamine systems is to provide the drive and motivation for the activities that make such nutrients available to the animal and to restrain such activities when necessary. If so then it is also plausible that these systems must interact in intimate ways. Therefore destroying different components of these interdependent systems, or interrupting the connections between them, could give rise to similar even if not identical impairments of behavior. It is thus not surprising that both interruption of the nigrostriate fiber bundle and destruction of the cells of the lateral hypothalamus result in hypophagia. Parenthetically it should be added that the presumed role of the serotonin system in evoking feelings of contentment and also suppressing appetite has become known widely enough to prompt the recent fad of eating tryptophan (the amino acid presursor of serotonin) as a dietary supplement. That excess dietary tryptophan promotes good feelings and weight loss has, however, not been proven conclusively.

In Table 17.2 are presented some of the better known consequences of experimental stimulation and of lesions made in the hypothalamus. The list is by no means complete, and it should be interpreted with the just discussed reservations in mind.

Table 17.2.

Results of Stimulation and Consequences of Lesions in the Hypothalamus

Nucleus or Area	Effect of Stimulation	Effect of Lesion
Supraoptic nucleus and paraventricular nucleus	Release of ADH-vasopressin and/or oxytocin	Diabetes insipidus
Periventricular area, suprachiasmatic nucleus, arcuate nucleus	Secretion of releasing factors into pituitary portal circulation	Various endocrine deficiencies
Preoptic nuclei, anterior nucleus	Cutaneous vasodilatation, sweating, panting Secretion of gastric acid	Hyperthermia when exposed to warm environment
Posterior area	Cutaneous vasoconstriction, increased muscle tone, shivering General arousal,* rage	Loss of temperature regulation, loss of fever response to pyrogens†
Area dorsolaterally adjacent to paraventricular nucleus	Drinking, seeking of drinking water	
Ventromedial nucleus	Cessation of eating; placidity	Excessive eating, obesity; aggressive behavior
Lateral hypothalamus: area lateral of ventromedial nucleus	Voracious eating	Weight loss due to insufficient food intake
Area lateral of mamillothalamic tract	Defensive behavior; rise of arterial pressure Increased cardiac output, vasodilatation in muscle	Adipsia; diminished exploratory behavior, hypoactivity‡

* General arousal may be mediated by fibers that pass through this region and are addressed to the ascending reticular formation; see Chapter 19.

† Pyrogens are substances that cause fever when injected.

‡ The hypoactivity may or may not be due to interruption of the nigrostriate pathway; see Section 18.2c.

17.5a. THE CENTRAL REGULATION OF TEMPERATURE

Heat is produced by all work, physical and chemical. In the resting body of an animal most heat comes from the liver and the intestines; in the working body, from the skeletal muscles. Were it not for physiological regulation, in a warm environment the heat produced by the organs would raise the body temperature; in the cold, the body would cool down. To keep temperature constant, heat must flow to the environment as fast as it is produced by the tissues.

However, not all parts of the body are kept at equal temperatures. Inside the abdominal and thoracic cavities, the temperature does not vary by more than about ±0.5°C, at least in good health and with the subject resting. Inside the skull the range is narrower. The surface temperature of the skin does vary quite markedly, although not equally with that of the surrounding air. The tissues of the limbs and walls of the body cavity form a shell or buffer zone, kept at a temperature intermediate between that of the surface and the core. The temperature gradient is interposed between the core and the surface of the body, perhaps as a matter of fuel economy. In a cold environment it takes less energy to keep the central body temperature within the physiological range if the tissues of the shell are allowed to cool to an intermediate temperature than it would take to keep the entire body mass equally warm, insulated by the skin alone.

To conserve heat the vessels of the skin contract and so keep hot blood away from the cool surface. Within the limbs, heat is transferred from the blood in the large arteries to that in the large veins which lie beside them. In this manner the large vessels form a *countercurrent heat exchanger*. Thus, arterial blood loses heat continually as it flows toward the extremities, and venous blood gains heat as it returns from the extremities toward the body cavity. In this way a continuous gradient of temperature is set up from shoulders to fingertips and from thighs to toes.

If heat conservation cannot keep the body core warm, heat production is stepped up, first by increasing the tone of skeletal muscles, then by shivering. In both instances, skeletal muscle fibers contract without doing mechanical work but producing heat that is transferred to the blood and distributed throughout the body by way of the circulation. If exposed to a cold climate for a prolonged period, the body acclimatizes by increasing its basal metabolic rate. This, however, is a function of the endocrine glands, not of the nervous system.

In a warm environment the problem is to dissipate excess heat. There are three ways to convey heat: radiation, conduction and evaporation. Heat loss can be increased greatly by the former two methods if the blood vessels of the skin dilate. Cutaneous blood flow can exceed the metabolic needs of the skin by several fold so that small veins fill with almost fully oxygenated blood, and the skin takes on a flushed appearance. Under these conditions the surface of the skin becomes quite warm, and can lose much of its heat to the environment.

When the air and the objects around an animal become warmer than its body, then heat will be gained instead of lost by conduction and by radiation. Evaporation then is the only method of heat loss left. Some water evaporates from the skin and from the airways under all conditions, but the amount can be much increased either by sweating or by panting. If the air is not only hot, but also saturated with water vapor, or if the body is submerged in water at a temperature higher than the body's, then heat loss by sweating fails too, and the body temperature rises. This can be dangerous.

Cutaneous blood vessels and sweat glands are controlled by sympathetic nerves. Shivering and panting are functions of skeletal muscles controlled by spinal ventral horn cells. Metabolic rate is controlled by the thyroid gland and influenced by other hormones such as adrenaline and insulin. With the possible exception of the islands of Langerhans, all these neuronal and endocrine mechanisms are influenced by neurons in the hypothalamic region which weave the many threads of temperature control into a coherent pattern.

Electrical stimulation of the preoptic and anterior nuclei of the hypothalamus can initiate the coordinated autonomic responses by which the body loses heat, for instance increased blood flow through the small vessels of the skin and either panting or sweating, depending on the species. Stimulation of the posterior hypothalamus causes cutaneous vasoconstriction and increased muscle tone or shivering, in other words both the conservation and the production of heat. From these observations arose the concept of the two reciprocally antagonistic centers, the one serving to adapt to a hot, the other to a cold, environment. Indeed if the preoptic and anterior nuclei are destroyed, an experimental animal will not be able to keep its body cool in a warm environment, but it will be able to maintain body temperature when exposed to cold. Uncontrolled hyperthermia (rise of body temperature) is also a clinical sign of hypothalamic damage in man.

When the posterior hypothalamus is destroyed by experimental lesion, all temperature regulation is impaired so that the animal is unable to adapt either to cold or to heat. This has been interpreted to mean that such a lesion destroys not only the cells in the posterior nucleus that coordinate heat conservation and heat production, but also the fibers that pass from anterior hypothalamus through this region to the brain stem and spinal cord. By losing the cells coordinating adaptation to cold, and at the same time the output fibers of the cells coordinating adaptation to warm, the animal loses all ability to adapt to changing temperature.

More recent research has demonstrated that there are neurons in the anterior hypothalamus, the firing of which are influenced by temperature changes. Some of these cells respond to cooling or heating the skin; others to cooling or heating the hypothalamus itself. No such temperature-sensitive cells were found in the posterior hypothalamus. This and other observations have led to a suggested modification of our ideas concerning hypothalamic heat regulation, which is illustrated in Figure 17.3*A*. According to this scheme, the anterior hypothalamus processes

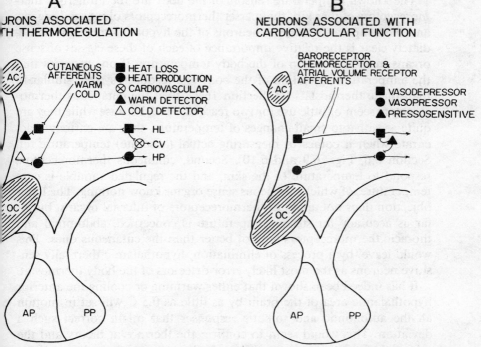

A

JRONS ASSOCIATED
H THERMOREGULATION

CUTANEOUS
AFFERENTS
WARM
COLD

■ HEAT LOSS
● HEAT PRODUCTION
⊗ CARDIOVASCULAR
▲ WARM DETECTOR
△ COLD DETECTOR

B

NEURONS ASSOCIATED WITH
CARDIOVASCULAR FUNCTION

BARORECEPTOR
CHEMORECEPTOR &
ATRIAL VOLUME RECEPTOR
AFFERENTS

■ VASODEPRESSOR
● VASOPRESSOR
▲ PRESSOSENSITIVE

Figure 17.3. The location and presumed interconnections of cell groups in the hypothalamus concerned with temperature regulation (*A*) and control of circulation (*B*). *AC*, anterior commissure; *OC*, optic chiasma; *AP*, anterior pituitary; *PP*, posterior pituitary. (Reprinted with permission from J. N. Hayward: *Physiological Reviews* 57:574–658, 1977.)

the incoming information relating to temperature, and the posterior hypothalamus programs thermoregulatory responses. A similar division of the tasks relating to the control of the circulation has also been suggested (Fig. 17.3*B*). These schemes, like their predecessors, are still hypothetical.

The question of how the body's thermostat is set has been asked. The set point is around 37.5°C, slightly higher in waking hours than during sleep, in women higher after ovulation than before, and higher during work than at rest. The set point is raised in fever, but is still under control. Failure of temperature control due to environmental heat stress is not called fever, but heat stroke, and is a life-threatening condition.

The known temperature sensors of the body are the numerous thermoreceptors of the skin, the sparser thermoreceptors of internal organs, and the temperature-sensing neurons of the hypothalamus. Not immediately clear is the relative importance of each of these classes of sense organs in the regulation of the body temperature. If one assumes that the temperature regulation of the body is a feedback system similar to man-made thermostats (cf. Section 16.1), then the cutaneous thermoreceptors seem of little use for two reasons. First, because while they are quite sensitive to small changes of temperature, they are entirely inaccurate when it comes to measuring actual (absolute) temperature (cf. Section 6.6, Figs. 6.9 and 6.10). Second, cutaneous thermoreceptors respond to temperature of the skin, and the regulated variable is core temperature, of which cutaneous sense organs know nothing. The latter objection does not apply to thermoreceptors of internal organs, but as far as accuracy for steady temperature is concerned, abdominal and thoracic thermoreceptors are not better than the cutaneous ones. This would leave, by a process of elimination, hypothalamic thermally sensitive neurons as the most likely error detectors of the body thermostat.

It has indeed been shown that either warming or cooling the anterior hypothalamic area of the brain by as little as 0.5°C will set in motion all the autonomic and somatic responses that might correct such a deviation. This would seem to confirm the thermostat theory and the role of the hypothalamic neurons as both sensors and regulators of the thermostat. More recently, however, it became possible to implant small electric thermometers into the hypothalamic region of the brain and allow the experimental animal to recover from surgery. Now if the negative feedback thermostat theory were correct, then whenever the animal was exposed to cold or heat the hypothalamic region should undergo detectable changes of temperature which may be small, but not smaller than the ones which have been shown to initiate the appropriate defense mechanism of the body; for without an error signal negative feedback control will not operate (cf. Section 16.1 and Fig. 16.2).

In actual fact, the hypothalamic temperature did not significantly change when animals were placed in either a hot or cold environment (Fig. 17.4). This shows that compensatory mechanisms have forstalled changes of intracranial temperature. The hypothalamus was therefore shown not to operate as a negative feedback thermostat. Rather, it behaved *as though* it "knew" both the heat flow between body and environment and the rate at which heat was produced by the body, and

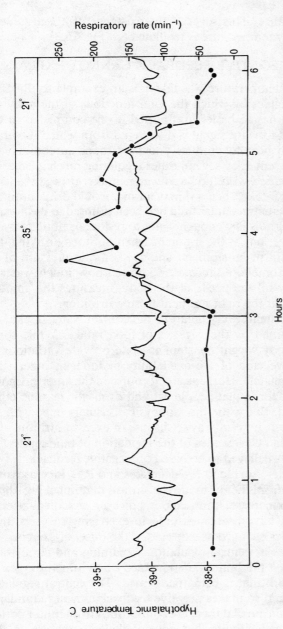

Figure 17.4. Temperature of hypothalamic tissue during exposure to heat. The *continuous line* is the recording of the output of a small temperature gauge implanted in the hypothalamus of a rabbit. The *solid circles* show the respiratory rate. Numbers at *top* of graph show room temperature in degrees Celsius. Note that during exposure to heat the rabbit pants. During such exposure hypothalamic temperature does not fluctuate more than previously, when the animal was in a cool environment. (Reprinted with permission from R. F. Hellon: *Federation Proceedings* 40:2804–2807, 1981.)

kept the two in balance. This suggests the existence of a *feed-forward* signal by which body temperature is regulated (cf. Fig. 16.3).

17.5b. WHAT NEGATIVE FEEDBACK CANNOT EXPLAIN

The regulation of temperature was taken as an example to illustrate certain general principles by which the vital functions of the body are governed. The story has to be left unfinished, to be completed in the future when the feed-forward signal is discovered from which the brain estimates how much heat to produce and how much to conserve. A similar enigma is presented by several other regulating mechanisms, for example those concerned with food and water intake. If negative feedback governed water intake, then a thirsty animal would drink until the osmotic pressure of its extracellular fluid had been restored to the normal level. A dog indeed drinks just enough water to restore osmotic pressure to what it ought to be, but at the moment when he stops drinking, the water he drank is still in its stomach and the osmotic pressure of its blood is still high. Somehow the brain "knows" how much water is needed to eventually fill the needs of the body, measures the amount taken in, and signals at the right moment to stop drinking.

If we do not understand every detail of the control water intake, we are even more mystified by the vagaries of food intake. While some species keep their body weight constant in spite of wide variations of muscular activity level and of the availability of food, in others this control is much less reliable. Humans are of course in the latter category. One complicating factor is that people eat and drink for reasons other than hunger or thirst. But while the kidneys can usually cope with an excess of water, there is no easy way to dispose of excess nutrition.

We have a somewhat clearer idea of the regulation of blood gases. At one time this also was believed to be based on negative feedback. It was thought that as we exercise, blood P_{O_2} decreases and P_{CO_2} increases and that these deviations from the norm are the stimuli that impel breathing and cardiac output to increase. It turned out, however, as soon as arterial gas tensions and pH have been measured in exercising subjects, that none of these variables changed as expected at the onset of exercise. As in the other examples of central regulation, breathing and circulation are adjusted *as though* the brain "knew" exactly how much oxygen is demanded by the work that is being performed. The central regulator *anticipates* demand and so makes negative feedback almost redundant. Experimental data indicate that there are connections from motor cortex and the other neuronal circuits that control skeletal muscles to the hypothalamus. From the information it receives, the hypothalamus apparently estimates the adjustments necessary to compensate for additional oxygen demand. Signals from the posterior hypothalamic region are then issued to the autonomic centers of the brain stem to appropriately increase respiration, cardiac output, and to change the distribution of vasomotor tone.

The puzzling fact is not that the brain can anticipate that there will be additional demand for oxygen, or for heat, or for drinking water, but that it knows exactly how much the demand will be. Now even though we know of no measuring devices that could meter, for example, heat flow or total oxygen consumed, from the information the brain receives it is in principle possible to compute these quantities. Heat flow, for example, could be estimated from (1) the time integral of the rate of cooling of the skin and (2) the area of skin exposed. It is, however, unlikely that the brain achieves this in the manner of a well-programmed man-made computer. More probably there is a process at work that is akin to learning of other behaviors. Temperature regulation is unreliable in an infant. In the early postnatal months the brain may be learning, by trial and error, how much heat production and conservation is appropriate to how much cooling of the skin; more precisely, to how much of vasoconstrictor signals to send in response to how many cold-receptor nerve impulses. Trial and error may play a similar part in learning to adjust oxygen delivery to a given muscular effort.

Does this then mean that the classical homeostatic reflexes, all of which are in essence negative feedback mechanisms, are of no physiological significance? This, of course, would not be a sound conclusion at all. Many reliable and reproducible experiments have demonstrated negative feedback in the autonomic and somatic divisions of the nervous system and chemical negative feedback in the endocrine system that must be of functional significance. The most likely use for these reflexes is second-line defense mechanisms that operate when primary regulation fails.

In mild or moderately severe exercise the oxygenation of arterial blood remains normal. But in efforts that test the limit of endurance, for example running or swimming in competition, hypoxemia certainly can occur. It is then, that signals of the carotid body begin to drive the respiratory centers and the protective value of negative feedback mechanisms becomes obvious. Such maximal effort is accompanied by respiratory distress, or *dyspnea*, until pain restrains the effort, and one must hope before self-inflicted damage occurs. There has been some difference of opinion concerning the nature of the physiological signals that cause respiratory distress. At one time it was widely held that low P_{O_2} acting on the carotid body, or the high P_{CO_2} or low pH acting on neurons in the brain stem, convey the feeling of conscious "air hunger." Many investigators, however, are of the opinion that this feeling arises from mechanoreceptors of the airways. According to this theory, hyperpnea is a reflex evoked by the known peripheral and central stimuli that drive respiration. The *subjective* feeling would be *secondary* to the reflex. In other words, we feel suffocated because we breathe harder, and not the other way around. This theory blames the dyspnea of altered blood chemistry (low P_{O_2} or high P_{CO_2}) on the same physiological mechanism as that of airway obstruction: the stimulation of airway mechanoreceptors.

17.6. Chapter Summary

1. Preparation of the organism for flight or fight is mediated in large part by the sympathetic division of the autonomic nervous system, but sympathetic efferent fibers also participate in many discrete adjustments when the organism is not faced by an emergency.
2. General visceral afferent units share many properties of cutaneous afferent units and have similar adequate stimuli.
3. The adequate stimulation of vascular baroreceptors is deformation of the nerve terminal produced by stretching of the arterial wall caused by the pressure of the blood.
4. Afferent fibers of the carotid body respond to lowering of P_{O_2}, of pH, and to rising P_{CO_2}.
5. In autonomic ganglia preganglionic fibers form nicotinic cholinergic junctions with the cells of origin of postganglionic fibers. Most preganglionic fibers are myelinated B fibers, postganglionic fibers unmyelinated C fibers. Small intensively fluorescing (SIF) cells of autonomic ganglia are catecholaminergic short-axon inhibitory interneurons.
6. The triple response of Lewis consists of the local red response, the wheal (edema) and the flare. The flare is caused by vasodilatation mediated by axon reflexes.
7. The submucous plexus of Meissner contains neurons of receptor function. The neurons of Meissner's plexus supply input to the myenteric plexus of Auerbach. The latter contains the neurons that transact the local reflexes of the gut wall: for example, peristalsis.
8. While the ureters fill the bladder with urine, the detrusor muscle relaxes as a consequence of reflex inhibition by sympathetic efferents so that intravesicular pressure rises only slightly. When the bladder wall is distended beyond a certain critical degree, stretch receptors in the wall initiate reflex contraction of the detrusor muscle mediated by parasympathetic efferents. Detrusor contraction elevates the pressure inside the bladder, and this causes a sense of urgency. Then, if the external sphincter, which is under voluntary control, is allowed to relax, voiding takes place.
9. In paraplegic patients not only is voluntary control over the bladder lost, but also both receptive relaxation and emptying tend to be impaired. Consequently the bladder can neither fill nor empty completely.

10. The distribution of functions among hypothalamic structures has been investigated by the complementary techniques of electrical stimulation by stereotactically inserted focal needle electrodes and by observations of functional deficits consequent to lesions inflicted by stereotactically placed probes. The best known results of such investigations are summarized in Table 17.2.

11. In healthy mammals under ordinary circumstances, body temperature, extracellular osmotic pressure and oxygen content of arterial blood are regulated without resorting to negative feedback (homeostatic) reflexes. It is assumed that these functions are governed by as yet ill-understood feedforward signals. Negative feedback mechanisms act as lines of last defense in stress or disease.

Further Reading

Books and Reviews

Appenzeller O: *The Autonomic Nervous System: An Introduction to Basic and Clinical Concepts.* Amsterdam, North Holland, 1976.

Brooks CM, Koizumi K, Sato A (eds): *Integrative Functions of the Autonomic Nervous System.* Tokyo, University of Tokyo Press, and Elsevier, 1979.

Cannon WB: *Bodily Changes in Pain, Hunger, Fear and Rage.* New York, Appleton, 1929.

Hess WR: Das Zwischenhirn. Translated: *The Functional Organization of the Diencephalon* (translated by J. R. Hughes). New York, Grune & Stratton, 1957.

Martin JB, Reichlin S, Brown GM: Neurologic manifestations of hypothalamic disease. In *Clinical Neuroendocrinology: Contemporary Neurology Series,* vol 14. FA Davis, Philadelphia, 1977, pp 247–273.

Morgane PJ, Panksepp J: *Physiology of the Hypothalamus: Handbook of the Hypothalamus,* vol 2. New York, Marcel Dekker, 1980.

Rushmer RF, Smith OA: Cardiac control. *Physiol Rev* 39:41–68, 1959.

Sernka T, Jacobson E: *Gastrointestinal Physiology: The Essentials.* Baltimore, Williams & Wilkins, 1979.

Smith JJ, Kampine JP: *Circulatory Physiology: The Essentials.* Baltimore, Williams & Wilkins, 1980.

West JB: *Respiratory Physiology: The Essentials,* ed 2. Baltimore, Williams & Wilkins, 1979.

Articles

Andersson B, McCann SM: A further study of polydipsia evoked by hypothalamic stimulation in the goat. *Acta Physiol Scand* 33:333–346, 1955.

Ono T, Oomura Y, Nishino H, et al: Neural mechanisms of feeding behavior. In Katsuki Y, Norgren R, Sato M (eds): *Brain Mechanisms of Sensation.* New York, John Wiley, 1981, pp. 271–286.

chapter 18

Control of Movement by the Brain

Motor functions of the cerebral cortex, the basal ganglia, the cerebellum and the brain stem.

18.1. Motor Cortex

In 1870 two young doctors in Berlin, Fritsch and Hitzig, published the results of an experiment which in one stroke refuted three ideas widely if not generally held up to that time. It is said that the epoch-making experiments were performed in Dr. Hitzig's bedroom on Mrs. Hitzig's dressing table. Mrs. Hitzig's comment has not been recorded. Fritsch and Hitzig reported for the first time that electrical stimulation of a certain region, but not others, of the cerebral cortex of a dog evokes movements of muscles of the contralateral body half. This proved the following ideas wrong: (1) that the only functions of the neocortex were the storage of "engrams" or elementary memory traces and the formation of associations between them; (2) that all parts of cortex are similar and there is no specialization of function among the various regions; and (3) that the cortex is electrically inexcitable.

Hughlings Jackson actually suggested earlier that there is a brain region commanding the movement of muscles. Jackson inferred this from observing convulsive movements of the type we today call *Jacksonian fits* (see Section 4.11a). Few believed him, however, until the report by Fritsch and Hitzig was published. Shortly thereafter Betz of Kiev described the "giant" neurons which are found only in the motor cortex and today bear his name. Betz also suggested that these cells are the ones sending excitation from motor area to spinal cord and thence to skeletal muscles. We should add that these cells are giants only among the lesser neurons of the mammalian nervous system, for in lower animals, for example squid or goldfish, we find nerve cells many times larger than any in mammalian nervous systems.

18.1a. MOTOR AREAS OF THE NEOCORTEX

Contractions of skeletal muscles can be evoked by electrical stimulation of not just one, but several, areas of the cerebral neocortex. Brodmann's cyoarchitectonic area 4 is usually referred to as the *primary motor area*, M-I or MS-I. In man and other primates it occupies the precentral gyrus. In physiological experiments this region may be distinguished by its low threshold to electric stimulation and because the movements evoked by near-threshold stimuli are limited to one or a few muscles of the opposite body half. By systematically exploring the surface of the primary motor cortex by electric stimulation, maps of the body musculature have been drawn that resemble the somatotopic maps of the sensory receiving area of the postcentral gyrus (see Section 7.7 and Fig. 7.5 and 7.6). Thus stimulation of the most lateral part of the precentral gyrus evokes movements of the tongue; then, as the stimulating electrode is moved medially, movements are successively produced in muscles of the face, the upper extremity, the trunk, the lower extremity, and finally the perineum and the tail. The lowest spinal segments are represented on the medial aspect of the hemisphere.

In front of Brodmann's area 4 lies area 6. Here electrical stimulation also evokes movements, albeit of a somewhat different character. Movements are less brisk and involve larger muscle groups even when the stimulus is only slightly above threshold. Muscles of the trunk, in general muscles related to posture, occupy more of area 6, those of the extremities more of area 4. Area 6 is sometimes referred to as *premotor*. Some authors reserve the term "premotor" for the rostral half of area 6 and consider its caudal half to be indistinguishable from area 4. The rostral part of area 6 has also been called the "motor association cortex" (see also Section 21.2).

A so-called "*supplementary*" *motor area* is located on the medial aspect of the hemisphere in the posterior cingulate gyrus and adjacent to it. Electrical stimulation here often evokes movements in symmetrical muscles of both sides of the body, although the contralateral response is usually stronger than the ipsilateral effect.

A specialized motor area is found in front of area 6, in the lateral frontal cortex, mostly in Brodmann's area 8. Electrical stimulation here causes both eyes to be turned away from the stimulated side. This part is known as the *frontal eye field* (Fig. 7.5*B*).

Finally, stimulation of the somatic sensory areas (see Section 7.7) also evokes movements. In this case, stronger currents are required, and the latency of the response is consistently longer than when motor cortex is stimulated. Many investigators believe that the motor effects evoked from sensory cortex are indirect, conducted by corticocortical connections from the sensory to the motor area. It will be recalled that many output fibers of area 3a project to area 4. Area 3b projects to area 1, which projects to area 2, which also projects to area 4 (Fig. 18.1). By shorter or longer paths, all parts of the first sensory receiving area send input to the primary motor cortex, and activation of these projections may in part be responsible for the motor effects evoked by electrical stimulation in areas 3, 1 and 2.

18.1b. OUTPUT OF THE CORTICAL MOTOR AREAS

The classical motor pathway of the cerebral cortex is the *corticospinal* or *pyramidal* tract. These fibers connect the cerebral neocortex with the spinal gray matter without synaptic interruption. The term "pyramidal" refers to the bulges of white matter at the base of the brain stem known as the medullary pyramids, and *not* to the pyramidal cells of the cortex. Pyramidal cells are all the neurons the axons of which leave any part of the cortex. Thus, besides those forming the pyramidal tract, all corticocortical, corticocommissural, corticostriate, corticodiencephalic and other corticofugal fibers are pyramidal cell axons.

The primary motor cortex is but one of several areas contributing fibers to the pyramidal tract. The premotor and supplementary motor areas also add a share. More unexpectedly, the parietal cortex, including specifically the sensory receiving areas, also send fibers through the pyramidal tracts to the spinal cord. But not all of these have motor function. The fibers from sensory cortex, or many of them, terminate in the dorsal gray matter of spinal segments. Many of these have been shown to inhibit transmission across the synapses between primary afferent fibers and neurons of the spinothalamic and spinocervico-thalmic projection cells. These corticospinal fibers are, then, components of the efferent mechanisms which control afferent input (cf. Section 7.2e).

While not all the fibers in the pyramidal tract are motor, most are. Some corticospinal fibers of motor function make direct synaptic contact with ventral

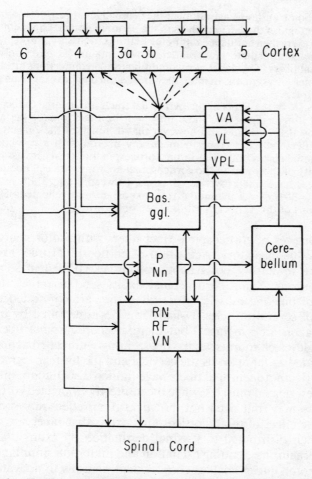

Figure 18.1. Flow chart of signaling in some of the main pathways connecting components of the motor system. Cerebral cortical areas: *6*, premotor area *4*, primary motor area; *3a*, *3b*, *1* and *2*, primary somatosensory receiving area (see also Figs. 7.5 and 7.6); *5*, anterior part of parietal association cortex (see Section 21.2c). *VA*, *VL* and *VPL*, ventroanterior, ventrolateral and ventroposterolateral nuclei of the thalamus; *Bas. ggl.*, basal ganglia; *P. Nn*, pontine nuclei; *RN*, red nucleus; *RF*, reticular formation; *VN*, vestibular nuclei. Note that output of VA is addressed mainly to area *6*, output of VL mainly to area *4*.

horn cells. Some authors have adopted the distinctive term *corticomotoneuronal* fibers to distinguish these from others in the pyramidal tract. Other corticospinal tract fibers exert their influence on motor neurons indirectly, through interneurons in the intermediate gray matter. Lower mammals have only indirect corticospinal fibers. The direct corticomotoneuronal connections are a privilege of primate nervous systems. In man, they are assumed to have taken an especially important role.

About 2–3% of the fibers in the pyramidal tracts are of large caliber, between 10 and 20 μm in diameter. These may well be the axons of the giant cells described by Betz. I should add however that in much of the current literature the term "Betz cell" has come to mean any neuron with a cell body in the primary motor cortex and axon in the corticospinal tract, regardless of its size. The majority of these and of the corticospinal neurons with cell bodies in other cortical areas have small myelinated axons, between 2 and 5 μm in diameter. Roughly 20–30% of the pyramidal tract axons are unmyelinated. The origins and functions of this C fiber contingent are unknown.

The synapses of corticospinal tract fibers with motor neurons need not always be excitatory. Activation of corticospinal tract axons may also evoke inhibitory postsynaptic potentials (IPSPs) in some alpha motor neurons. Some corticospinal axons send terminals to motor neurons of but one muscle. More often they are connected to motor neurons of several muscles. Usually muscles innervated by one corticospinal axon are synergists, but there are corticospinal fibers whose effect is addressed to muscles having seemingly unrelated action, sometimes located as far apart as the cervical and the lumbar segments. The direct corticomotoneuronal fibers have limited distribution, influencing one or a few related muscles, while the indirectly connected corticospinal tract fibers may, but need not, broadcast their effect more widely. Of course, the effect of those corticospinal axons that innervate interneurons is then distributed to its final destination by axons branches of those interneurons. Sending excitation and inhibition simultaneously to several motor nuclei enables corticospinal neurons to activate coordinated movement patterns. These corticospinal tract fibers seem to call up complete subroutines of motor programs.

The muscles of the face are innervated by the motor nuclei of the cranial nerves. These receive connections from motor cortex through the fibers known as the *corticobulbar tract*. Corticobulbar and corticospinal fibers are quite similar.

Of all the output pathways of the cerebral cortex corticospinal and corticobulbar tracts have been studied the most. These are, however, by no means the only fibers originating in the primary motor area, and they may not even be the most important ones. Among others area 4 sends connections to: (1) the ventrolateral (VL) nucleus of the thalamus; (2) the pontine nuclei and thence to the cerebellum; (3) the striatum, especially the caudate nucleus; (4) the reticular formation of the brain stem (Fig. 18.1). The output tracts of the other motor areas of the cortex are at least as varied as those of area 4. The motor pathways not contained in the corticospinal tract often are referred to as the corticoextrapyramidal system, and are believed to be responsible for much of the programming of normal motor activity.

18.1c. INPUT TO THE MOTOR CORTEX AND ITS COLUMNAR ORGANIZATION

One of the important input pathways to the motor area of the cerebral cortex originates in the ventrolateral nucleus of the thalamus. This part of the thalamus receives much of its input from the cerebellum. In return, the motor cortex sends signals to the cerebellum by way of the corticopontocerebellar path (Fig. 18.1).

As has already been mentioned, the sensory receiving area of the cortex is also connected to the motor area (see Section 7.7). By these corticocortical connections information can reach the motor cortex after it has been processed by the sensory cortex. There is at this moment controversy over whether a direct input also exists from the sensory thalamus (ventroposterolateral, VPL) to the motor area. Whether straight, or over a detour through the sensory cortex, signals from peripheral receptors do reach the cortical motor area by a rapidly conducting pathway. Some originate in tactile receptors of the skin, but many of them come from muscle stretch receptors. Generally speaking, any point in the motor cortex where stimulation causes contraction of a given muscle receives signals from receptors in that muscle and in the skin overlying it.

Like the somatic, visual and auditory sensory cortical areas, the motor cortex has a *columnar functional architecture* (cf. Section 7.8). Evidence for a predominance of vertical connections is found in both morphology and physiology of this region. Neurons lying above and below one another receive information from and send signals to the same muscle or group of muscles. Incoming afferent fibers and outgoing efferent axons run predominantly at right angles to the surface. It is plausible that each column contains the subroutine or the elementary program for a simple movement, and that input fibers to that column either activate or inhibit that particular subroutine.

The arrangement of inputs and outputs in the motor cortex may be the basis for so-called cortical reflexes. Earlier (Section 16.3b) we have mentioned the long-latency stretch reflex that presumably is cerebral. The afferent limb of this reflex arc may be the cortical projection of muscle spindles, and the efferent limb the corticospinal fibers originating in those cortical columns to which the stretched spindles send their signals.

Other cortical reflexes are the "placing" and "hopping" reactions of dogs and cats, which will be described in Section 18.4b. Experimental removal of the primary motor cortex abolishes these responses, and they do not recover even many months after the lesion.

18.1d. THE MOTOR CORTEX AND VOLUNTARY MOVEMENTS

In the five or six decades following the discovery of the motor area of the mammalian neocortex, there has been much speculation concerning the possible function of this part of the brain. Opinions voiced in this period have not always been founded on fact, and today may sound overly simplistic. For example, at one time many believed that all voluntary movements are controlled by the corticospinal fibers originating in the primary motor cortex. The corticospinal tract cells have for this reason been christened "upper motor neurons" and the cells we today call alpha motor neurons became known as "lower motor neurons." These expressions survive in clinical terminology even now, although their meaning has changed (see Section 18.1f).

Diametrically opposing the view that the primary motor cortex is the command center for voluntary movements was the opinion that it is not a "motor" area at all, but the cortical analyzer of movement. In other words, area 4 would be the sensory cortex for kinesthesia.

Truth, as it turns out, lies between these two extreme positions. The primary motor cortex does participate in the control of movements, both voluntary and involuntary, although it is by no means the master switchboard without which no movement would be possible. And the motor cortex does receive sensory signals relating to movement, albeit in conjunction with the sensory area, especially 3a. Its function is thus both "sensory" and "motor," though it probably is fair to say that it is more the latter than the former.

Another long-vexing question has been whether the primary motor area has a "high" or a "low" position in the chain of command for movements. Is it the seat of the intention to move, or is it an outflow channel concerned only with the execution of movement and not its initiation? Although the division of tasks among the many cerebral motor subsystems is by no means clear, the weight of current evidence indicates that the cortical motor areas form an executive system, not a decision-making center. Moreover, as we have seen already, they have to do not only with voluntary but also with involuntary motor acts. (For a discussion of voluntary *versus* involuntary acts, see Section 4.2.)

18.1e. THE ACTIVITY OF CORTICOSPINAL NEURONS DURING MOVEMENTS

In the 1960s an experimental procedure was developed for recording the impulses discharged by individual neurons in the motor cortex of awake and alert monkeys. Although partially restrained, the animals were able to move their limbs freely. The method has been adopted by several investigators, and it has now been applied not only to motor cortex, but to other central nervous system (CNS) areas as well. In the great majority of these investigations the animals were trained to respond to specific sensory signals by performing prescribed movements. These movements may be classified as voluntary in that they required choices based on the recognition of sensory signals, choices which a human subject could make only by conscious decision.

An early result of these experiments was the discovery that neurons in motor cortex discharge well in advance of alpha motor neurons of the spinal cord (Fig. 18.2). This refuted once and for all the notion that area 4 is a purely sensory area. That question settled, more difficult ones were attempted. Research centered on two questions, both originally posed by pioneers in the research of this area, Ferrier and Sherrington. (1) Do corticospinal neurons (a) control muscles (or muscle groups) or (b) represent movement patterns? If the former were true, then one cortical neuron's discharge would invariably activate one and the same group of alpha motor neurons and never another, regardless of, which of the other muscles moved, or of the purpose of the movement. In the latter case, the discharge of a given cortical neuron would trigger a certain movement in which now one, then another group of spinal motor neurons may participate. To give an example, in order to grasp a peanut, an animal may have to either flex or extend the elbow, depending on the distance of the object to be grasped. If the cortical signal would represent the command "grab," then the discharge of a cortical neuron may evoke either flexion or extension depending on the starting position and the relative distance. (2) Does the signal emitted by the motor cortex (a) govern the force of a contraction (or of a movement) or (b) determine the extent (the path) of a contraction (or of a movement), regardless of the load (that is, regardless of the force required to make that movement)?

Experiments to enable a choice of one or the other of these two pairs of alternative hypotheses are still being conducted. Reports published so far contain no decisive evidence. It may be that different cortical neurons or different cortical columns control different aspects of movements. Electromyographic (EMG) discharge of muscles is strongly coupled to the discharge of impulses of some of the cortical neurons; in these cases the cortical neuron may indeed exert a direct influence on the contraction of that one muscle. In other cases no such coupling was

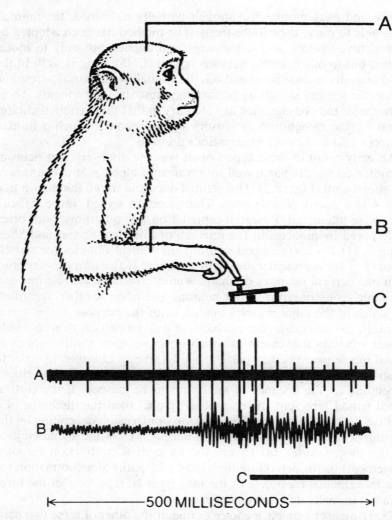

Figure 18.2.   The recording of the discharge of a neuron in primary motor area of a monkey. *Top*, the experimental arrangement; *bottom*, the recordings. *A*, recording from cortex; *B*, electromyogram; *C*, line indicates closing of telegraph key. (Note that tracing *A* contains impulses of two neurons. The cell generating the impulses of larger amplitude fired before the onset of the EMG discharge; this cell may be connected to motor neurons involved in the movement. The cell firing the smaller impulses was inhibited before the onset of the movement; its output may be addressed to the antagonist muscle). (Reprinted with permission from E. V. Evarts: *Scientific American* 229:96–103, 1973.)

shown and the cortical cell seemed to have some other, more subtle function. The one tentative conclusion, then, is that corticospinal neurons form a team whose members have different roles in the common task of controlling discrete, skilled movements.

18.1f. DEFECTS OF THE MOTOR CORTEX AND OF ITS OUTFLOW TRACTS

The catastrophic consequences of complete disconnection of all motor areas of the cerebral cortex from subcortical parts are evident after strokes caused by a major bleeding into the posterior crus of the internal capsule. Such an accident leaves the patient *paralyzed* and, after an initial period of muscle hypotonia, *spastic* on the side of his face and body contralateral to the site of the bleeding. A typical, readily recognizable attitude is taken by the paralyzed limbs: the arm remains flexed, the leg extended. This is the *hemiplegic posture*. With time, there may be some recovery, and the patient may learn to walk. To take a step, he must learn to swing around his stiff leg from the hip. The technical term for this movement is *circumduction*.

We have become acquainted with the term *spasticity* when discussing the paraplegic state (see Section 15.7), and defined it as *hypertonia* of skeletal muscle with *hyperreflexia* and the *clasp knife* response. Spasticity is much more powerful in a hemiplegic than in a paraplegic patient. While the extensor muscles of the legs of a paraplegic cannot support his body weight, those of a hemiplegic leg often can.

Since their corticospinal tracts are interrupted, hemiplegic patients show Babinski's sign and they lose the cutaneous abdominal and cremaster reflexes on the affected side (see Section 15.5c).

The decerebrate state, as we have seen earlier, is characterized by extensor hypertonia in all four limbs (see Section 15.6), the hemiplegic posture by flexor hypertonia of the affected arm and extensor hypertonia of the leg. The reason for this difference is not entirely clear. The reticulospinal and vestibulospinal systems have been blamed for the hypertonia of decerebrates. Normally, so the theory goes, facilitatory neurons in the descending reticular formation and in the vestibular nuclei are inhibited from higher levels of the CNS. After decerebration the inhibitory reins are removed and the unbridled excitatory drive of brain stem neurons takes control over the gamma motor neurons of the extensor muscles. The flexion of the arms of the hemiplegic are believed to be the result of interplay between vestibular input and neuronal circuits that are destroyed in decerebration but remain intact in hemiplegia. The influence of vestibular input is demonstrated when the patient bends forward. Changing position in this way often causes the previously bent arm to extend stiffly. The location, and the normal function, of the neuronal circuits involved has, however, not been discovered.

When stroke destroys the fibers of the posterior crus of the internal capsule, all the corticofugal connections are interrupted, not just the corticospinal ones. Considerable effort has been expended to discover the different roles of the component parts of such a lesion. In experimental animals it is possible to interrupt the corticospinal tract without damaging other descending systems. This is achieved by a knife cut in the pyramids of the medulla oblongata, either on one side or on both. This experiment was first performed by Sarah Tower in the late 1930s. When first published, the results seemed astonishing. They have been confirmed in most essential respects by several investigators since then.

In cats, the handicap caused by a carefully made lesion in the medullary pyramids was minimal. A casual observer would not notice that anything was wrong with such an animal; only careful testing of its motor ability revealed a deficit. In monkeys and apes the disorder was more severe, especially immediately after the lesion, but primates were not totally paralyzed either. They were able to carry out many seemingly voluntary motor acts, and their motor performance improved steadily for several months after the lesion. The lasting deficits of monkeys consisted of: (1) clumsiness and weakness of the distal muscles of the extremities; (2) inability to move digits independently; and (3) abnormal reflexes, such as a traction reflex of the hands (see Section 18.4c). These animals were not spastic, however.

In human patients damage limited to the medullary pyramids is extremely rare. Larger lesions of the lower brain stem usually are fatal, for obvious reasons. Nevertheless five cases have been described in which the corticospinal tract was damaged without much harm to other structures in the medulla. The clinical picture of these human patients was similar to that of the subhuman primates subjected to the experimental lesion, except that some muscle hypertonia did develop with time in some of them.

Hemiplegia can be a consequence not only of a lesion of the internal capsule, but of any level in which descending fiber systems of one hemisphere can be interrupted. Examples include the cerebral peduncle or the motor cortex itself.

The deficiencies caused by lesions of the motor cortex are variable, and they change as time passes. Penfield writes of a patient in whom a small epileptogenic focus had to be removed from the motor area. The patient was right-handed, and the excision included the hand area of the primary motor cortex of the left hemisphere. Immediately after the operation the patient suffered a severe spastic paresis of the right hand, but a year later she was able to play the piano with a finesse approaching her skill before the operation.

Of course not all cortical defects recover this well. The larger the lesion, the more severe the handicap, and the less the chance of complete rehabilitation. Age also has much to do with cerebral plasticity. The prospects of younger patients are better than of older ones. And, bilaterally symmetrical cortical lesions are always much more devastating than unilateral ones. Fortunately, they also are much rarer. The nature of the recovery process from the effects of cerebral lesions is discussed in Section 20.5.

Lesions of the motor cortex and of its output tracts are, traditionally, called "upper motor neuron lesions" in the clinical literature. The diagnostic rule is as follows: "Paresis with hyperreflexia: upper motor neuron lesion; paresis with loss of tendon reflexes: lower motor neuron lesion."

The expression "upper motor neuron" is a legacy of the era when corticospinal tract neurons were believed to issue all motor commands, which then were executed by the "lower motor neurons" in the ventral horns. While this view of the organization of the motor system has been obsolete for quite some time, the terms remain useful to clinicians as a sort of shorthand. "Upper motor neuron lesion," then, should be understood to stand for "lesion of the descending motor pathways," "lower motor neuron lesion" for "lesion of ventral horn cells or their axons."

18.2. The Basal Ganglia

The largest part of the forebrain of birds consists of basal ganglia, with but a small cortex to top it off. In mammals the proportions are reversed, but even here the basal ganglia represent a sizeable mass of gray matter. Judged by their size and by their central position, these structures probably have many functions. Unfortunately the many experiments aimed at discovering the functions of these structures have produced, in Henneman's words "a bewildering array of results and few reliable conclusions."

The most striking signs of disease of the basal ganglia are disturbances of movement (see Sections 18.2c and 18.2d). For this reason these structures are usually described with the motor system of the brain. Recent experiments in which the discharge of individual neurons was recorded while the animal was executing some trained voluntary task seem to support the view, that neurons in the basal ganglia participate in the programming of movements.

While there is thus good reason to believe that the basal ganglia do have motor functions, to regard them as purely motor in function may be too limited a view. First, the striatum receives input not only from the motor areas, but from many other parts of the cerebral cortex. Second, electrical stimulation of this region sometimes evokes relatively simple acts, such as turning of head and body, but at other times also more complex behavioral responses. For example, it has been reported that stimulating some points of the caudate nucleus at an appropriately low frequency causes animals to lapse into sleep. Third, this region receives manifold sensory input. Fourth, the tail of the caudate nucleus is anatomically continuous with the amygdala in the temporal lobe, suggesting a possible relationship to limbic functions. These four sets of facts do not by any means contradict the idea that the basal ganglia are important for the execution of movements, but they do underscore the likelihood that this region has other, as yet ill-defined functions as well.

18.2a. DECORTICATE PREPARATIONS

F. Goltz is credited with having first succeeded in 1892 in removing almost all the neocortex of both hemispheres of a dog and keeping the animal alive for 18 months. In Goltz's dog the thalamus and corpus striatum were also damaged, but others have subsequently succeeded in removing the cortex without hurting underlying structures. Decorticate cats and dogs have been studied extensively by Bard and by Pavlov, among others.

Decorticate cats and dogs have normal body posture and walk with normal strides. They can find food and water and eat and drink normally. Body temperature and other autonomic functions remain within normal limits. The deficiencies of the decorticate are in the "higher" functions.

Decorticate dogs do not seem to recognize people or other animals as individuals. They cannot be taught the tricks that normal dogs learn so readily. Pavlov had maintained that no conditional reflexes can ever be established in decorticates. It later became clear that conditioning of a very simple kind is possible not only in decorticate but even in spinal preparations (that is without brain or brain stem). It is true, however, that this is much more difficult and takes many more trials without a cortex than it would with cortex intact. Decorticates show no signs of communication or of forming affective bonds. Also, they are prone to fits of aggressive behavior. These outbursts have been termed *sham rage*, in the belief that the decorticate is not capable of conscious emotions. The aggression released by decortication is distinguished from the aggression triggered either by lesion or by stimulation of the hypothalamus in that it is less goal-directed. Decorticate animals attack anything that happens to come in their way. Hypothalamically aroused animals (see Section 17.5 and Table 17.2) that have otherwise intact brains seek out and attack other animals or people, often the experimenter, in a more deliberate manner. More detailed experimentation revealed that sham rage is not the result of removal of the neocortex, but of certain older parts of the telencephalon. To release it, the transitional cortex of the midline (cingulate gyrus), as well as the pyriform cortex and the amygdala must be destroyed in addition to the neocortex.

After removal of the cortex, what remains of the forebrain consists of the limbic system, the basal ganglia and the diencephalon. The complex behavior patterns of decorticate animals must be controlled by these structures. The specific role of the basal ganglia in these behaviors is not known. It generally is assumed that the subcortical gray matter of the brain enjoys less autonomy in primates, especially in man, than in lower mammals. Nonetheless, there can be little doubt that these masses of gray matter have important functions in our nervous systems as well.

18.2b. COMPONENT PARTS OF THE BASAL GANGLIA AND THEIR CONNECTIONS

In neuroanatomy, the basal ganglia are defined as the following structures: the caudate nucleus and the putamen, which together form the corpus striatum, or *striatum* for short. The globus pallidus is often referred to as the *pallidum*. Striatum and pallidum together form the largest main part of the basal ganglia. Whether or not the claustrum belongs is not clear. The *subthalamic nucleus* (corpus luysi), the *substantia nigra* and the *red nucleus* (nucleus ruber) of the midbrain are anatomically separate yet closely connected and functionally related and therefore usually described together with the basal ganglia.

All of the above, plus the parts of the reticular formation from which the reticulospinal fibers take their origins (the *descending reticular formation*) form together the *extrapyramidal system*. This term was invented by Wilson in 1912 to mean the system of neurons that control the movements that are not under direct cortical control and are performed without deliberation, such as postural contractions and other automatic movements. The pyramidal system was at that time believed to initiate all voluntary movements. As already indicated, the equation of all voluntary acts with the corticospinal system and all involuntary acts with the extrapyramidal system is incorrect. Not all function that is cortical is conscious, and not all conscious functions are cortical. Moreover, pyramidal and extrapyramidal systems do not operate independently, but perform different aspects of a shared job. The numerous corticostriate, corticorubral and corticoreticular fibers, which collectively are referred to as the *corticoextrapyramidal* connections, enable this cooperation (Fig. 18.1).

Generally speaking, the striatum receives signals, and the pallidum emits them (Fig. 18.3; also Carpenter, Figs. 11.8–11.16). Most massive and best described are the connections that reach the striatum from the cortex, the thalamus and the substantia nigra. The output of the striatum is, in large part, directed toward the pallidum. The pallidum in turn sends signals to certain of the thalamic nuclei and to the tegmentum of the midbrain and pons including, among others, the red nucleus. There

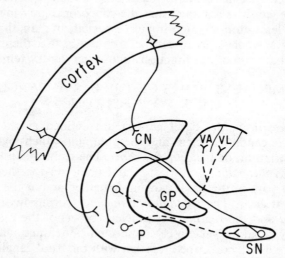

Figure 18.3.   Some of the main connections of the basal ganglia. *CN*, caudate nucleus; *P*, putamen; *GP*, globus pallidus; *VA* and *VL*, ventroanterior and ventrolateral nuclei of the thalamus; *SN*, substantia nigra.

also is a two-way connection between pallidum and the subthalamic nucleus of Luys. Not all the output of the striatum is directed toward the pallidum. Between substantia nigra and the striatum impulse traffic is two-way, for there are nigrostriatal as well as striatonigral fibers.

18.2c. PARKINSON'S DISEASE

In the preceding section emphasis was placed on the close cooperation between the cerebral cortex and the extrapyramidal nuclei in the control of normal movements. The signs and symptoms which are caused by defects of the motor cortex and of the corticofugal fiber tracts are nevertheless very different from those caused by diseases of the basal ganglia and associated extrapyramidal structures. Thus while these diverse parts of the brain cooperate in programming and controlling normal movements, each has a distinct job.

In general the diseases of the extrapyramidal system cause three kinds of malfunction: (1) disorders of muscle *tone*; (2) abnormal *posture*; and (3) uncalled-for *involuntary movements*. Generally there is no weakening of voluntary movements (paresis) and there are no abnormal reflexes of the kind typical of pyramidal lesions.

Parkinson's disease is the most prevalent of the extrapyramidal syndromes. Parkinson, a 19th-century English physician, is said to have recognized the disease as a separate entity by watching residents of a nearby old people's home shuffle past his window. Indeed, when fully developed, parkinsonism is easy to diagnose, even at a distance. The patient shuffles on stiff legs with partly flexed arms and a bent back. The arms do not swing with the rhythm of walking, but are held rigidly. When the patient sits quietly, there often is a characteristic coarse *tremor at rest* of the fingers and hands. The tremor is traditionally likened to pill-rolling. The tremor diminishes when the patient deliberately moves his arm and hand, and it disappears during sleep. When asked to stand up and walk, the patient is slow to start, but speeds up somewhat when in action. There also is a slowing of speech. There is very little of the small purposeless extra movements that most people make. Blinks of the eye are rare. The face is mask-like in its immobility. The overall spareness of motion is referred to as akinesia.

The tremor of parkinsonian patients is usually maintained by an alternating contraction of antagonist muscles. Some other forms of tremor are caused by co-contraction of antagonists. With tungsten microelectrodes, recordings have been obtained from group IA afferent fibers from muscle spindles of the muscles participating in tremor. The spindle afferents discharged bursts of impulses twice in each tremor cycle: once when the muscle contracted, and again when it relaxed. The first burst showed that intrafusal muscle contracted in phase with the extrafusal muscle; the second burst was caused by the stretching of the spindle as the muscle elongated. The intrafusal contraction indicates alpha-gamma coactivation and, therefore, that the tremor, unlike clonus (see Section 15.7), is not reflexly driven but paced by the CNS.

In neurological examination of such a patient the most conspicuous sign is a generalized hypertonia of skeletal muscles, described as *extra-pyramidal rigidity*. It can be distinguished from spasticity in several ways. A spastic limb usually offers more resistance to passive manipu-lation in one direction than in others. For example, in the arm of a hemiplegic patient the flexors are more hypertonic and therefore the arm resists passive extension more than flexion. If forcibly moved out of its characteristic posture, a spastic limb tends to return to it. The limbs of a parkinsonian patient resist passive movements in all directions equally; that is, all muscle groups are more or less equally hypertonic. When forcibly moved, a rigid limb tends to remain where the examiner left it, at least for a while. But perhaps the most reliable differential signs are these: when forcibly stretched, *spastic* muscles are characterized by the *clasp knife* response (see Section 15.7); *rigid* muscles by *cogwheel resistance*. Cogwheel resistance got its name because it feels as though cranking a coarse unoiled gear. This alternation of yield-resist-yield-resist has the same frequency as the tremor exhibited by the patient's hand when he is resting. Many neurologists believe that the tremor and the cogwheel are different manifestations of the same underlying mech-anism.

In the past many parkinsonian patients had been treated by stereotactic surgery. Such an intervention consists of making a lesion in a subcortical cerebral structure. Justification for the treatment was the realization that what disturbs parkinsonian patients most is the unbridled excitation of certain neuron groups that have lost inhibitory restraint. The added lesion inflicted by the surgical intervention was expected to extinguish the brain circuit, the activity of which was out of control. The anatomical target of the stereotactic procedure was initially the globus pallidus and in later years the VL nucleus of the thalamus.

Stereotactic surgery has in recent years been largely supplanted by medical treatment with *l*-DOPA (see below), although the operation is sometimes still performed as a last resort, when drug therapy has failed. The procedure is mentioned here because patients who came to stereotactic surgery afforded an opportunity to explore deep-lying nuclei with microelectrodes. During explora-tion groups of neurons were found that discharged bursts of impulses with the same rhythm as the tremor of the patient. These neurons were probably the central pacemakers of the tremor. Finding such pacemaker cells confirmed that the surgeon's instrument was on the right track for making the relief-bringing lesion. If, in a diseased brain, these cells drive abnormal involuntary movements, then it is reasonable to assume that in a healthy brain the same cells may be involved in the programming of normal movements.

The first breakthrough in understanding Parkinson's disease came when it was realized that the substantia nigra was paler in the brains of patients dying of this disease than in other cadavers. The normally dark color of the substantia nigra is due to the presence of the pigment melanin. Subsequently, it became clear that the lack of melanin was associated with a deficiency of 5-hydroxytryptamine (serotonin, 5-HT) and, most importantly, also of dopamine. Histochemical study aided by the fluorescence microscope then revealed the dopaminergic pathway leading from substantia nigra to striatum. This series of discoveries had lifted dopamine from the status of a laboratory curiosity to that of a clinically important compound in brain chemistry. From recognition of dopamine deficiency it was a logical step to try to improve the condition of Parkinson's patients by feeding them *l*-DOPA, the precursor of dopamine. These attempts were unsuccessful until it was realized that truly large amounts must be given to derive any benefit.

The proper drug to give is not dopamine itself, but its precursor, *l*-DOPA, for two reasons. First, dopamine does not cross the blood-brain barrier, and therefore is ineffective when administered either orally or parenterally. But even if a clinically applicable method could be devised to administer the compound directly into the brain substance, there would remain an advantage to giving a precursor and not the transmitter itself. The *l*-DOPA is taken up by dopaminergic neurons, which convert it into the active form and release it as they see fit. If the transmitter itself were administered, it would react with all receptor sites throughout the brain tissue, regardless of whether particular synapses need the compound at that moment or not. This consideration should be kept in mind whenever a new treatment utilizing presumed transmitter agonists is devised. Not all patients respond to *l*-DOPA, suggesting that deficiency of dopamine may not be the only possible cause of parkinsonism.

Long before the discovery of the role of dopamine, there has been another medical treatment for Parkinson's disease, using one or other of the analogs of atropine, which block muscarinic cholinergic synapses. The first to use such drugs, in the form of belladonna extract, was Charcot, the 19th-century French neurologist. The fact that both *antagonists* of acetylcholine and *agonists* of dopamine are effective in the treatment of Parkinson's syndrome has led to the idea that in the corpus striatum cholinergic and dopaminergic synapses form balanced and mutually antagonistic systems. Parkinson's disease, according to this hypothesis, is the consequence of the normal balance being upset, tilting in favor of the cholinergic influence. This would explain why either blockade of cholinergic synapses or the bolstering of dopaminergic transmission could restore the lost balance.

18.2d. OTHER EXTRAPYRAMIDAL DISORDERS

The etiology of Parkinson's disease is not known, but certain known poisons sometimes cause a disturbance resembling it. Carbon monoxide is one of them. We should add parenthetically that the nigrostriate system is but one of several that can fall victim to this poison. Reserpine is another compound that can cause similar symptoms, and this is a well known side effect of overdosing patients with this drug. This is understandable, since reserpine owes its very action to the depletion of catecholamine stores in nerve terminals, and dopamine is one of the catecholamines. It is customary to distinguish Parkinson's *disease* (of unknown etiology), from Parkinson's *syndrome* or, in another terminology, *idiopathic* from *symptomatic* parkinsonism. In the latter a known agent causes the disorder.

There are many other disorders of the basal ganglia which, however, are much rarer than Parkinson's disease (and syndrome). The clinical picture of these conditions is dominated by abnormal involuntary movements and abnormal postures. *Chorea* is the name given to brief, phasic movements that appear at irregular intervals and in unpredictable sequence in different limbs and muscle groups. In advanced cases the patient's limbs are in almost ceaseless, bizarre and purposeless motion. Medical historians believe that St. Vitus' dance was what today we would call chorea minor, a sequela of scarlet fever. *Athetosis* is similar to chorea, except that its movements are of a slower, more writhing character. *Ballismus* is the least common; it means sudden movements of a whole arm, as in throwing a ball. It is called hemiballismus if, as is usual, it occurs on one side only. Similarly, we speak of hemichorea and of hemiathetosis when the disorder is one-sided. Ballismus is attributed to damage to the subthalamic nucleus of Luys.

A more detailed description of the numerous disorders that can affect the basal ganglia belongs in clinical medical texts, but one of them merits a brief mention here, because of its presumed pathophysiological mechanism. This is *Huntington's chorea*, a hereditary disorder of the striatum. In these cases the imbalance of brain chemistry is believed to be the opposite of that causing parkinsonism. While in the parkinsonian patient the cholinergic system gains the upper hand because the dopamine system is deficient, in Huntington's chorea, the dopamine system overpowers a weakened acetylcholine system. Consequently, while the parkinsonian patient has trouble initiating a movement, the choreatic patient cannot stop moving. It follows that Huntington's chorea should be treated either by bolstering cholinergic transmission or by suppressing dopaminergic synapses, the purpose being the reverse of that for Parkinson's disease (and syndrome). The condition is complicated, however, because the basal ganglia of the Huntington patient is often also deficient in γ-aminobutyric acid (GABA).

18.2e. TRANSMITTERS IN THE STRIATUM

Dopamine, administered by a microdelivery system directly to individual neurons in the caudate nucleus of cats or rats, inhibits most cells, excites a minority, and leaves a few unaffected. Stimulation of the nigrostriate pathway causes similar effects. When time and again the effects of dopamine and of nigrostriate impulse volleys were compared on cell after cell, the pharmacological and synaptic actions were often but not always identical. This supports the idea the dopamine is the transmitter of many of the fibers in the nigrostriate pathway, but also indicates that it may not be the only one.

That acetylcholine and cholinesterase are present in unusually large amounts in the caudate nucleus has been known for many years. Because of the seemingly mutually opposing action of dopamine and of acetylcholine inferred from clinical observation, the question is whether cells that are inhibited by dopamine are the ones excited by acetylcholine and *vice versa*. Unfortunately this simple hypothesis turned out not to be correct. An alternative, which enjoys the support of several investigators, suggests that acetylcholine is the transmitter of short-axon interneurons in the striatum, and that dopaminergic input from the substantia nigra holds these cholinergic interneurons under tonic inhibition. When there is a shortfall of dopamine, the cholinergic cells are released from inhibition and become excessively active. This scheme could explain the success of treatment with both *l*-DOPA and atropine.

Dopamine and acetylcholine are not the only transmitter substances of the synapses in the corpus striatum. Fibers that originate in the raphe nuclei and terminate here have serotonergic nerve endings. GABA, glutamate, and substance P are other suspected transmitter agents, and this may not yet be the end of the list. In the case of GABA, a consensus has developed that this is the main transmitter of the fibers running from striatum to substantia nigra, which reciprocate the dopaminergic nigrostriate fibers.

18.3. The Cerebellum

Noting the position of the cerebellum astride the brain stem, Descartes suggested that it was the gatekeeper of the animal spirits which animated the organs of the body. In Descartes' view, animal spirits flowed from the brain through the brain stem, spinal cord, and nerves toward the many parts of the body. They also returned through the same route to the brain. The brain stem was their funnel and gateway. The cerebellum, by the action of its brachia (arms; or peduncles, little feet) which seem to embrace the brainstem, controlled the floodgates through which the spirits flowed. As Lashley remarked in another context (see Section 20.1), if we substitute "nerve impulses" for "animal spirits," Descartes' ideas have a remarkably modern ring.

The cerebellum receives a massive flow of information by way of numerous pathways, among them the dorsal and ventral spinocerebellar tracts and the spinoolivocerebellar paths (Fig. 18.4). The massive input from the spinal cord is not reciprocated. Except for sparse fastigiospinal fibers to the cervical spinal cord, no direct cerebellospinal tract exists. Yet clinical and experimental evidence unequivocally points to the cerebellum as the main organ for the guidance and the coordination of movement carried out by skeletal muscles. This the cerebellum achieves not by controlling motor neurons, but by influencing other cells that act on motor neurons. The output of the cerebellum is directed to the ventrolateral nucleus of the thalamus, and through it to the cerebral motor cortex; also to extrapyramidal structures, chiefly the nucleus ruber; and also to the vestibular nuclei. Truly, the cerebellum does direct the flow of vital spirits from brain to spinal cord, and thus into the motor nerves.

18.3a. INPUT AND OUTPUT OF THE CEREBELLUM

Signals from sensory receptors in muscles, joints and skin are conducted in an orderly fashion to the cerebellum, so that two receiving areas are formed in the cerebellar cortex. These areas are somatotopically arranged, with different points of the cortex receiving input from different points of the body. Two complete pairs of body "maps" have been described, one contiguous pair in the cortex of the anterior lobe, the others in the two paramedian lobules. These body representations are interconnected.

Electrical stimulation in these somatic receiving areas of the cerebellar

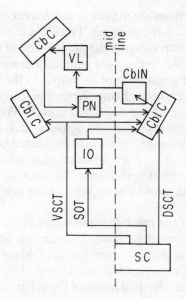

Figure 18.4. Crossed, uncrossed and double-crossed connections of the cerebellum. *Cb C*, cerebral cortex; *VL*, ventrolateral nucleus of the thalamus; *PN*, pontine nuclei; *Cbl N*, deep cerebellar nuclei; *Cbl C*, cerebellar cortex; *IO*, inferior olives; *SC*, spinal cord; *VSCT*, ventral spinocerebellar tract; *DSCT*, dorsal spinocerebellar tract; *SOT*, spino-olivary tract.

surface can evoke movements, always of muscles of the same body region from which sensory information is received at the stimulated cerebellar cortical point. Since there is no direct path from cerebellar cortex to motor neurons, the effect must be mediated through the motor systems of the forebrain and/or brain stem. Confirming this notion, electrical stimulation of the cerebellar cortex facilitates the effect of appropriately timed electrical stimuli applied to the cerebral cortex. That points in the somatic area of the cerebellar cortex are connected to the corresponding somatic projection points in the motor area of the cerebral cortex has also been confirmed by electrical stimulation of the former and electrical recording of the response from the latter. The path from cerebellum to cerebral cortex goes through the *VL nucleus* of the thalamus, from cerebral cortex to cerebellum by way of the *pontine nuclei* (Figs. 18.1 and 18.4).

It should be well remembered that each *cerebellar* hemisphere receives and sends signals mainly to the *ipsilateral* body half. Since the *cerebral* hemispheres' connections are mainly *contralateral*, the cerebellocerebral connections must cross the midline. Thus, for example, the left hemisphere of the cerebellum connects to the left side of the body and to the right cerebral hemisphere; the right cerebral hemisphere receives most of its input from and sends most of its output to the left side of the body and also to the left cerebellar hemisphere. The body representations in the paramedian lobule of the cerebellar cortex, like the so-called "second" and "supplementary" somatic sensory and motor areas of the cerebral cortex are, however, *bilaterally* connected. Also remember that the dorsal spinocerebellar tract remains entirely on one side of the midline, but each ventral spinocerebellar tract is partly crossed and partly double-crossed, providing input to both cerebellar hemispheres (Fig. 18.4).

The gray matter of the cerebellum is found in its cortex and in three pairs of nuclear masses at its core. The surface area of the cortex is vastly expanded by the multiple deep parallel folds of the folia. Research, especially of the last two decades, combining electrophysiological and anatomical techniques, clarified many of the synaptic connections found in the cerebellum.

Input to the cerebellum comes by way of three types of fibers. The *climbing fibers* are the axons of cells, the perikarya of which lie in the inferior olives. Other afferent fibers, from spinal cord, pontine nuclei, vestibular nuclei, and the rest have the distinctive morphology of the so-called *mossy fibers.* Both climbing and mossy fibers give off branches to the deep nuclei of the cerebellum and then proceed to the cerebellar cortex (Fig. 18.5). Sparser and less well characterized are catecholaminergic afferent terminals of probably inhibitory action. Most of these seem to originate in the locus coeruleus and convey their effect by releasing noradrenaline.

There are only five types of cells in the cerebellar cortex (Fig. 18.5). Four of these cell types are intrinsic to the cortex, that is all their axon terminals remain within it. Only the *Purkinje cells* send their axons out of the cerebellar cortex. These large neurons were first recognized by Purkinje in unstained specimens. The axons of these cells do not reach very far either. Most end in the deep cerebellar nuclei; some (from the nodulofloccular lobe) terminate in the lateral vestibular (Deiters') nucleus.

The main output pathways of the cerebellum are formed by the axons of cells with cell bodies in the deep nuclei, not in the cortex. These are

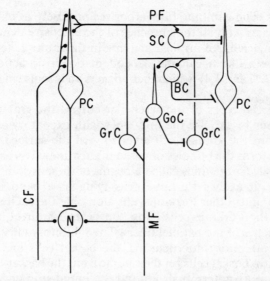

Figure 18.5. Excitatory and inhibitory synapses in the cerebellum. *Round terminals* symbolize excitatory boutons, *flat terminals* inhibitory boutons. *PF*, parallel fibers; *SC*, stellate cell; *PC*, Purkinje cell; *BC*, basket cell; *GoC*, Golgi cell; *GrC*, granule cell; *CF*, climbing fiber; *N*, neuron in deep cerebellar nucleus; *MF*, mossy fiber.

the fibers that form the efferent tracts already mentioned: to the VL nucleus, the red nucleus, and other motor centers.

18.3b. SYNAPTIC CIRCUITS OF THE CEREBELLUM

One of the surprises of the recent past was the discovery that all Purkinje cells are of inhibitory function. Their transmitter is very probably GABA. With the cerebellum in an apparent resting condition, the output cells of the cerebellar nuclei emit a steady stream of impulses. This steady background excitation is modulated by excitation of collateral branches of the climbing and mossy fibers and by the varying degrees of inhibition exerted by Purkinje cells (Fig. 18.5).

Purkinje fibers can be excited in two ways: by climbing fibers and by parallel fibers. The former, as we have seen, are the axons of cells in the inferior olive. The latter are the axons of granule cells in the cerebellar cortex. There is one climbing fiber for each Purkinje cell, implying a one-to-one relationship between cells of the inferior olive and the

Purkinje cells. The climbing fiber arborizes profusely to make multiple synaptic contacts with all the branches of the extensive dendritic tree of its one Purkinje cell. An impulse arriving in the multiple terminals of a climbing fiber evoke a calcium-dependent dendritic action potential (see Sections 3.11 and 4.4), which then triggers an impulse in the Purkinje cell axon.

Of the five cell types of the cerebellar cortex, the granule cells, the most numerous by far, are the only ones with excitatory action. Their axons rise from the granule cell layer toward the surface, where they bifurcate and form the bundles of white matter known as parallel fibers. If a tight bundle (sometimes called a beam) of these is stimulated by an electric pulse, it excites Purkinje cells lying in a band immediately below, and inhibits other Purkinje cells alongside the excited ones. The excitation of the Purkinje cells lying "on beam" is direct, through the multiple branches of the parallel fibers. The inhibitory effect is indirect, mediated by inhibitory interneurons, the basket cells and the stellate cells (Figs. 18.6). Basket cells get their name from the basket-like feltwork formed by their axon terminals around the initial segment of the axon of Purkinje cells, a strategic location to suppress the discharge of impulses, which normally originate there.

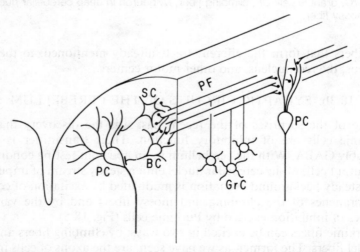

Figure 18.6.   Granule cells excite "on-beam" Purkinje cells directly and inhibit "off-beam" Purkinje cells indirectly. *PF*, parallel fiber; *SC*, stellate cell; *PC*, Purkinje cell; *BC*, basket cell; *GrC*, granule cell. *Round terminals* symbolize excitatory, *flat terminals* inhibitory connections.

The fifth type of cell of the cerebellar cortex, the Golgi cell, is also a short-axon inhibitory interneuron. But while basket and stellate cells inhibit Purkinje cells, Golgi cells inhibit granule cells.

Granule cells and Golgi cells are activated by mossy fibers. Synaptic contacts are made in intricate little structures called synaptic glomeruli (see Carpenter, Fig. 8.8). Each glomerulus contains the expanded terminal of a mossy fiber, several dendritic tips of granule cells and Golgi cells, and inhibitory axon terminals of Golgi cells.

The basic wiring diagram of the cerebellar cortex may seem deceptively simple (Figs. 18.5 and 18.6). The multiple synaptic contacts between the relatively few cell types allow, however, the formation of complex patterns of excitation and inhibition. The secret of the workings of the cerebellum, like that of other parts of the CNS, lies in the intimate details of which cell says what to which, when and why. Of these goings-on we know next to nothing.

Experiments have been performed in which the discharge of neurons in cerebellar cortex or in cerebellar nuclei was recorded while the animal was performing a previously learned motor task. The experimental arrangement was rather similar to that already described for the cerebral motor cortex (Fig. 18.2). One general conclusion was that some of the cerebellar cells regularly discharged before any of the muscles contracted. From this it seems that the cerebellum not only analyzes movement, but also participates in its planning or in the running of the program.

18.3c. PATHOPHYSIOLOGY OF THE CEREBELLUM

If we do not know how the cerebellum performs its job, we have a relatively clear idea what its assignment is. This knowledge is in large measure derived from observation of the disturbances of function after lesions of the cerebellum, both experimental and accidental.

The consequences of cerebellar disease fall into three groups: (1) an incoordination of movement referred to as *ataxia*; (2) *difficulty* of maintaining the *upright* position; and (3) in man but not in lower mammals, *hypotonia* of skeletal muscles. Of these three the second, relating to balancing the body, is the consequence of damage to the nodulofloccular lobe, or archicerebellum (see Section 18.3e). First the results of damage to the neo- and paleocerebellum which form by far the largest part of its mass will be discussed.

Cerebellar ataxia can be recognized by a large array of distinctive signs. All show, in one way of another, the lack of precision in carrying out simple movements. The victim of cerebellar disease, if the remainder of his CNS is intact, is not weak, has no sensory deficit, and suffers no impairment of intelligence, consciousness, or other mental functions. His only difficulty is in coordinating and controlling movements, but that can be incapacitating enough. Sensory ataxia (see Section 16.3c) differs from cerebellar ataxia in that someone who has suffered damage to primary afferent fibers can, to some degree, compensate for the disability by carefully watching what he is doing, substituting vision for lost proprioception. But the patient suffering from cerebellar ataxia cannot improve his performance by watching his own movements, since his difficulty stems not from insufficient information, but from losing the central coordinating organ, the "computer" controlling his movements.

A conspicuous sign of cerebellar disease is a *tremor of action* sometimes incorrectly referred to as intention tremor. A parkinsonian patient shows the characteristic tremor most when sitting quietly. Nothing about a cerebellar patient reveals his defect as long as he sits still. When he starts to walk, his gait resembles that of one who is drunk. When reaching for an object, his hand follows a zig-zag path, and the oscillations increase as the movement progresses. This is because as he deviates from the intended trajectory, he corrects and then overcorrects his course, then overcorrects the previous overcorrection. Engineers call this behavior "hunting," and it is typical of an inappropriately adjusted servo-control system (see Section 16.2). The classical example is the patient who tries to take a glass of water to his lips, but by the time the goal is reached, the glass is empty.

To analyze the specific disability caused by cerebellar impairment, experiments have been conducted in which a small-diameter cooling probe was inserted into one or other of the deep cerebellar nuclei of trained monkeys. Temporary cooling caused a suppression of all neuronal activity in the nucleus, followed by recovery. During cooling, for example the dentate nucleus, movements of the arm on the affected side became abnormal in that movements were initiated too late, then accelerated too much for too long, and did not stop at the right point. The result was overshooting the target, dysmetria, similar to that seen in human patients with cerebellar disease.

18.3d. NOTES ON MOTOR SKILLS AND MOTOR LEARNING

Most readers will remember how they learned new motor skills, such as riding a bicycle or staying up on skates or skis. At first each move was consciously planned, before each turn a decision was made. Then, with practice, the routine became more and more automatic. There are those who attribute the ability to automatize motor skills to the capacity of the cerebellum to learn. By this they mean a plasticity of synaptic connections that allows modification of the pattern of excitation in the neuronal circuits. Others, with equal emphasis, deny this. Their view is that the cerebellum is a computer with a fixed repertory of programs. If so, then it must be the plasticity of the motor circuits of the brain and/or of the brain stem that allows motor learning. In colloquial terms, the cerebellum analyzes and presents the facts, and the remainder of the brain learns to adapt to the facts reported by the cerebellum.

Whichever way this argument will turn out, this much seems clear: Before any move is made, the CNS must generate a plan, whether consciously or unconsciously. This includes a "sketch" of the task at hand; and an internal "model" of the sequence of muscle contractions required to carry out the intended move. Then, as the program is "run" the CNS is informed of the progress of the motor output, and of the degree to which the desired result is accomplished. Presumably another internal "model" is generated, representing the outcome of the action. Achievement is compared to plan, and the degree of success is noted and laid down in memory. There is a subjective counterpart to this: if the movement was performed as intended, there is a feeling of satisfaction, and one of ill ease if it was not. This is so even if a wrong move does not result in a bruise, as it may with bicycling or skiing. Training succeeds to the extent that the brain circuits learn to estimate in advance exactly how much correction is required for how much deviation from the goal, and to do so without the subject having to think about it consciously. The difference between servo-controlled and pre-programmed movements was mentioned earlier (Section 16.2), the difference being that servo-controlled movements can be corrected while in progress, whereas pre-programmed (ballistic) movements can only be improved from one try to the next. The learning process may otherwise be quite similar in both cases.

18.3e. THE VESTIBULOCEREBELLUM

Damage limited to the *nodulofloccular lobe*, also known as the archicerebellum or vestibulocerebellum, impairs the victim's ability to balance his body. Such damage, if it spares the remainder of the cerebellum, causes no ataxia. This part of the cerebellum receives input from and sends output to the vestibular nuclei, and its function evidently is closely linked with them.

In the next section I will briefly summarize the postural adjustments collectively known as the righting reflexes of the body. The nodulofloccular lobe has a role in coordinating these movements. It also participates in the other functions of the vestibular nuclei, such as the coordination of eye and head movements during turning of the body or of the head. The adjustments of the "gain" of the vestibuloocular reflex when wearing prismatic glasses was already mentioned in Section 13.3. These adjustments cannot occur if the vestibular nuclei are disconnected from the archicerebellum. All these facts indicate that vestibular nuclei and the nodulofloccular lobe form an integrated functional system.

Pathological nystagmus can be a sign either of vestibular or of cerebellar disease. It is, however, not limited to nodulofloccular lesions, but can occur as a consequence of damage to other parts of the cerebellum as well.

The intimate connection between vestibular and nodulofloccular systems became evident also in investigations of motion sickness. Dogs are often prone to this condition, as those who have traveled with pets know well enough. They lose this sensitivity if the archicerebellum has been ablated in an experimental operation. This obviously is not a practical method of preventing motion sickness, but it does pinpoint the anatomical sites of its pathophysiology. Monkeys are naturally immune to motion sickness, which is hardly surprising considering their way of life in the trees. Humans show a wide spectrum of varying sensitivities, some more like monkeys, others more like dogs in this respect. The widely varying response to protracted stimulation of the vestibular organs raises interesting but unanswered questions concerning its mechanism.

18.4. Reflexes of the Brain Stem and Brain

A number of stereotyped behavior patterns have been described that fit the definition of unconditional reflexes given in Section 4.2b, and are controlled in part by neuron circuits in the brain stem, the cerebellum and the forebrain. Since these responses are carried out by trunk and limb muscles, they must be mediated through and be integrated with motor programs of the spinal cord. They differ from spinal reflexes in that they cannot be performed by a paraplegic or a quadriplegic spinal cord.

18.4a. RIGHTING REFLEXES

When awake, most mammals prefer a head-up body position. There are a few obvious exceptions such as bats and sloths, but we need not deal with those.

To right itself, an animal must know up from down. Sensory clues to find the vertical are made available to the CNS by the labyrinths, the eyes, and the cutaneous tactile senses. Input from any one of these suffices for the animal to right itself.

The sequence of movements by which an animal gets up from the prone or the recumbent position is typical for the species and relatively invariant. If, for example, a cat is laid on its side (against its will), it will first turn its head upright, then follow with the upper trunk, then the rest of its body, and then finally it will stand up. People have more varied patterns than lower mammals; we rely less on inborn, stereotyped movement patterns.

As we have seen earlier, an acutely decerebrate cat does not right itself, but if such an animal is kept alive for a number of weeks, this ability returns. This suggests that in the normal animal righting reflexes are "directed" or "shaped" by the forebrain, but also that the basic program is wired into the brain stem. High spinal (quadriplegic) organisms never right themselves: the spinal cord alone cannot perform the complex sequence of movements required.

18.4b. PLACING AND HOPPING RESPONSES

If a normal cat is held by an experimenter and lowered toward a table, it will extend its legs in anticipation of landing. If the dorsum of the foot is touched to the edge of the table, the cat will lift the leg and place it on the tabletop. This latter movement is performed even if the animal is blindfolded. These are the so-called limb-placing responses, the former called *visual placing*, the latter *tactile placing*.

If a cat is held so that one foot rests on a tabletop, and if he then is moved sideways, he will re-place his leg again and again, always so that, should the experimenter let go, the leg would support the body. This is the *hopping response*; and "hopping" accurately depicts the movement.

These responses, although unconditionally reflexive, require intact somatosensory and motor cortical areas. They are permanently lost in decorticate or decerebrate animals.

18.4c. GRASP REFLEX; FORCED GRASPING; TRACTION REFLEX

Placing and hopping responses cannot be evoked in humans and are therefore perhaps less interesting than the various grasping reactions. Grasping is an easily evoked reflex in healthy human infants, and in them it is quite powerful and quite typical. Healthy adults will not automatically grasp objects without intention; that is to say, without either being specifically requested to do so — or without being interested in the object. An automatic *grasp reflex* does occur, however, after certain injuries of the forebrain.

There are actually three related responses that differ in certain details. *Grasp reflex* means the automatic closing of the hand upon tactile stimulation of the palm. *Forced grasping* is a stronger response in which the object grasped is not let loose, even when examiner tries to pull it away. In fact the patient's hand can then be led around by the examiner with the aid of a pencil or other object that has been grasped. The *traction response* differs from the two grasp responses in that it requires proprioceptive stimulation, not just touching of the palm. Proprioceptive stimulation in this case is the stretching of the hand muscles or a movement of the finger joints. The response itself consists of contraction of finger flexors.

Grasp and traction responses are the consequence of cortical lesions. Grasp responses are likely after lesions of the frontal cortex, the traction reflex after lesion of the primary motor cortex (area 4). Massive stroke interrupting white matter coming from frontal and parietal regions can release a combined grasp reflex and traction response.

The opposite of grasping is tactile avoidance, consisting of moving the hand away from an object that touches the skin. Automatic tactile avoidance is a sign of parietal cortical lesions and will be discussed in Sections 21.2c and 21.3.

These automatic responses, grasping and avoidance, seem to represent motor programs that are controlled by neuron circuits located in structures below the cortex but above the spinal cord. Ordinarily these programs are activated only when cortical control directs them. But after a cortical lesion they are released from control and they then can be dominated and triggered by stimulation of peripheral sense organs.

18.5. Chapter Summary

1. The primary motor area of the cerebral cortex receives input from somatic sensory cortex, from the VL nucleus of the thalamus and through it from the cerebellum and the basal ganglia, and probably also from proprioceptive mechanoreceptors of the limbs by way of VPL nucleus.
2. Output of primary motor cortex is addressed to the spinal cord, the basal ganglia, the cerebellum and the motor nuclei of the brain stem.
3. Of those neurons in motor cortex that send their axons to the spinal cord, many consistently discharge in advance of the contraction of one particular skeletal muscle during voluntary movements. It is likely that these cells influence firing of the motor neurons innervating that muscle. Other motor cortex neurons are less tightly coupled to spinal motor neuron function.
4. Interruption of corticospinal tract without damage to other fibers causes impairment of discrete movements, especially of the digits of the hands, but no paralysis and only mild or no spasticity.
5. Hemiplegia caused either by damage to the motor areas of the cerebral cortex or by interruption of their outflow tracts is characterized by severe spastic paresis or paralysis and typical posture consisting of flexion of the upper limb and extension of the lower limb.
6. From the connections of the basal ganglia with other parts of the CNS, from the disorders caused by basal ganglia disease, and from the firing

patterns of neurons in the basal ganglia during voluntary movements, it is established that these structures are important in the programming of certain types of movements. It seems likely that they also have functions other than motor control.

7. Parkinson's syndrome is characterized by muscle hypertonia of a rigid (not spastic) type; by coarse tremor that is maximal at rest; by difficulty in initiating movements and paucity of expression; and by a typical posture.

8. Parkinson's disease is caused by deficiency of the dopaminergic input from substantia nigra to corpus striatum. Most patients are helped either by augmenting dopaminergic transmission through administering *l*-DOPA or by suppressing cholinergic transmission by atropine-like drugs. From this and other observations it is believed that an indirect antagonism exists between dopaminergic and cholinergic effects in the striatum.

9. In Huntington's chorea the dopaminergic system overwhelms the cholinergic system.

10. The cerebellum receives massive input from cutaneous and proprioceptive mechanoreceptors, but sends no output directly to the "lower" motor centers of the spinal cord and brain stem. Instead, the cerebellum interacts with the remainder of the motor system by connections addressed to the nucleus ruber, motor cortex (by way of VL nucleus of the thalamus), premotor cortex (by way of VA nucleus); and to brain stem structures such as the reticular formation, the vestibular nuclei and others.

11. Input to the cerebellum comes by way of the climbing fibers which originate in the inferior olives and the mossy fibers which are the final segment of the spinocerebellar and pontocerebellar fibers.

12. The output of the cerebellar cortex is formed by the axons of Purkinje cells. These are GABA-ergic inhibitory fibers.

13. Of the interneurons of the cerebellar cortex, the granule cells are excitatory, the stellate, basket and Golgi cells are inhibitory.

14. At rest the projection neurons of the deep cerebellar nuclei are continually and seemingly spontaneously active. This discharge is modulated by the excitatory effect of collaterals from climbing and mossy fibers, and the inhibitory effect of Purkinje cells.

15. Cerebellar disease in man is characterized by ataxia, one of the manifestations of which is tremor of action. Other cerebellar signs include muscle hypotonia and difficulty in balancing the body. The last named disorder is due to damage to the noduloflocular lobe (vestibulocerebellum).

16. The righting reflexes of lower mammals do not require an intact cerebral cortex, only the brain stem and vestibulocerebellum. Chronically decorticate or decerebrate cats can right themselves.

17. Release of grasp reflexes in adults is usually a sign of damage to either the frontal cortex or the motor areas of the cerebral cortex.

Further Reading

Books and Reviews

Brooks VB (ed): *Motor Control*: section 1, vol 2, part 2, of the *Handbook of Physiology*. Bethesda, American Physiological Society, 1981.

Carpenter MB: *Core Text of Neuroanatomy.* Baltimore, Williams & Wilkins, 1978.

Dray A: The physiology and pharmacology of mammalian basal ganglia. *Prog Neurobiol* 14:221–235, 1980.

Eccles JC, Ito M, Szentagothai J: *The Cerebellum as a Neuronal Machine.* Springer, Berlin, 1967.

Magnus R: Studies in the physiology of posture. *Lancet* 211:531–536 and 585–588, 1926.

Phillips CG, Porter R: *Corticospinal Neurons.* London, Academic Press, 1977.

Talbott RE, Humphrey DR (eds): *Posture and Movement.* New York, Raven Press, 1979.

Articles

Hägbarth KE, Wallin BG, Lofstedt L, et al: Muscle spindle activity in alternating tremor of parkinsonism and clonus. *J Neurol Neurosurg Psychiatry* 38:636–641, 1975.

Pellionisz A, Llinas R: Tensorial approach to the geometry of brain function: cerebellar coordination via metric tensor. *Neuroscience* 5:1125–1136, 1980.

Tower S: Pyramidal lesion in the monkey. *Brain* 63:36–90, 1940.

chapter 19

The Cycle of Sleeping and Waking

Although little is known about the biological reasons for the need to sleep, there are both data and theories concerning the control of the normal sleep-wake cycle in the mammalian brain.

19.1 The Need to Sleep

It is obvious enough to all, especially to those in the medical and scientific professions, that sleeplessness can be distressing, and that we need sleep in order to function well, but the physiological reasons for this need are not known. Some hold the opinion that the problem is falsely stated; sleep, they say, is the normal state of the organism, and animals wake up only to find food, or a mate, or to eliminate waste, to then lapse again into natural slumber. The trouble with this ingenious point of view is that it does not explain why feeling sleepy can be so compelling.

It is clear that certain functions are measurably disturbed after sleep deprivation. The most obvious difficulty is of course caused by the tendency to doze at odd moments, which interferes with any task requiring a presence of mind. Among the other deficiencies caused by extended sleeplessness is impairment of learning and of motor skills. Most sleep-deprived persons are, however, able to gather their strength for brief periods of time and thus to perform tests of short duration up to normal standards. There are also changes of perception, emotion and mood.

Extreme sleep deprivation is said ultimately to lead to a psychotic state. A famous case, recounted by Luce and Segal and reprinted in the textbook by R. F. Thompson (see list of further reading) concerns Peter Tripp, a disc jockey in New York, who in 1959 undertook to remain awake for a record length of time. The purpose of the stunt was to raise funds for a worthy cause. To prove that he was alert, Tripp stayed on the air to broadcast his program for most of a total of 200 continuous hours. Neurologists and psychologists examined his vital functions and his mental status in the intervals in which he was off the air. Toward the end of his ordeal, Tripp was disoriented, experienced delusions, and showed signs of overt paranoia, but nevertheless managed to continue his broadcasts up until the very last. Then he slept for 13 hours, after which he seemed fully recovered.

Not allowing prisoners to sleep is a method of torture used to confuse the victim and to extract confessions. It has been claimed that laboratory rats eventually die if kept awake, even if their other bodily needs are met. The experiments upon which this conclusion was based have subsequently been criticized, and there has been at least one more recent report that contradicted this conclusion. In that experiment cats were kept awake by stimulation of the midbrain reticular formation through implanted electrodes. Apparently these animals went without sleep for two weeks without obvious ill effects. Complex brain functions requiring vigilance or learning have, however, not been tested in these animals, and of course we have no sure way of knowing whether or not cats experience hallucinations.

It is well known that young children need more sleep than older ones or adults need, and that there are wide variations among individuals. Cases have been documented in laboratories specializing in sleep diagnostics and sleep research, of some people doing well sleeping just one or two hours regularly per 24-hour period. Some people who complain of habitual insomnia in fact get enough sleep, they just need less sleep than the average; one of the tasks of practicing physicians is to recognize this condition and to reassure the patient. Of course many others truly cannot sleep as much as they need, but they can be recognized because they show adverse signs of sleeplessness such as difficulty in paying sustained attention and an increased tendency to fall asleep during the day.

Even though our sleeping and waking is keyed to the sequence of night and day, it is not dependent on it. Living in isolation rooms under constant lighting and heating, without clocks and without means of communication with the outside, people develop a so-called free-running sleep-wake cycle which, on the average, is about an hour longer than the 24-hour rhythm normally dictated by the rotation of the earth. Tradition has much to do with sleeping habits. Peoples of central, western and northern European ancestry prefer to limit sleep to the hours of darkness, even if it means less than optimal performance in the early afternoon. Most other nationalities allow for a *siesta* at the appropriate time of day, and make up for it by staying awake part of the night. There is no proof that efficiency at work requires 16 or 17 continuous hours of waking.

The need to sleep has been explained as a trait that evolved because it gives a competitive advantage as it compels animals to rest periodically and so ensures recovery from bodily fatigue; it also obliges animals to avoid predators by remaining hidden when not required to forage for food. Both theories are at best only partial explanations. Resting without sleeping can restore physical vigor after exhausting exercise; on the other hand, people do need to sleep even if confined to bed around the clock for many days or weeks. Moreover, sleep comes naturally to predator and prey alike. Therefore, while it may be perfectly valid to count as secondary benefits of sleep the recovery of tired peripheral organs, or the behavioral advantage of staying out of sight of enemies, the evidence seems compelling that sleep is primarily required for the health of the brain, not of the other parts of the body.

In very general terms one can think of two ways in which sleep can serve cerebral function. It could be that during sleep materials are recovered or resynthesized that were consumed during waking; or it may be that during sleep waste products are eliminated that have accumulated in the waking state. These two classes of function are of course not mutually exclusive. More specific theories on ways in which sleep, and especially the state known as rapid eye movement (REM) sleep, may serve brain function have been postulated, and we shall briefly mention some of these shortly.

The sleeping brain is not inactive. The total amount of energy expended by brain tissue can be estimated from the oxygen consumption, measured as the difference between the amounts of oxygen contained in unit volumes of arterial and cerebral venous blood, multiplied by the cerebral blood flow. (For methods of measuring regional blood flow, see e.g. Smith and Kampine, pp. 69–70 and pp. 185–187.) When cerebral oxygen consumption was first measured in healthy human volunteers, no significant difference could be detected between the sleeping and the waking states. However, with the more sensitive method of estimating glucose metabolism in animal brains from the accumulation of radioactively labeled deoxyglucose, it has recently been shown that overall metabolic activity is in fact about 30% lower during deep sleep than in the waking state. This difference is, however, small compared to other organs, especially muscles and glands, the metabolic activity of which can increase several fold between the resting and the fully active states. To use a crude analogy, from the point of view of power consumption the brain is like a radio receiver that is constantly turned on. Whether it is tuned to a station (awake) or not (asleep), makes only a small difference in the amount of current it draws. Cerebral metabolism may change more than normal under pathological conditions and under the influence of drugs. Thus total oxygen consumption of the brain is substantially decreased in most forms of coma and during surgical stage general anesthesia, and it is increased by generalized seizures.

Sleep alters not so much the overall activity of the brain as the distribution and the patterning of neuronal activity. Although the brain consumes energy, it does not perform physical work on the environment. Instead, it processes information. Information processing does not cease during sleep, it is only somewhat reduced in certain neuronal circuits and takes on a different general format.

19.2. The Phenomenon of Sleep

19.2a. SLEEP STAGES

Apart from the investigation of seizures, no area of neuroscience has benefited more from the invention of electroencephalography (EEG) than has sleep research. With EEG the seemingly uniform state of sleeping can be subdivided into distinct stages. To conduct an experiment concerning sleep processes, subjects move into a specialized laboratory for several consecutive night-long sessions. Several channels of EEG are recorded along with other variables such as the electrocardiogram, eye movements (electrooculogram, see Section 9.4b) and the electromyogram of certain muscles, usually of the neck and the shoulder. With such instrumentation the following sleep stages have been defined (Fig. 19.1).

Awake. Subject responds to stimuli. EEG either low-voltage fast (sometimes designated LVFA or beta activity: see Table 4.1), or alpha rhythm.

Stage 1. Drowsy, or dozing off, a transitional state. Subject might sluggishly respond to questions, but usually does not remember afterwards what has been said. The EEG is irregular in rhythm and variable low to medium voltage in amplitude.

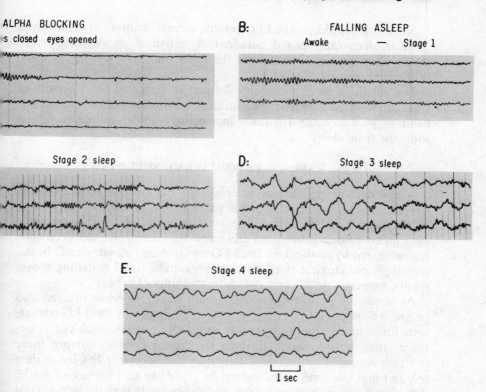

ALPHA BLOCKING
s closed   eyes opened

B: FALLING ASLEEP
      Awake   —   Stage 1

Stage 2 sleep

D: Stage 3 sleep

E: Stage 4 sleep

1 sec

Figure 19.1. EEG tracings typical of sleeping and waking. *A*, initially alpha waves, maximum in the second tracing (see also Fig. 4.5), then transition to desynchronization when the eyes are opened. The tracings are contaminated by inadvertedly recorded electrocardiographic waves. *B*, transition from relaxed wakefulness (with alpha activity) to stage 1 sleep. *C*, stage 2 sleep, showing sleep spindles; on the *bottom tracing* two "K complexes." *D*, stage 3 sleep with delta waves and sleep spindles. *E*, pure delta waves, typical of stage 4 sleep. (Courtesy of Mr. Victor Hope and Dr. James McNamara of the Duke University Veterans Administration Hospital Epilepsy Center.)

Stage 2. Light sleep. EEG shows sleep spindles (bursts of 10–14 cps waves; see p. 129 and Figs. 4.7 and 19.1*C*), interspersed in electrical activity similar to that seen in stage 1. Also seen are "K complexes": large characteristic biphasic waves of unknown origin, frequent in this stage, but occasionally seen in other stages as well.

Stage 3. Moderately deep sleep. Sleep spindles interrupted by large, irregular, slow (0.5–2 cps) waves (delta waves).

Stage 4. Deep sleep. The EEG tracing consists entirely of delta waves.

REM sleep (also called paradoxical, activated or desynchronized sleep). This stage is distinct from the other four, and will be discussed in the next section.

The depth of sleep is usually defined in terms of the intensity of stimulation, usually of a sound stimulus, required to awaken the sleeper. From stage 1 to stage 4 it takes increasingly louder sounds to arouse someone from sleep.

19.2b. REM AND SLOW-WAVE SLEEP (SWS)

A few decades ago it was noticed that EEG waves recorded from sleeping cats sometimes changed in pattern from spindles or delta waves to desynchronized low-voltage fast activity. Because of the accepted association of desynchronized EEG and the alert state, the sleep state characterized by low-voltage fast EEG was termed "paradoxical." In this seemingly paradoxical sleep state animals make small twitching movements, especially in the face, whiskers and upper limbs.

At about the same time another team of investigators noticed that people who seemed to be in stage 1 sleep, as judged by the EEG tracing, sometimes made rapid movements with their eyeballs. Such eye movements may be noticeable through the closed eyelids, but are more precisely recorded by electro-oculography (see Section 9.4b). It was then realized that the state characterized by *rapid eye movements*, or *REM*, differs from ordinary stage 1 sleep, and its similarity with the paradoxical sleep state of cats was established. The eyeballs can move somewhat in other sleep stages, also, but REM means characteristic rapid conjugate movements from side to side as though scanning a scene. If subjects are awakened from REM sleep and asked if they had a dream, 8 of 10 can recall having had one. When awakened from other sleep stages, the incidence of dreaming is much lower, and it is lowest in stage 4 sleep.

REM sleep occurs in all mammals, but not all the manifestations of REM sleep are exactly alike in all species. It has already been mentioned that in man the EEG in REM sleep resembles stage 1 sleep, whereas in cats it is more like the desynchronized pattern of an alert animal. Cats are more difficult to arouse from REM than from other sleep states, but people can be awakened from REM state about as easily as from stage 1 or 2.

The EEG of the REM state has two other characteristic features: a so-called saw-tooth pattern and the occurrence of pontogeniculooccipital (PGO) waves. The latter are sharp waves that can appear before the onset of REM and are correlated in pons, lateral geniculate nucleus and occipital cortex. Of course, in human subjects only the occipital cortex is ordinarily accessible for recording by EEG leads.

The notion disseminated by popular science literature that dreams occur only during REM sleep is not quite correct, although it is true that in REM sleep people almost always dream, and apparently only rarely in the other sleep stages. Dreams of the REM state have a distinct flavor. They are more "eventful" and visually vivid than non-REM dreams. The dreamer is not likely to incorporate into the dream content stimuli reaching his sense organs while in REM sleep, whereas it is common for such stimuli to influence the content of non-REM dreams.

Heart beat and breathing tend to be more irregular and on the average faster during REM than during non-REM sleep. Penile or clitoral erection occur frequently. Even though phasic movements are common, postural muscle tone diminishes, especially in the muscles of the trunk, neck and shoulder. While the rate of cerebral metabolism is slightly lower in non-REM sleep than in the awake state (see preceding section), in REM sleep it is slightly higher.

This constellation of multiple changes in cerebral and somatic functions have suggested that REM sleep is in some fundamental way different from the other sleep stages. Thus the concept arose that the brain can function in three distinct states: *awake* (W), in *slow-wave sleep* (SWS or NREM), and in *REM* state. Slow-wave sleep in this context includes all four sleep stages described in the preceding section. It has been suggested that in REM state the forebrain is aroused, although disconnected from the outside world. "Disconnection" implies that sensory stimuli are less readily registered, for example, are less likely to enter the dream content. It is also implied that motor commands are not reaching "lower" motor circuits. This is shown by the decreased muscle tone and also by the distressing feeling of being paralyzed that is sometimes experienced when waking from REM sleep. The brief movements frequently made in REM sleep are considered to originate from CNS structures other than the forebrain, probably from the brain stem, and therefore do not contradict this hypothesis.

Young children not only sleep more than older ones and adults, they also spend a larger fraction of their sleep time in REM. The amount of time spent in REM varies among adults as well, as does total sleeping time, but it is relatively stable for any one individual if of regular habits. If in an experiment a subject is prevented from having REM phases during a night by being awakened immediately each time REMs (or PGOs) are registered, he will make up for the loss by having more REM sleep the following night. If the same subject is awakened an equal number of times from non-REM sleep, his sleep pattern during the subsequent night is not affected. It has also been claimed that people deprived of the opportunity to have REMs during several consecutive nights become irritable and distressed, more so than people awakened an equal number of times during non-REM sleep. Not all investigators agree that REM deprivation has a specific effect on mood, but the phenomenon of making up for lost REM time has repeatedly been confirmed in human as well as in animal subjects.

There is thus some reason to believe that REM sleep is in some specific way important. It is also thought that sleep assisted by drugs, especially by those of the barbiturate class, is less restful than drug-free sleep, because it is deficient in REM periods. Pychoanalysts have of course much to say about the need to dream, and perhaps REM dreams are more beneficial for mental hygiene than are non-REM dreams. On a more biological level, it has been suggested that brain tissue in the REM state performs some essential function for which it has no opportunity in either the waking or in the SWS state. Perhaps the circuits engaged in the waking hours in other functions have a chance to process a backlog of data in REM state. Hypothetically, it has for example been suggested that in REM state the traces required for long-term storage of memory are being consolidated (see Chapter 20). Three types of observations in support of this hypothesis have been reported. First, the amount of time spent in REM sleep increases during nights following sessions in which animals are trained to perform a complex task. Second, certain types of learning can, under certain specifiable conditions, be hindered by depriving an animal of REM sleep. And third, protein synthesis of the kind assumed to be associated with the consolidation of memories is enhanced in the brain during REM state. While this hypothesis has not yet found general acceptance, it certainly is intriguing, and it is supported by a number of investigators.

19.2c. THE PATTERN OF SLEEP STAGES

Sleep research and the diagnosis of sleep disorders have become the province of specialists working in specialized laboratories. A night of recording yields hundreds of yards of chart paper. It is customary to condense the results in the form shown in Figure 19.2. Such a diagram shows the time spent in the various sleep stages.

While no two nights of sleep are quite identical, certain general trends seem to be fairly uniform. As people fall asleep, they pass in succession through the stages from 1 to 4. Then the sequence is reversed, but often instead of re-entering stage 1, a REM phase may follow stage 2. Each night contains several cycles of deepening and lightening sleep, with cycle lengths varying between 60 and 120 minutes. As the night advances, REM periods extend and deep sleep phases shorten. In the late cycles stage 4 sleep occurs only rarely. The first REM phase is almost

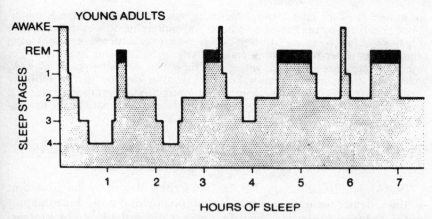

Figure 19.2. The succession of sleep stages in a night of sleep in a healthy subject. (Reprinted with permission from A. Kales and J. D. Kales: *New England Journal of Medicine* 290:487–499, 1974.)

always reached after at least an hour has elapsed and sleep has first progressed at least once through all four non-REM stages. This rule is broken, however, in REM-deprived subjects. After REM deprivation a sleeper may slip into a REM phase shortly after falling asleep. Many normal sleepers wake up for brief periods once or twice each night; this is more likely near dawn than in the initial hours of sleep.

Charts such as the one of Figure 19.2 are somewhat misleading, because the transition from one sleep state to another may in reality not be a sudden as suggested by the graph. Also sleep researchers emphasize that the character of sleep progressively changes throughout the night, so that for example stage 2 sleep of the evening is not quite the same as stage 2 sleep at dawn.

19.3. The Neuronal Control of the Sleep-Wake Cycle

A little more is known about the control of the sleep-wake cycle than about its biological function. While the issues are by no means settled, many interesting observations have been made, and several theories have been proposed that can account for part if not all the observations. The most conspicuous feature of sleeping is of course its regular alternation with waking. Consequently much research was aimed at identifying the biological clock that drives the sleep-wake cycle. Some researchers sought the clock that periodically "turns on" the alert state, and assumed that while it is not "on," the brain would automatically lapse into sleep. Others assumed that sleep itself is induced by the active engagement of some neuronal circuit. Among the latter was the theory of "internal inhibition" postulated by the Pavlovian school, and various hypotheses suggesting the existence of "sleep centers" or sleep circuits which when turned on would bring about sleep, either by inhibiting brain activity or by changing its pattern. Yet other investigators sought a synthesis of these two opposing points of view. According to them the sleep-wake cycle is controlled by two reciprocally interacting centers or neuron circuits, one for waking and the other for sleeping, and the two are alternately engaged see-saw fashion, somewhat like the inspiratory and expiratory neuron circuits.

19.3a. THE THEORY OF THE ASCENDING RETICULAR ACTIVATING SYSTEM

Best known is the theory that the forebrain is alerted by the excitation of the reticular formation of the mesencephalon and pons. Formulation of this theory was preceded by a discovery made in the 1930s by Bremer. He performed two kinds of operation on the brains of cats. In the first series he had cut through the midbrain, separating forebrain from brain stem. In the second set he similarly transected the lower medulla cleaving the entire brain from the spinal cord. Bremer called the former preparation a *cerveau isolé* or isolated forebrain, and the latter an *encéphale isolé* or isolated brain. In these preparations all long tracts of the white matter are interrupted, so that the lower neuraxis detached from a cerveau isolé behaves as a decerebrate (see Section 15.6), while the disconnected spinal cord of an encéphale isolé is like a decapitate or high spinal animal (see Section 15.5). Artificial ventilation is necessary to keep the latter alive.

For our discussion the most important of the observations made by Bremer was that the EEG tracing of a cerveau isolé resembles that of an animal in permanent slow-wave sleep, whereas the EEG of an encéphale isolé shows periods of desynchronization alternating with sleep patterns. The significance of this observation became clearer after Magoun, Moruzzi and a number of others performed in the 1940s and 1950s a series of investigations revealing the importance of the reticular formation of the midbrain.

The key findings of these studies can be summed up as follows. In one series of experiments large electrolytic lesions were made in the brain stem. If such lesions destroyed the reticular formation of the upper midbrain of both sides, the animals did not wake up from general anesthesia, but remained comatose* with EEG dominated by sleep

* *Coma* is the clinical term for pathological loss of consciousness defined as *unarousable unresponsiveness*.

spindles and delta waves. Other animals had stimulating electrodes implanted in the midbrain reticular formation, but their brains remained otherwise intact. Low-intensity, high-frequency electrical stimulation through these electrodes easily woke these animals not only from natural sleep, but also, transiently, from light general anesthesia induced by a low dosage of barbiturates. In yet another set of experiments evoked potentials (see Section 2.2) were recorded from both the midbrain reticular formation and also from the cerebral cortical sensory receiving areas. When a general anesthetic drug was administered to these animals, the potentials evoked in the midbrain reticular formation disappeared at the time when, judged by their behavior, the animals became unconscious; but in the cerebral cortex potential waves could then still be evoked by sensory stimulation. Primary cortical sensory evoked potentials are suppressed only in very deep anesthesia, when respiration is also depressed.

All these studies were performed with appropriate control experiments. It was, for example, shown that electrolytic lesions of comparable magnitude placed in other brain areas, as in the white matter containing ascending sensory tracts, did not interfere with apparently alert behavior or the EEG pattern of animals. The outcome of this investigation was to focus attention on the reticular formation, which up to this time was neglected in research. Much effort was then expended to trace its input and output connections. Signals are conducted from cutaneous and also from other sense organs to the midbrain and pontine reticular formation (see Section 4.8 and Fig. 7.1B). A neuron in the reticular formation may be influenced by input from more than one sense modality. This multimodal convergence is very different from the arrangement of the nuclei in primary sensory pathways, where projection cells are connected to one type of sense organ only. Output from the reticular formation is addressed among others to the so-called non-specific thalamic nuclei, those near the midline and the intralaminar group (see Section 4.8). Circuits in the lower parts of the reticular formation, namely in the pons and medulla, are concerned with autonomic functions such as the control of breathing and integration of signals governing the circulation. Muscle tone is also influenced by output from the lower reticular formation. In other words, the reticular formation is a very large area, different parts of which have different connections and varied functional significance.

The circuits believed to be involved in controlling the alert state of the animal became known as the *ascending reticular activating (or arousal) system*, sometimes abbreviated ARAS. Excitation of this system was believed to put the forebrain in the alerted state. Left to its own devices, the forebrain would lapse into sleep (normally) or coma (pathologically), characterized by the spindle bursts generated by the thalamocortical circuits (see Section 4.8 and Fig. 4.7) and the delta waves generated by the cortex itself. Excitation in the ascending reticular system would act first on the non-specific midline and intralaminar thalamic nuclei, and through them on the cerebral cortex, causing the desynchronization of the EEG, behavioral alerting, and subjective awakening of the subject.

In the healthy organism some clock-like oscillator would engage and disengage the reticular activating system, allowing the forebrain sleep overnight and alerting it for the day. Sleep could, however, also be interrupted by sensory input insofar as such sensory input can excite neurons in the ascending reticular system. The reason that sensory stimuli cannot arouse someone from general anesthesia is because anesthetic drugs block synapses carrying signals to the midbrain reticular system.

Any condition that interferes bilaterally with the functioning of the midbrain reticular formation or with its ascending connections would be expected to cause coma. This prediction of the theory is fulfilled in clinical experience since it has been known for some time that lesions affecting this part of the brain stem indeed render patients unconscious. The slow-wave pattern of the EEG of cerveau isolé preparations is also explained, because in these the forebrain is separated from the midbrain, whereas in the encéphale isolé the two remain connected.

19.3b. THE RELATIONSHIP OF HIPPOCAMPAL AND NEOCORTICAL EEG PATTERNS

In the 1950s the rather intriguing observation was made that in alert animals with neocortical EEG in typical desynchronized state, the electrical activity of the hippocampal archicortex consisted of regular oscillations of relatively high voltage and of a frequency between 4 and 8 cps, the *theta rhythm* or regular slow activity (RSA). The idea was launched that there is some kind of reciprocity between neocortex and archicortex: when the former is desynchronized, the latter is synchronized, and *vice versa*. This attractively simple scheme later proved to be only partly correct. It is true that hippocampal theta rhythm occurs only when the neocortex is desynchronized, but not all desynchronized states of the neocortex are associated with hippocampal theta activity. There have been numerous attempts to define exactly the behavioral correlate of hippocampal theta waves. For example, it has been suggested by different authors that hippocampal theta waves are related to one or more of the following behavioral states: (1) orienting and exploring; (2) active locomotion of any kind (walking, swimming); (3) any purposive, voluntary movement; (4) high emotional arousal, with or without movement. In other alert states, while the neocortex may show either low-voltage fast activity or alpha rhythm, the hippocampal EEG consists of irregular waves. One difficulty of finding general agreement in this matter seems to be differences among species. Thus primates seem to display less theta activity than other families of mammals, and some (not all) neurologists deny that theta waves exist in man. In human subjects the opportunities to record from hippocampal cortex are of course limited, and during such recordings the patients are usually bedridden. If it is true that theta rhythm is associated with locomotion, it would not be seen in a subject lying in bed. Furthermore, when such recordings are performed it often is from diseased tissue or adjacent to it.

During slow-wave sleep the hippocampal electrical activity consists of large but irregular waves (LIA), interrupted by brief periods of small irregular waves (SIA) similar to the low-voltage fast activity (LVFA, desynchronization) of the neocortex. During neocortical desynchronization of REM sleep, theta waves appear in the hippocampal formation of rats, cats and rabbits.

Hippocampal theta rhythm, like neocortical desynchronization, can be evoked by high-frequency electrical stimulation of certain points in the reticular formation of the upper brain stem.

19.3c. CRITIQUE OF THE RETICULAR AROUSAL THEORY

During REM sleep, as we have seen, the EEG of the forebrain in some species of animals is like that in the alert and attentive state, even though the animal behaves as though deeply asleep. As has already been mentioned, this seeming paradox has led to the suggestion that in REM state the forebrain is aroused sufficiently to be conscious, but the circuits that process sensory input and those of the lower motor centers are disconnected from the circuits that elaborate conscious experiences. Dreams replace perceptions based on input from the outside world.

In a similar vein it has also been suggested that while in the REM state the forebrain is alert and the rest of the neuraxis is asleep. During sleepwalking the forebrain is asleep and the brain stem plus spinal cord are partially awake. In agreement with this supposition, sleepwalking apparently occurs only in slow-wave sleep, never in REM state.

Critics of the reticular arousal theory have cited a number of situations where under the influence of drugs, or correlated with particular behavior, EEG patterns can deviate from what the simplest interpretation of the reticular theory would predict. For example, while a cat is drinking milk, parts of its cerebral cortex show a slow-wave pattern, while other parts remain in the pattern more typical of the waking state. No essential information will be omitted if we do not discuss here the arguments surrounding these "anomalous" findings. There are however two important sets of experiments with a bearing on clinical practice, and those I should describe briefly.

In one set of experiments the forebrain of animals was separated from the brain stem and the animal was then kept alive for several months. Initially the forebrain was in slow-wave sleep and the body in decerebrate rigidity, as originally described by Bremer (see Section 19.3a). After some time the animal resumed a cycle of active and inactive periods, as also occurs in the chronic decerebrate state (see Section 15.6a). While "resting" the body of these animals assumed postures typical of normal sleep for the species, and its body underwent periods in which it showed signs typical of the REM state, such as decreased postural tone with twitching movements of limbs and whiskers, and rapid eye movements. In the same stage of recovery when the lower neuraxis started the cycle of activity and rest, the forebrain began to show cyclic changes of EEG pattern. The slow-wave periods were interrupted by desynchronized low-voltage fast activity. The periods of rest and activity of the lower neuraxis were, however, dissociated from the periods of slow-wave and desynchronized patterns of the EEG of the chronically isolated forebrain. This shows that the "sleep-wake" cycle of the disconnected parts of the central nervous system was not driven by oscillations in the concentration of a hormone or metabolite circulating in the blood.

The other important experiment consisted of making lesions in the reticular formation and then keeping the animals alive for weeks or months instead of the few days allowed in the original experiments of Magoun and collaborators. After some time such animals recover from coma and resume what appears to be a nearly normal sleep-wake cycle, with all the usual behavioral and EEG correlates. Cases in which people wake up after prolonged coma due to midbrain injury do occur, and the question is whether in them the neurons in the injured tissue survived and eventually resumed function, or whether in some cases at least consciousness was regained in spite of an irreversible lesion, just as in the experimental cats. Perhaps even more intriguing was the fact that if the experimental midbrain lesion was made in two separate sessions, first the one side and then the other, with a week's interval, then no coma was caused at all. The animals woke up from the anesthesia of the operations in normal time.

Do we then conclude that the ascending reticular formation has no function whatever, related to the maintenance of the alert state or to the control of the sleep-wake cycle? That would mean disregarding a great deal of accumulated positive evidence, of which only the most important has been described earlier in this chapter. While a complete theory that would account for all known facts has not yet emerged, the following principles seem to be solidly founded.

Under normal conditions neuron circuits located in the reticular formation do seem to be important in coordinating the sleep-wake cycle. If this circuit is put out of commission by injury or disease, an initial state of coma ensues. Eventually, however, the forebrain can develop its own rhythm of sleeping and arousal. As long as the forebrain remains connected to the brain stem, it imposes its rhythm on the lower parts of the neuraxis, but if the lower brain stem is detached, then it can develop its own cyclic pattern of activity and rest independently of the forebrain.

An analogy with the heart suggests itself. The reticular formation of the upper brain stem is similar to the sinoatrial node in that it is the normal pacemaker of the sleep-wake cycle. If, however, the normal pacemaker is destroyed or is disconnected, other parts of the system can become pacemakers. Thus in the chronic cerveau isolé as in total heart block, the forebrain (atrium) and the brain stem (ventricle) assume rhythms that are completely dissociated. The beat of the ventricle can be felt as the pulse, and the cycle of activity and rest of the animal can be observed in its overt behavior; but the rhythm of the atrium, as that of the forebrain, can only be detected by means of, respectively, electrocardiographic (ECG) or EEG tracings.

19.3d. ELECTRICAL INDUCTION OF SLEEP

Hess made the early discovery that animals can be put to sleep by stimulating certain points in the posterior dorsal hypothalamus at a low frequency with permanently implanted electrodes. He assumed that this revealed a normal function of this region, and the concept of a hypothalamic sleep center became popular for a while. It later turned out that there are several parts of the subcortical gray matter including certain of the thalamic nuclei and some points in the caudate nucleus where low-frequency stimulation can induce sleep. For this reason some authors, perhaps today a majority, consider the effect non-specific, and assume that such stimuli engage the circuits responsible for thalamo-cortical synchronization, and by that effect promote sleep. Sites have been found in the upper brain stem, where at one and the same point low-frequency stimulation induces synchronization, and high-frequency stimulation induces desynchronization of the EEG activity of the neo-cortex.

Possibly related to the induction of sleep by electric stimulation are twin phenomena known as the *augmenting and recruiting responses*. These responses are evoked by the stimulation of certain thalamic nuclei at a frequency between 5 and 13 Hz. Both augmenting and recruiting responses (or recruiting waves) consist of EEG waves which follow the stimulating frequency and are between 50 and 100 msec in duration, but with amplitude modulated in a waxing and waning pattern even though the stimulating pulses applied to the thalamus are of constant intensity. The amplitude modulation of these electrically evoked responses resembles that of sleep spindles, except that the bursts of increasing and decreasing amplitude follow one another more frequently than natural sleep spindles do. Augmenting responses are evoked by stimulation of specific sensory nuclei, for example the ventroposterolateral and ventroposteromedial, and can be recorded from the cortical receiving area to which that nucleus projects. The augmenting waves are "grafted" onto the primary evoked potentials that are also evoked by stimulating these nuclei, but can be distinguished by their size and shape. Stimulation at lower frequency, for example 1 Hz, evokes primary evoked potentials only; at 10 Hz both the primary response and the augmenting response are evoked. Recruiting responses are evoked by stimulating the non-specific thalamic nuclei (midline and intralaminar nuclei), and they can be recorded over wider areas of cortex, for these nuclei project widely especially to the so-called association cortex. The shape of recruiting and augmenting responses is not identical, but the mechanism of their generation is probably similar, and both may be related to the mechanism of naturally occurring sleep spindles.

19.4. Chemical Agents and Sleep

If the idea of a hypothalamic sleep center is not widely accepted today, there is much discussion of another theory that also holds that sleep can be induced by the activity of a specific neuron group. This concerns the serotonergic neuron system originating in the raphe nuclei of the brain stem (Fig 2.16*B*). We have already met with the descending output of certain parts of this nuclear group in connection with the efferent control of afferent synapses in the spinal dorsal horn (see sections 7.3 and 7.9b). It is the ascending connections of some seroto-nergic neurons that are suggested to induce sleep, specifically slow-wave sleep.

The evidence favoring a sleep-inducing serotonergic system results from experiments in which serotonergic neurons were destroyed by lesion or by specific poisons, and other experiments in which their activity was enhanced by pharmacological means. Generally serotonin-deficient animals were shown to sleep little, or at least less than normally, and interventions that enhanced the activity of central serotonin systems caused increased sleep. It has also been suggested that central noradrenergic circuits, with cells originating in the locus ceruleus, are responsible for REM sleep. A hypothetical circadian clock would engage the serotonin system which initiates slow-wave sleep, and once slow-wave sleep is in progress, the noradrenergic system would begin a cycle of its own, with a cycle length of about 90 minutes. Each time the noradrenaline cycle reached its high point it would interrupt slow-wave sleep and induce a REM period. A variant of this hypothesis suggests that waking and alerting are also functions of the noradrenergic systems, or perhaps of a separate circuit of noradrenergic neurons. Interactions of the REM-driving noradrenaline cycle and the noradrenergic alerting system are not quite clear.

The theories of aminergic driving of the sleep-wake cycle are not yet firmly established. Nor is the relationship between the aminergic brain stem systems and the reticular formation clarified, but connections between them do exist. Especially, the hypothesis that noradrenergic neurons caused REM sleep has been criticized. It is, however, in keeping with the role of monoamines in regulating the overall level of alerting the forebrain that monoaminergic fiber terminals often do not form proper synapses with individual neurons, but end in a series of beads or varicosities apparently broadcasting transmitter substance among many cells (see Section 2.5e).

Even before the monamines were suspected of playing a part in the sleep-wake cycle, acetylcholine was proposed as a transmitter mediating the desynchronizing response of the cerebral cortex. In Chapter 2 the presence of cholinergic excitatory synapses in the cerebral cortex was mentioned. These synapses are "muscarinic," that is, they are blocked by atropine and related drugs. Moreover, instead of depolarizing cells by enhanced Na^+ permeability, they achieve that effect by decreased K^+ permeability (see Section 2.5b). This is a relatively slow action, and its significance is not so much in causing cell discharge but in enhancing the effect of other excitatory inputs converging on the same cell. This is referred to as a *modulatory effect*. Several investigators are of the opinion that the desynchronizing effect of the ascending reticular formation on the cortex is mediated by the modulating effect of these muscarinic cholinergic synapses, although the pathways taken by these inputs have not been accurately mapped, nor the manner in which they achieve desynchronization determined.

In keeping with this suggestion, atropine and related drugs induce slow-wave activity and suppress low-voltage fast desynchronized activity of the cerebral neocortex. They do not cause overt coma, although in the dosage large enough to cause EEG synchronization they strongly modify cerebral function. Before the invention of tranquilizing drugs, scopolamine (an atropine analog) was used extensively to subdue psychiatric patients and to reduce responsiveness and cause amnesia during childbirth.

Cholinergic input originating in the brain stem is also believed to be responsible for inducing the rhythmic slow oscillations known as theta rhythm in the hippocampus. Two separate mechanisms are believed to operate in causing theta waves. One can be blocked by atropine, the other is atropine-resistant.

From what we know today it would seem, then, that the forebrain is perhaps alerted by a cooperation between noradrenergic and cholinergic input, and that slow-wave sleep may be induced when serotonergic input to the forebrain predominates. This, however, may not be final word in this matter.

Working along different lines, other investigators succeeded in extracting from cerebrospinal fluid tapped from sleep-deprived animals a peptide which, when injected into the lateral ventricle of control animals, causes them to sleep more than the usual amount. The cells that produce this sleep-inducing peptide have not yet been identified, nor is anything known about its usual function. It is, however, at least possible that accumulation of this material in the brain is what causes us to feel sleepy, and that sleep gives the brain a chance to inactivate it.

19.5. Chapter Summary

1. The most obvious consequence of sleep deprivation is discomfort and the tendency to fall asleep, and hence impairment of performance in tasks requiring vigilance. In extreme cases transient but severe psychotic signs occur. The biological function fulfilled by sleeping is, however, not understood.
2. For a summary of the definitions of the stages of sleep turn to p. 486.
3. In REM sleep skeletal muscle tone is minimal but occasional movements do occur, and the forebrain shows desynchronized EEG and somewhat elevated metabolism. Dreams are much more frequent and more vivid in REM stage than in slow-wave sleep stages.
4. A night of normal sleep consists of several cycles of deepening and lightening slow-wave sleep, each culminating in a REM state.
5. High-frequency electric stimulation of the upper brain stem reticular formation causes desynchronization of the neocortical EEG, hippocampal theta activity and behavioral alerting. Bilateral destruction of the midbrain reticular formation causes coma with slow-wave and spindle activity of the neocortical EEG, from which, however, an animal can recover in a number of weeks.

6. After transecting the upper spinal cord of a cat the neocortical EEG of the isolated brain alternates between desynchronized and slow-wave patterns. After transection of the midbrain, the isolated forebrain remains in a slow-wave pattern for several weeks, but then resumes alternation between slow-wave and desynchronized states. After such an operation the musculature is in a state of decerebrate rigidity, but normal posture and the ability to walk are recovered after a few weeks. After midbrain transection the cycle of activity and rest in the brain stem-spinal cord and the EEG cycle of slow waves alternating with desynchronization in the forebrain are independent of one another.

7. Serotonergic neurons with cell bodies in the raphe nuclear complex and ascending axons are believed to play a part in controlling the normal sleep cycle. Noradrenergic neurons of the locus coeruleus, with axons addressed to forebrain targets, may have some role in initiating REM sleep as well as in alerting the forebrain during waking hours. A cholinergic system of neurons originating in the brain stem may also have a role in desynchronizing the neocortical EEG and in inducing theta oscillations in the hippocampus. The exact roles played by these three presumably interacting systems is not yet clear.

Further Reading

Books and Reviews

Akert K, Bally C, Schadé JP (eds): Sleep mechanisms. *Prog Brain Res* Vol. 18, 1965.

Kleitman N: *Sleep and Wakefulness.* Chicago, University of Chicago Press, 1963.

Magoun HW: *The Waking Brain.* Springfield, Ill., Charles C Thomas, 1958.

Petre-Quadens O, Schlag JD: *Basic Sleep Mechanisms.* New York, Academic Press, 1974.

Smith JJ, Kampine JB: *Circulatory Physiology: The Essentials.* Baltimore, Williams & Wilkins, 1980.

Vanderwolf CH, Robinson TE (with comments by 32 other authors): Reticulo-cortical activity and behavior: a critique of the arousal theory and a new synthesis. *Behav Brain Sci* 4:459–514, 1981.

Articles

Adametz JH: Rate of recovery of functioning in cats with rostral reticular lesions. *J Neurosurg* 16:85–98, 1959.

Aston-Jones A: Activity of norepinephrine-containing locus coeruleus neurons in behaving rats anticipates fluctuations in the sleep-wake cycle. *J Neurosci* 1:877–886, 1981.

Kennedy C, Gillin JC, Mendelson W, et al: Local cerebral glucose utilization in non-rapid eye movement sleep. *Nature* 297:325–327, 1982.

Villablanca J: Behavioral and polygraphic study of "sleep" and "wakefulness" in chronic decerebrate cats. *Electroencephalogr Clin Neurophysiol* 21:562–577, 1966.

chapter 20

Physiological
Mechanisms of Learning

Facts and speculation about the way in which the brain acquires and stores information.

20.1. Types of Memory

The regulation and control of any complex process requires information that must be stored in one form or other. Plant life for the most part depends on information contained in the genetic code. Animal behavior is guided, to a degree that increases with evolutionary differentiation, by information acquired during an individual lifetime. The human brain is unique in the amount and complexity of information it can store. Making and using tools, spoken and written language, indeed culture defined in the widest sense, all depend on learning.

Until not long ago psychologists divided memory processes in two classes: *short-term* and *long-term*. The former is the kind by which we remember a telephone number from the time we look it up in the directory until we dial it. The latter is used, one hopes, in recording information such as that contained in this text. Other investigators prefer the terms *working memory* and *reference memory*. The two pairs of terms are defined somewhat differently, but the basic idea behind them is similar. Short-term or working memory is thought to be (1) of small capacity, holding a maximum seven items—plus or minus two—

at any one time; (2) labile and disrupted if attention is diverted; (3) automatically erased within a minute or two. One can hold items in short-term memory for longer than this time limit only by continual verbal rehearsal in one's mind: rehearsal re-enters the contents and so counteracts erasure. Long-term memory traces are more difficult to acquire, but once laid down they endure for a long time, perhaps the lifetime of the individual. Long-term memory has a very large capacity. Difficulty in recalling an item arises not because the memory trace fades, but because access to it may be hindered. The very size of the store may make finding items difficult. We have well-practiced access routes to the items we recall often, but whatever has been stored and then not used will become increasingly difficult to remember. If retrieved, such seemingly forgotten memories become once more accessible—an experience all of us past a certain age have now and then had—with joy or otherwise.

It is a widely held view that items can be stored in long-term memory only after they have been first held in short-term memory. The postulated passage from labile, short-term storage into stable, long-term store is also called the consolidation of the memory trace. There are, however, others who regard the two processes as independent, functioning side by side without interaction. In part the argument has centered around the following observations. If brain function is globally disrupted, for example by a generalized seizure, by unconsciousness due to cerebral concussion, or by general anesthesia, the subject, after recovery, cannot remember events that occurred immediately before the disruption (*retrograde amnesia*). Events farther in the past are not forgotten. From this it has been inferred that short-term memory depends on some dynamic process, such as the continued circulation of impulses in a certain pattern, which when disrupted is erased. Long-term memories are stored by some enduring change in the neurons or in the connections between them which would be unaffected by such upheavals.

There are certain observations at variance with this classification of memory processes. One of them is this; if animals are trained to perform a certain task and training is interrupted at an early stage by electrically induced generalized seizure (electroconvulsive shock), they may seem to have forgotten what they have learned. If, however, training is then resumed, the animals learn faster than when first learning a new task. This so-called "saving" in the re-training suggests that the original memory has not completely been erased, but access to it has been disrupted. This is taken to mean that the consolidation of the trace is not the passage from one method of storage into a radically different one, but the gradual strengthening of one and the same process.

In recent discussions of this topic, some investigators have held the opinion that there are several qualitatively different classes of memory storage, perhaps three (short, intermediate, long) or perhaps as many as five. Memories are registered by a different mechanism, each requiring a different method of entry, each having different storage capacities, lifespan and accessibility. On the opposite side there are investigators who regard all memory functions manifestations of a fundamentally uniform basic mechanism, differing only in secondary characteristics.

Subjectively and intuitively we seem to recognize several differences in ways of learning and remembering. To recall something into the conscious mind does not seem to be the same as using a learned motor skill. We feel that to recall a face is different from recalling a melody, and that both differ from reciting a poem. Learning the rules of German grammar does not necessarily enable one to converse with an inhabitant of Munich. Similarly, understanding the laws that determine the speed and force of the wind seems to be achieved in a manner different from learning to sail a vessel.

In spite of such striking differences, the various forms of learning may depend on certain common elementary processes. In very general terms, learning anything that is complex probably involves generating a model, or a program, in a format suitable to be stored in memory. A face may, for example, be recalled by exciting neurons in a pattern that is similar to the one generated when that face was actually perceived. The processes of seeing and of remembering cannot be identical, of course, for a fully conscious normal person readily distinguishes the two. Nevertheless it seems likely that the two functions employ neuronal patterns that are congruent in certain essential features. If so, then the memory of a face is laid down in the form of a program or a model for generating that particular neuronal excitatory pattern. That this may be so occurred first to Descartes, although he spoke of "animal spirits" whereas we speak of "nerve impulses," and "pores through which the spirits pass," instead of "synapses" (Lashley). In a similar sense the ability to, for example, swing a tennis racquet implies the existence of the program for activating muscles in the proper sequence and each to the proper degree.

To acquire such neuronal programs it must be possible to impress certain changes on the functioning of neurons or of the synpases between them. The postulated elementary form of information storage in the brain is usually referred to as a *memory trace* or *engram*. From what we know today it is not possible to decide whether all forms of learning depend on variants of a single kind of elementary biophysical or biochemical change, or whether there exist several basically different mechanisms of memory trace formation in mammalian nervous systems.

20.2. Theories of Memory Trace Formation

Many theories of the physiological basis of learning have been proposed. They can be placed in groups, according to the central principle that inspired them. I will summarize only the core ideas that have been most influential.

The classical engram concept. Originally an engram was defined as the trace in the brain of an elementary idea, as it were the "atom" of mental content. One engram was supposed to be stored in one cortical neuron. It was estimated that we have many more neurons than we would need to store all the memory traces acquired in a lifetime. Engrams of related content would be stored close to one another; the shorter the distance between engrams in the brain, the stronger the mental association between the ideas they represent.

This concept of a one-to-one relationship between ideas and neurons is now considered obsolete and is mentioned here only to show the origin of the word "engram," which is still used, although in a different sense, to mean simply and generally the material storage of information, leaving the specific mechanism to be discovered by future research. Ironically, magnetic memories of digital computers operate on a principle similar to the one originally proposed for the storage of engrams. This is ironic because at the time when the original engram theory was proposed, digital computers had not yet been invented.

Synaptic plasticity. That learning may have to do with enduring alteration of the transmission characteristics of synapses occurred to several writers toward the end of the 19th century, and they in turn have undoubtedly been influenced by Descartes, whose earlier ideas have already been quoted. The hypothesis of synaptic plasticity became more popular when the Pavlovian and behaviorist schools of thought made the establishment of conditional responses the favored method of studying learning in animals (see Section 4.2b). Pavlov proposed that conditional reflexes are established by forming *new connections* between those cortical neurons that receive the conditional stimulus and those that receive the unconditional stimulus. Once such a new pathway has been established, the conditional stimulus would acquire the same power of evoking the response that only the unconditional stimulus originally possessed.

Pavlov's idea of a new connection then became fused with that of a plastic change in synaptic efficiency. Since it was generally believed that new fibers could not grow in an adult mammalian central nervous system, another method of establishing new connections had to be considered. The long-term facilitation of anatomically preformed but initially functionally ineffective synaptic connections seemed the likely alternative. This implied that at birth vast numbers of redundant and ineffective synaptic connections exist, each of which can be brought into service as the organism gains experience.

There was also a rival notion, almost the mirror image of the foregoing. According to it, at birth excitation can pass between any two points in the central nervous system (CNS) through a random network of connections. As the organism matures, synaptic inhibition gradually sculpts usable patterns by suppressing the unwanted interconnections. To support this idea, it has been pointed out that infants begin to move by simultaneously waving all four limbs, and then gradually learn to use just one at a time. Also, the closing and opening of a fist precedes separate movement of individual fingers. As a corollary, it was postulated that seizures are the consequence of regression to the original immature mass discharge pattern.

In the light of more recent research it is easy to find fault with any of these early speculations about the nature of the learning process. The basic notion of synaptic plasticity, that is of some form of long-term change in synaptic efficiency, does however persist (see next section).

There is one concept that has become more acceptable today than it was 50 years ago: that of the formation of new connections in the literal sense of the word. There is now good evidence that after localized brain lesions surviving axons can sprout new terminals that replace degenerated ones (see Section 20.5). In the adult mammalian CNS such new axon branches apparently grow only short distances. And, so far, no one has succeeded in showing that axons sprout new branches also in healthy adult brains. Nevertheless there are some who now think it possible that the growth of new connections is the substrate of long-term memory storage.

Theories of equipotentiality and of mass action. In a famous article summing up much of his life's work, Lashley wrote that 30 years of searching for the location of the engram in the brain convinced him that "... learning is just not possible ... Nevertheless, in spite of such evidence against it, learning does sometimes occur."

Lashley searched for the engram in experiments in which various parts of the cerebral cortex of animals were surgically removed and the animals painstakingly tested for (1) retention of habits learned before the operation; (2) ability to re-learn what they appeared to have forgotten; and (3) ability to learn new tasks. In very simplified terms the overall conclusion from this work was that memory function is disturbed in proportion to the amount of cortex destroyed, irrespective of which part of the cortex had been removed. As far as learning is concerned,

Lashley felt that all parts of the cortex are equipotent. An exception was made for the specific sensory receiving areas: what had been learned through vision is lost after lesion of the visual cortex (although some of what was lost can be re-learned), while responses learned by using certain kinds of auditory cues are disturbed by lesion of the auditory cortex. But the so-called association areas are not assigned either to the acquisition or to the storage and recall of any specific categories of memory, although these areas do participate in a general sense in memory function. Lashley also denied the existence of conditional reflex pathways with anatomically fixed locations (that is, new connections in the Pavlovian sense).

Instead of localized storage of memory traces or of spatially fixed conditional reflex pathways, Lashley proposed a new concept. He agreed that recall involves reactivating a previous pattern of neuronal excitation. But he insisted that the pattern representing any one memory could be evoked not just in one specific set of neurons, but in many sets in many places and perhaps anywhere in the regions of the brain that have to do with memory function. Lashley compared these manifold cortical excitatory patterns to the spread of interference patterns on the surface of a liquid disturbed at several points at once.

Lasley's concept of interference patterns inspired a new theory proposed just a few years ago. It was suggested that the brain stores information in a manner analogous to laser holography. In a hologram the interference patterns of laser light reflected from an object or a scene are stored on a photographic plate. The original image can be restored by illuminating the plate, using a point source of light. This theory of memory storage has lost some of its appeal since its publication, because no one can as yet think of a physical process by which the brain could store a hologram.

Theories of chemical coding of memories. After the nature of the genetic code had been discovered, the idea arose that the experiences acquired through learning by an individual could be stored in the brain in a manner similar to that by which the experiences of the species are laid down in genetic information in cell nuclei. Thus the theory of encoding memories in the structure of macromolecules was born. Only nucleic acids or proteins could serve as chemical encoders, for no other molecule produced by living organisms has the size and complexity of structure required to carry the necessary amount of information.

If this theory proved correct, many secondary problems would arise. For example how would the sensory information which is originally encoded in neuronal signals be translated into the chemical code, and how would the memory traces stored in chemical form be re-translated into neuronal signals when they are recalled? Furthermore, would all neurons of the brain contain all the information the individual has learned, or is learning the province of specialized groups of cells? Are certain kinds of memories stored in certain kinds of neurons? It has also been suggested that glial cells are the ones containing memory traces and that the storage and the retrieval of information involves the exchange of macromolecular material between neurons and glia (see also Section 5.9).

Before these questions could be solved, it was necessary to prove the cornerstone of the hypothesis, namely, that brains indeed produce memory-coding molecules. Many experiments have been performed to decide the issue. The most critical ones have involved the training of a group of animals, preparing an extract of their brains, and injecting that material into untrained animals. Such experiments have been performed on planaria (flatworms), fish, rats and others. The theory would have been confirmed if the untrained recipients had immediately known what the trained donors had learned. Many investigators claimed that recipient animals gave the expected response in a larger number of times than could be attributed to chance, or that they could be trained more easily than untreated ones, but the difference between treated and control groups was never very large, and many of the experiments have been criticized on other grounds. In many other experiments there was no statistically significant difference between treated and control groups. Therefore the issue must be judged still undecided.

Another controversial claim is that inhibiting protein synthesis in brain tissue hinders learning. This would be expected if memory traces were coded in the structure of protein molecules, but there could be other reasons. If, for example, the consolidation of memory traces depended on the growth of new axon terminals, or on the increased synthesis of transmitter substance by certain terminals, these functions would also be interfered with by drugs that inhibit protein synthesis.

20.3. Mechanisms of Synaptic Plasticity

Neurophysiologists generally understand by the term "plasticity" an enduring change in synaptic function. Such a plastic change could be caused either by preceding activation of the same synapse, as in *long-term* or *homosynaptic potentiation* (see Section 4.3) or under the influence of input from another synapse (*heterosynaptic potentiation*, Fig. 20.1). Plastic changes have been shown to occur in simple nervous systems and also in the mammalian brain. The question is whether they can explain the storage of memory traces. If we accept that the conditioning of certain simple reflexes mediated by the vertebrate spinal cord or in the nervous systems of snails and slugs are the simplest forms of "remembering," then the answer is a tentative "yes." As far as more complex learning is concerned, the doubts and reservations raised first by Lashley and since then by many others have not yet been resolved.

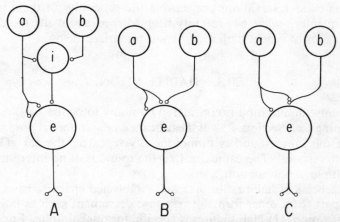

Figure 20.1.   Hypothetical mechanisms of synaptic plasticity that could explain simple associative conditioning. *A*, the effect of long-term homosynaptic potentiation in a shared pathway. Suppose that afferent neuron *a* can synaptically excite both interneuron *i* and efferent neuron *e*. Suppose that excitation from afferent neuron *b* is also transmitted to *i*; but firing by *i* causes only subthreshold excitatory postsynaptic potentials in *e*. Suppose also that the junction *i–e* is capable of long-term potentiation. Then, initially, input from *a* will cause an output from *e*, but input from *b* will not. Following high-frequency repetitive activation of *a*, however, since it will result in repetitive firing of *i* also, the junction *i–e* will increase in potency; thereafter input from *b* will be able (by mediation of *i*) to evoke an output from *e* even though earlier it did not. *B*, heterosynaptic potentiation based on a postsynaptic mechanism. Assume that axons of afferent neurons *a* and *b* terminate side by side in synaptic contact with efferent neuron *e*, and that they release the same transmitter. Assume also that *a* releases more transmitter than *b*. Assume finally that receptor sensitivity in the subsynaptic membrane of *e* is enhanced if a sufficient amount of transmitter acts upon it; this critical amount is reached when *a* and *b* fire in rapid succession. Then, after repeated pairings of firing in *a* and *b*, receptor sensitization will progress until input from *b* alone will be sufficient to evoke an impulse in *e*. *C*, Heterosynaptic potentiation by a presynaptic mechanism. Assume that afferent neuron *a* has axon terminals in synaptic contact with axon terminals of *b*, and that the arrival of impulses in the terminals of *a* and of *b* in rapid succession causes an enduring enhancement of the ability of *b* to release transmitter. Then, after repeated joint firing of *a* and *b* there will be a lasting increase in the effectiveness of input from *b* causing output from *e*. (Modified and redrawn after E. R. Kandel: *Cellular Basis of Behavior*. San Francisco, W. H. Freeman, 1976.)

Keeping these reservations concerning the generality of these mechanisms in mind, what has recently been learned about the biophysical mechanisms of synaptic plasticity are summarized below.

20.3a.   HABITUATION

Response habituation is considered by many to be the simplest form of learning (see Section 4.5). If a cat hears a new sound, it pricks up its ears. If the same sound is monotonously repeated, the cat gradually ceases to respond. The cat learns that the sound is of no interest; this is an example of habituation.

The process of habituation has well-established characteristics which set it apart from other forms of response decrement such as fatigue or desensitization. (1) Habituation is specific for one stimulus. For example, after habituation to one tone, another tone still evokes a response. (2) Raising the intensity of the stimulus erases habituation (dishabituation). (3) If, after habituation, the stimulus is withheld for a period of time and then presented again, the response reappears. (4) There is no habituation to noxious stimuli. (5) If a noxious stimulus is presented together with a non-noxious one, there is no habituation to either of the two. Such pairing of two stimuli is in effect a form of conditioning; the result of this form of conditioning is, then, to prevent habituation.

The mechanism of habituation has been studied in detail in the marine slug *Aplysia*. This animal withdraws its gill when the skin of its syphon is mechanically stimulated. This response shows habituation, dishabituation and several other features typical of some more complex responses of mammals. The neuron network mediating the reflex has been mapped, and the functioning of the participating synapses has been studied by electric recordings. The habituation of gill withdrawal could, in principle, have been the result of a number of processes, including for example synaptic inhibition. In fact it was shown to be the result of decreased output of excitatory synaptic transmitter substance at the presynaptic axon terminals mediating the withdrawal reflex (*homosynaptic depression*). It has also been shown that this depression is different from ordinary fatigue and does not involve exhaustion of available transmitter.

From available observations it seems possible that the apparent habituation of the flexor reflex seen under certain conditions in mammalian spinal cords may be the result of similar homosynaptic depression. Whether the habituation of the much more complex behaviors of mammals, such as for example the orienting response, which are mediated by the forebrain, are also dependent on a similar mechanism, is uncertain. There is evidence that habituation of the orienting response of mammals is mediated by inhibition originating in the hippocampus (see Section 20.4).

20.3b. LONG-TERM POTENTIATION

In Chapter 4 (Section 4.3) long-term potentiation was described as a property of synapses in the hippocampal formation. This is a form of synaptic plasticity: repeated use of a synapse makes transmission through it increasingly easy. In the synapses of the hippocampal formation the effect endures for many hours, sometimes for days.

If two pathways share an interneuron, then under certain conditions long-term potentiation could enhance transmission also through the pathway not originally excited. To understand this, consider the arrangement in Figure 20.1A. Suppose that the synapse between interneuron i and the efferent neuron e is capable of long-term potentiation. Then, if afferent neuron a is repeatedly activated, then input through it, as well as input through afferent neuron b will have an increased excitatory effect on e as long as the i–e synapse remains potentiated.

20.3c. HETEROSYNAPTIC POTENTIATION

If activity on one synapse changes the efficiency of transmission in another, we speak of heterosynaptic effect. Such effects could be achieved either by a change in the sensitivity of the postsynaptic neuron to the transmitter or by a change of the amount of transmitter released, as illustrated in Figure 20.1B and C. In the hypothetical scheme illustrated in Fig. 20.1B it is assumed that fibers of two afferent neurons, a and b terminate on the efferent neuron e adjacently, with no glial partition between them (cf. Section 5.9a). It is further assumed that both release the same transmitter, and that under the influence of that transmitter the postsynaptic membrane incorporates increasing numbers of receptor molecules. It will be recalled that there is some evidence that long-term potentiation may in part or in whole be due to increased numbers of receptors in postsynaptic membranes. In the case illustrated in Figure 20.1B, potentiation by input from afferent neuron a would then also potentiate input from neuron b, even if b had not previously discharged.

Fig. 20.1C illustrates heterosynaptic potentiation by a presynaptic mechanism. In this case the firing of impulses by afferent neuron a is assumed to cause a change in the presynaptic terminal of afferent neuron b, resulting in increased output of transmitter by b. In such a case, unlike the ones illustrated in Fig. 20.1A and B, potentiation of transmission from neuron b could be achieved without simultaneous potentiation of input from a.

Heterosynaptic potentiation has been demonstrated at some combinations of synapses of *Aplysia*, and it has also been claimed that it may operate at some, not all, regions of the mammalian hippocampus. The presynaptic form apears to depend on calcium; either more free Ca^{2+} is present in the potentiated terminal, or more enters with the arrival of each presynaptic impulse. Heterosynaptic potentiation, (Fig. 20.1*B* and *C*) and potentiation of shared pathways (Fig. 20.1*A*) have been suggested to be synaptic mechanisms mediating simple conditional reflexes (classical associative conditioning). There is, however, one more feature of conditioning for which the underlying biophysical mechanism must account. It is the requirement that in order for conditioning to be successful, the conditional and unconditional stimuli must be applied together or one after the other in rapid enough succession. As drawn in the schemas of Figure 20.1, activation of neuron *a* would potentiate transmission from *b* regardless of whether *b* has discharged in conjunction with *a* or not. To somehow incorporate this requirement into the hypothesis, we must postulate that it is a condition for potentiation to occur that afferent neuron *b* must discharge before the effect of a preceding discharge of *a* has terminated. For example, it may be necessary that *b* release its transmitter before all the transmitter released by a preceding impulse in *a* has been removed.

20.4. The Hippocampus and Memory Function

20.4a. THE AMNESTIC SYNDROME

In the early days of surgical treatment of epilepsy parts of both temporal lobes were ablated in a small number of patients to control severe complex partial seizures of bilateral origin. When such bilateral resections included the hippocampal formations on both sides, the patients developed a severe memory defect. They could not remember events that occurred in the days or weeks before surgery (*retrograde amnesia*) and had great difficulty in learning new events, faces, or data thereafter (*anterograde amnesia*). For example, after moving to a new address, one patient could learn the way to his new home, but not the names and faces of his new neighbors, not even after repeated meetings. But short-term memory function seemed intact. This defect was interpreted as an inability to transfer information from short-term into long-term memory, or, in other words, to "consolidate" memory traces.

The *amnestic syndrome* consequent to surgical resection of the hippocampal formations appears to be similar in certain respects to that of patients suffering from *Korsakoff's syndrome*, a severe toxic brain disorder, most frequently the result of chronic alcoholism. In patients suffering from Korsakoff's psychosis the hippocampal formations are extensively damaged, but lesions occur elsewhere as well. To the lesions outside the hippocampus are attributed certain disorders not shared by patients who lose only their hippocampi at the hands of the surgeon. Perhaps best known of these signs is confabulation: Korsakoff patients do not readily admit forgetting, but "fill the gaps" left by their memory disorder with tales they make up, often in vivid detail. Pure temporal lobe cases do not confabulate, but admit not remembering.

Patients in whom a hippocampal formation was ablated only on one side do not have the striking disability of memory typical of the bilateral lesion. Careful testing does reveal, however, diminished retention, different for the two brain halves. Hippocampal lesion in the dominant, usually the left, hemisphere impairs remembering of both heard and read verbal material. Lesion of the right hippocampus causes poor memory of faces, spatial patterns, and musical melodies. (See also Section 21.1).

To many investigators it seemed that experimental lesions made in the hippocampal formation of animals, including monkeys, did not interfere with learning. Even investigators who did find a memory defect described it as an impairment of working (short-term) memory, not of reference (long-term) memory, which is the exact opposite of the condition seen in human patients. Various explanations have been offered. For example, a significant difference is that in surgery for epilepsy not only the hippocampus is removed, but also overlying white matter and neocortex. But even when the same surgical procedure was replicated in monkeys, it was difficult to demonstrate a disorder corresponding to human amnesia.

It was then pointed out that human and animal memories are tested in fundamentally different ways. Even if the items to be remembered do not include words or numbers, conventional testing of retention by human subjects generally requires conscious recall and a verbal response. Animals are never asked for verbal responses; they are scored only on performance. Now it has been known for some time that conditional reflexes can be established in human patients suffering from the hippocampal amnestic syndrome and also that they can be trained in new manual skills. They will be able to perform the newly learned task without being able to remember that they have learned it. As already mentioned, they learn the way to a new home, but do not recognize new neighbors. People suffering from the amnestic syndrome can even be trained to repeat words if a cue is provided. If two words are repeated together several times in succession, then presenting the patient with the first word can elicit the second. In sum, the patients with hippocampal damage learn without being aware that they learn.

What, then, is the exact role of the hippocampus in learning? Is it the same in man and beast? Neither of these two questions has properly been answered. It is likely that the hippocampus, as also other major cerebral structures, does not have a single, unique function, but participates in several. To each of these several cerebral functions the hippocampus may contribute something which the synaptic organization of the hippocampal formation is specifically designed to do. What this contribution is has not yet been defined, but it may include one or both of the following two general categories.

It has been suggested that the hippocampus serves to suppress irrelevant and interfering input, while attention is directed to a specific set of signals. Intrusion by unwanted input interferes with learning. The habituation of the orienting response is considered to be an example of this general screening function. Such habituation is defective after bilateral hippocampal lesion. It should be noted that, for different reasons, the hippocampus has been implicated in both initiating and in suppressing (habituating) the orienting response (see Sections 19.3b and 20.3a). The two are not logically mutually exclusive: the same circuit may serve to switch a response on and off, or there may be parallel circuits for the two functions within the same brain area. But any final model of the orienting response must take into account the fact that destruction of hippocampal tissue does not abolish the response; but it does prevent its habituation. Perhaps related to deficient habituation is the observation that hippocampal lesion hinders animals from changing behavior as the occasion demands. Also, this deficit could be tied in with the one attributed to impairment of working memory (mentioned in Section 20.1): not remembering the immediately relevant and not noticing when the environment has just changed.

Another theory suggests that the hippocampus organizes "cognitive maps." By this is understood logical structures by which the interrelationship of items of information can be organized. Such cognitive maps could order spatial information in essentially the same way as geographic maps do: by replicating the interrelationship of objects in space. They could, however, also organize abstractions such as words by arranging them in a multi-dimensionally scaled logical array. According to this theory the hippocampus does not store information as such (it does not actually contain the engrams), but organizes the access to the filing system by which items can be stored and subsequently retrieved. The cognitive maps might be represented by the firing patterns of hippocampal neurons. In man, verbal material would be organized in the dominant hemisphere, spatial information in the non-dominant hemisphere. In animals such lateralization may not exist.

There is enough tissue in the hippocampus to mediate both functions. Both theories have been criticized; neither has, however, been refuted.

20.5. Improvement of Function After Injury to the Central Nervous System

"The patient is a 62-year-old professor of anatomy who was suddenly taken ill during a lecture trip abroad." So begins the first-hand account written by Brodal, the distinguished neuroanatomist, of a stroke he himself had suffered. His case history should be read by all who must take care of victims of cerebrovascular accidents and also by anyone interested in the theory of brain function, especially of the plasticity of brain function. Brodal's restrainedly objective yet vivid description drives home both aspects of the aftermath of major brain lesions: the power as well as the limits of functional recovery. For even when a patient's performance seems to an observer almost as it has been before the onset of illness, the patient himself is, in Brodal's words, "painfully aware that this is not so."

In the mammalian central nervous system neither lost neurons nor interrupted fiber tracts are capable of regeneration. The improvement seen after central lesions must therefore be explained by some other, essentially physiological, mechanism. A number of different processes may contribute to such functional recovery, and it is rarely clear which of the several alternatives is the most important one in any individual case. All explanations of recovery of cerebral function involve one form or other of plasticity of function, in other words learning in the widest sense of the word. It is for this reason that this topic has been included in this chapter. Only the briefest outline of some of the most discussed alternative mechanisms of functional recovery can be given here.

20.5a. IMPROVEMENT BY SUBSTITUTION OF FUNCTION

It is believed that in some cases the function of a lost component of the CNS can be "taken over" by the intact remaining parts. This could happen in different ways.

Redundant neurons. Some neuroscientists believe that the intact brain contains more neurons and more connecting fibers than are needed to perform the functions assigned to them. When some of the redundant cells or pathways are lost, the remaining ones can gradually assume a larger share of the task.

Re-learning of a lost skill. After injury, the surviving parts of the CNS may acquire functions originally performed by the damaged parts. This idea is easiest to accept if the damaged brain circuit and the one replacing its functions have similar structure and had related functions already before the injury occurred. As a crude analogy, think of a right-handed person learning to write with the left hand. This is easier than to learn to write or to paint with brush or pen held in the mouth after the loss of both arms.

Among the multiplicity of connections between any two points of the brain there is always more than one potential path from point A to point B. Thus, if information cannot be transferred through a direct route then, in principle, there always is a possibility to re-route it through a detour of multiple synaptic connections. There is good reason to believe that such re-routing actually does occur. The need to re-program the transmission could explain the time and the effort required to recover a lost skill, and also why such a re-learned task always remains more tiring for the patient than the same task has been before his injury or disease.

The method or strategy of solving a problem after brain injury is usually different from the one used before. Attention is paid to new details of sensory input in order to use new cues instead of those no longer available. Muscle groups are learned to be used in novel ways to compensate for the weakness or stiffness of some of the muscles.

20.5b. TRUE FUNCTIONAL RECOVERY IN DAMAGED CNS CIRCUITS

Recovery of transiently interrupted axonal conduction. Some of the most severe immediate signs of cerebral injury and disease, or of cerebrovascular accidents, may not be caused by destruction of tissue, but by temporary loss of axonal conduction. As long as continuity of the axons is preserved, there is hope for recovery. Fastest to heal are the consequences of pressure block, caused for instance by local cerebral edema. But even after demyelination of central axons, remyelination and restored conduction remain possible. Remyelination is the most likely explanation of the prolonged remissions that occur in the more favorable cases of multiple (disseminated) sclerosis.

Functional reorganization. If some but not all the axons in a fiber tract are interrupted, the target neurons of the tract lose part of their input. Several plastic processes may serve in the adaptation to such partial deafferentation. For example, the *balance* between *excitatory* and *inhibitory* input may be readjusted. If, for instance, all the lost neurons (or fibers) were excitatory, then the inhibitory restraint exerted on their target neurons from other undamaged sources may gradually be lessened to restore the balance between the remaining, now weakened, excitatory and the anatomically intact inhibitory input. An alternative mechanism may be a form of *denervation supersensitivity* (see Section 3.4f): the receptor molecules in the subsynaptic membrane of the surviving synapses may multiply, rendering the membrane more sensitive to the transmitter and restoring the power of transmission. Alternatively, the surviving presynaptic terminals may *hypertrophy* to manufacture and release increased amounts of transmitter. In either case, whenever a few synapses take over a function that many have performed before, while strength may be restored, finesse will deteriorate. The reasons are similar to those of the coarsening of the grading of contraction after reinnervation of partially denervated muscle (see Section 3.4f).

Collateral sprouting. In recent years it has become clear that intact axons sometimes sprout new branches which innervate synaptic sites vacated by degenerating terminals. It is unfortunately not yet certain that such new connections result in improved function. In fact the evidence for sprouting is clearest in cases where the synaptic sites vacated by the degenerating terminals of one tract are replaced by collaterals from another tract, the function of which need not be related to that of the lesioned tract. The freshly sprouted terminals may thus convey inappropriate signals, and consequently the function of the circuit may deteriorate instead of improving. Such malconnections could be the pathological substrate of some of the delayed sequelae of brain injuries.

As has been mentioned repeatedly, injured peripheral nerves do regenerate in favorable cases, but cut central fiber tracts do not. There has been much debate and experimentation to discover the reasons for this difference. Most probably it lies in a difference in the terrain into which the injured axons must grow. In the distal stump of an injured peripheral nerve the Schwann cells seem to provide some, presumably chemical, stimulus for the growth of the axon from the proximal stump (see Section 3.4g). The glial satellite cells of axons in the adult CNS do not seem to perform such a nurturing and guiding (trophic and tactic) function. Attempts at providing injured central axons of experimental animals with an appropriate artificial path and a stimulus for regeneration have met with some initial success. We can but hope that these ingenious attempts will eventually lead to a practical method of reconnecting severed central fiber tracts. For now the outcome of this quest is, unfortunately, quite unsure.

20.6. Chapter Summary

1. A well-known hypothesis is that we store memory traces in two separate registers: short-term or working memory that contains only a few items at any one time and is readily erased and easily disrupted; and long-term or reference memory that has a very large storage capacity and is very stable. Some believe that all items must first be stored in short-term memory before they can be transferred into long-term memory. Other schemes, some postulating more than two memory registers, others assuming a single mechanism for all types of memory storage, have also been proposed.
2. There have been four classes of theories of long-term storage of memory traces, postulating, respectively: (a) fixed sites for each engram; (b) plasticity of synaptic connections; (c) theories of equipotentiality and mass patterning

(the latest version being the theory of cerebral holography); and (d) chemical coding in macromolecules.

3. Response habituation has been considered to be the simplest form of learning. In sea slugs the habituation of the gill-withdrawal reflex was shown to be the consequence of decreased output of transmitter in synaptic terminals mediating the reflex. There are indications that habituation of the orienting response of mammals is the result of inhibition originating in hippocampal neuron circuits.

4. Long-term potentiation and heterosynaptic potentiation are elementary mechanisms of synaptic plasticity.

5. The mammalian hippocampal formation has been implicated by different investigators in one or more of the following functions: either initiating or suppressing the orienting response, or both; guarding against distraction during learning by the filtering of irrelevant input; consolidating long-term memories; storage in short-term working memory; organizing cognitive maps.

6. The amnestic syndrome caused by hippocampal damage involves impairment of cognitive learning, but it does not prevent the learning of new skills, and it does not erase previously consolidated memory traces.

7. Although neurons lost to disease or injury of the adult central nervous system of mammals are not replaced, and transected central axons do not regenerate, the functions that are impaired after injury to the CNS can often recover to a considerable degree. It is not known by what means functions are recovered, but among the various theoretical alternatives are: (a) substitution of function; the remaining intact components of the CNS "taking over" those tasks that the lost parts used to perform. This may be possible by re-routing information to bypass blocked pathways, and by a process of re-learning skills, using new strategies. (b) True functional recovery may occur by: recovery of conduction in axons that remained anatomically intact but were functionally blocked; functional reorganization by readjusting the balance of excitatory and inhibitory inputs, by denervation supersensitivity or by hypertrophy of surviving intact presynaptic terminals; and by the sprouting of new collaterals by surviving axons.

8. The inability of central axons to regenerate is probably due to the absence in the CNS of cells capable of performing the trophic and tactic functions served by Schwann cells in peripheral nerves.

Further Reading

Books and Reviews

Deutsch JA: *The Physiological Basis of Memory.* New York, Academic Press, 1973.

Eidelberg E, Stein DG: Functional recovery after lesions of the nervous system. *Neurosci Res Prog Bull* 12:191–303, 1974.

Goldberger ME: Motor recovery after lesions. *Trends Neurosci* 3:288–291, 1980.

Kandel ER: Calcium and the control of synaptic strength by learning. *Nature* 293:697–699, 1981

Olton DS, Becker JT, Handelman GE (with comments by 32 other authors): Hippocampus, space and memory. *Behav Brain Sci* 2:313–365, 1979.
Pribram KH, Broadbent DE (eds): *Biology of Memory.* New York, Academic Press, 1970.

Articles

Brodal A: Self-observation and neuro-anatomical consideration after a stroke. *Brain* 96:675–694, 1973.

chapter 21

Complex Brain Functions

Functions of the association areas of the necortex and limbic system; the electrical signs of cognitive processes.

At some time in the future psychiatry and neurology, psychology and neurophysiology will all become a single science. Until that fusion, the disciplines that deal with the physical and chemical aspects of brain function are separate from those dealing with its behavioral and mental manifestations. The border area between them is claimed by both or by neither, and it is this "no-man's land" that we have to discuss now. Our discussion must remain rather superficial, because not much is known about the physiological mechanisms upon which the so-called higher brain functions depend.

21.1. Hemispheric Specialization

Most of those who read this text probably already know that the ability to speak usually resides in the left hemisphere of the brain. This was discovered in the 19th century from case histories of patients who suffered one-sided brain damage. Such damage impairs speech in most cases when it affects the left side of the brain, and is unlikely to do so when it affects the right side.

It is possible to detect which hemisphere controls language functions also in persons who have not suffered brain damage. The most reliable method is known as Wada's test: a short-acting anesthetic drug, usually sodium amytal, is injected into the carotid artery of one side while the subject is counting or speaking. If the injection is made on the side controlling speech, the patient stops counting and is unable to respond to questions for a few minutes. This test revealed that 95% of right-handed persons and 70% of left-handers have language functions represented in the left hemisphere. Of the other left-handers 15% have speech controlled from the right hemisphere and 15% have bilateral representation.

The neurologists who contributed most to the early discoveries of language functions were Broca and Wernicke. The brain region known as *Broca's area* is located on the lateral aspect of the frontal cortex, rostrally of the representation of facial muscles in the motor area, usually on the left side. *Wernicke's area* lies on the same side but more posteriorly, on the posterior end of the superior temporal gyrus, not far from the auditory receiving areas.

Disorders of producing or understanding language, without impairment of hearing and without paresis or ataxia of the muscles of mouth, tongue, pharynx, larynx and respiration, are called *aphasias*. When impaired speaking is caused by paresis or ataxia, we speak of *dysarthria*. According to the original classification of aphasias, which was simple but is now unfortunately obsolete, injury to Broca's area was believed to cause motor or expressive aphasia, and injury to Wernicke's area to cause sensory or receptive aphasia. Motor aphasia was defined as an inability to speak with intact understanding of language. Patients suffering from sensory aphasia do not understand spoken language, but speak fluently, although they make frequent mistakes (paraphasia). The mistakes were attributed to the absence of self-control or feedback since sensory aphasics do not understand the words they themselves utter. Damage to the lateral parietal cortex, between Broca's and Wernicke's areas, was said to cause associational or conductive aphasia, believed to be due to an inability to link or to integrate the functions of the two main speech areas. As case histories accumulated and patients were studied more and more carefully, the inadequacy of this simple classification became evident, and others have replaced it. The various amended nomenclatures, and the theories behind them, fall outside the accepted boundaries of neurophysiology, and the reader should consult the short review by Goodglass listed at the end of this chapter or a recent edition of any major neurology textbook.

Impaired language function remains of course a reliable sign of damage to the so-called dominant hemisphere, and usually to the lateral aspect of the frontal, parietal or temporal lobes. Reading and writing may similarly be affected after unilateral brain damage, chiefly of the parietal cortex, on the same side as the one controlling speech. Disturbances of writing without paresis or ataxia of the hand are called *agraphia* or *dysgraphia*; those of reading, *alexia* or *dyslexia*. It should be pointed out, however, that reading and writing disabilities acquired due to brain damage are far less common than the apparently inborn developmental dyslexias that occur without overt neurological lesions to explain them. Such inborn dyslexias have statistically been linked to bilateral speech representation and to mixed cerebral dominance. The term *mixed dominance* means that hand dominance and speech are controlled from opposite hemispheres. The association of reading disorders with anomalous hemispheric specializations is, however, not absolute, and the relationship between the two conditions is controversial. Similarly uncertain is the supposed linkage between bilateral or mixed hemispheric dominance and stuttering.

It has become customary to refer to the brain half controlling both speech and hand dominance as the *dominant* or "major" hemisphere. It is, however, also clear that the so-called *non-dominant* or "minor" hemisphere has important functions that are its own. Among them are orientation in and perception of space. Generally, it seems that the dominant hemisphere is better at processing information sequentially, one item at a time. This is of course the way in which we speak, or listen to speech, and also read and write. By contrast the non-dominant hemisphere appears to be able to perceive many items simultaneously, in other words to process multidimensional information, as required for spatial perception. Also, the left brain is supposed to be more logical, the right more intuitive and also more emotional. Algebra, which requires chains of logical reasoning, belongs to the left, geometry to the right side. Visual arts seem to depend mainly on right hemisphere function. Music also depends more on the right hemisphere, although one might speculate that melody should belong to the left, harmony to the right. It has been asserted that of the two Japanese writing systems the one that uses signs representing syllables (*kana*) is controlled by the dominant hemisphere, the other which consists of ideograms (or morphograms) symbolizing concepts or words (*kanji*) by the non-dominant hemisphere.

Although hemispheric asymmetry is most conspicuous in the functions of association cortex, it extends beyond this area. For example, it will be recalled that lesions of the left hippocampal formation impair chiefly verbal memory, those of the hippocampus on the right side, visual memory (see Section 20.4a).

Research into hemispheric specializations has been aided by the exhaustively detailed study of almost 50 patients in whom the corpus callosum was surgically transected in order to prevent the generalization of seizures originating in multiple epileptogenic foci. In intact brains, information that is first processed in one hemisphere is then transferred to the other by the callosal fibers. In paients with surgically split brains such transfer can no longer take place. In them the functions of the two hemispheres can be tested separately, provided that stimuli are presented in such a way that information reaches one brain half only. For example, if an object is touched by just one hand, tactile input reaches only the hemisphere of the side opposite that hand. Similarly, stimuli presented in one half of the visual field reach only the contralateral visual cortex. Experimental psychologists have devised tricks that permit the separate testing of one hemisphere in subjects with intact brains as well. There are certain technical limitations to all these experiments, and to the possible inferences that can be drawn from them, either in split-brain or in normal subjects. For further details of this fascinating area of research the reader should consult the monographs by Gazzaniga and by Springer and Deutsch and the conference proceedings relating to this topic listed at the end of the chapter.

The functional asymmetry of the two hemispheres is not complete. Neurologists noticed early that severely aphasic individuals sometimes can sing, and also utter single words, especially emotional expletives. In some of the split-brain patients it appeared that the non-dominant hemisphere is capable of using language of a simple kind, and also that right hemisphere language can improve with time. Similarly, spatial orientation is not entirely limited to the non-dominant hemisphere. It is as though each hemisphere has a special talent, but neither completely lacks the skills of the other. And if unilateral brain damage occurs at an early age, the surviving hemisphere can to some degree learn to perform the lost functions. Thus if a young child suffers an extensive lesion in the dominant hemisphere, he need not remain aphasic for life.

21.2. Association Areas of the Cerebral Neocortex

Cortical association areas were originally defined as those which did not receive input from the dorsal thalamus. The theory was that sensory information arrives first in the primary receiving areas of the cortex, is further processed in the secondary sensory areas, and then is transferred by way of corticocortical fiber tracts to the sensory association areas where the objects represented by sensory input were recognized. In other words, sensation was supposed to be the function of the sensory receiving areas, perception of the association areas. Motor association areas were believed to make plans for movements which then were executed by the primary and secondary motor areas. The "will" was thought to reside in an unknown anatomical location and to link perceptions with motor acts.

It was along these lines of thinking that *agnosia* came to be defined as a neurological defect of perception with intact sensory function. Agnosias were thus attributed to defects of sensory association areas. Receptive aphasia and alexia are special forms of agnosias. Wernicke's area thus became defined as a specialized part of the auditory association cortex. Similarly, *apraxia* was defined as impairment of complex purposeful movements in the absence of paresis and of cerebellar ataxia. Apraxia was attributed to malfunctioning of the motor association cortex. Expressive aphasia and agraphia were considered special cases of apraxias, and Broca's area to be part of the motor association area.

In the decades that have elapsed since these theories were formulated our picture of the projections that connect the parts of the forebrain has been modified, and with it our concepts of the interactions of these parts. In our clinical vocabulary we have nevertheless retained the just-listed names for neurological deficiencies. They are still useful in describing the neurological state of patients, even if the theories which inspired the nomenclature are inaccurate.

From what we know today it seems still true that the association areas play a part in the types of functions originally ascribed to them, but it is also clear that they have other, more subtle, functions as well. And, of course, the simple unidirectional flow chart, according to which information is forwarded from peripheral input to sensory areas, then to the sensory association areas, then to motor association areas, and finally to motor areas, is false. There are many more corticocortical and corticosubcortical connections than was supposed and in most cases there are fibers conducting both to and from regions.

Of all the animals, man has the largest association areas, both in relative and in absolute terms. They occupy major portions of the frontal, temporal and parietal cortices. The association areas are now defined in two ways. By cytoarchitectonics as the *homotypical* parts of the cortex they are neither granular (as the sensory areas) nor agranular (as the motor areas), but are intermediate in structure with all 6 cell layers well marked. The other definition relates to thalamic input. Contrary to what had once been thought, most parts of the association areas do receive specific thalamic afferent fibers but these come from the so-called intrinsic thalamic nuclei and not from the sensory "relay" nuclei. For example, frontal association cortex has two-way connections with the dorsomedial nucleus (nucleus medialis) of the thalamus; parietal association cortex with the dorsolateral nucleus and with the pulvinar. Recent research has confirmed that association areas are richly and reciprocally connected with many other parts of the cerebral cortex, including the sensory areas (for example Fig. 18.1). In addition, many connections exist with other subcortical regions; for example between frontal cortex and certain nuclei of the amygdala and septum.

Much of what we know about the association areas is derived from observations of deficits consequent to clinical or experimental lesions. To these essentially negative data are more recently being added the recordings of impulse discharges of neurons in association cortex of relatively freely behaving, unanesthetized experimental animals.

21.2a. FRONTAL ASSOCIATION CORTEX (PREFRONTAL AREA)

That the frontal lobes of man are involved in controlling certain complex and specific aspects of behavior was first suspected after Harlow's 1848 report and 1868 follow-up of the much quoted case of Phineas Gage. This man had an accident in which an iron spike was driven through his forehead. He recovered his general health, but a profound change in his behavior became evident to those who knew him well both before and after the accident. He became unreliable at work, given to profanity, ill-tempered and generally slothful. The sad opportunity to study many more cases of extensive bilateral frontal lobe damage came in the two world wars. To these observations were added the psychiatric reports of patients in whom the fibers connecting the frontal lobes to subcortical gray matter were surgically cut (frontal lobotomies or leukotomies).

The behavior of monkeys has also been studied in great detail after experimental ablations of the association areas of the two frontal lobes. Left to themselves after such an operation, monkeys become hyperactive, restlessly pacing back and forth and touching and palpating objects in their way. Yet these animals become socially isolated and do not interact with others in their cage. In standardized psychological tests they show characteristic deficiencies. They fail at tasks which require them to do something some time after the presentation of a stimulus. Some investigators attributed this to a failure of short-term memory (see Section 20.1). Yet these animals can learn to differentiate between complex cues and to remember their meaning, provided that they are allowed to make the required choices between test stimuli at the time the stimuli are shown. If it is true that items can be stored in long-term memory only after previous entry into short-term memory, then both short- and long-term memory function of the frontal-lobe-ablated animals must be intact (cf. Section 20.1). If so, then the deficit is a specific difficulty of the timing or of the planning of acts that must be performed with a delay after sensory cues have disappeared. In addition, these monkeys fail in tasks in which stimuli are not shown side by side, but are spatially discontiguous. There is also perseveration, a tendency to repeat responses that were once successful but have in the meantime become inappropriate.

The changes of behavior of people after frontal lobe damage are extremely variable from individual to individual, even if the anatomical lesions are similar. Generally such patients do quite well on standard intelligence tests. Their performance in their professions and also in their households nevertheless often becomes unsatisfactory. The most disturbing change in most of these patients seems to be an inability to organize tasks in time and to plan for the future.

Most frontal lobe damaged patients also undergo a restriction of emotional life. A few develop a persistent and unmodulated mild euphoria, but in most, affect simply becomes flat, neither positive nor negative. One of the purposes of frontal lobotomies was, of course, to relievé the anguish of pathologically extreme affective responses. Another was to decrease the suffering caused by pain in incurable diseases, usually cancer. After frontal lobotomy patients still felt pain. If they had been psychotic, they retained cognitive disorders. But after the operation they seemed not to suffer anymore from these ills. This flattening of affect has been attributed to the interruption of the connections between frontal association cortex and limbic nuclei of amygdala and septum (see Section 21.5). Whether the price paid in functional loss was worth the relief afforded by these operations I must leave to others to discuss. Radical frontal lobotomy is rarely performed nowadays, but other, much less extensive psychosurgical operations are used in some centers for certain limited cases.

There have been attempts to find a single defect that could explain all the diverse consequences of frontal lobe lesions. The frontal association area is, however, rather large, and it contains more than one cytoarchitectonically distinct region. It may therefore be impossible to find a single functional principle that is common to the entire area. Nevertheless several of the most conspicuous deficiencies of frontal lobe lesions have one feature in common: a diminished appreciation of, and orientation in, time. This defect could perhaps link even some of the affective with the cognitive changes: if a person knows no future, then he has nothing to worry about and nothing to look forward to.

21.2b. TEMPORAL LOBES

The consequences of complete ablation of both temporal lobes in monkeys are known as the Klüver-Bucy syndrome after the two investigators who first described them in the 1930s. Like monkeys whose frontal association areas have been removed, those with temporal lobe lesion also become agitated and hyperactive. However, instead of the incessant tactile exploration of the frontally lesioned animals, the monkeys without temporal lobes explore by vision. One after another they pick up each object in their way and look at it, apparently without recognizing what it is and without making any use of it. These animals can see well: their visual threshold and visual acuity appear normal, nevertheless they seem to make no sense of complex visual stimuli. Klüver and Bucy described this defect as visual agnosia.

Another sign of bilateral temporal lobe lesions is loss of aggressiveness. This is evident in macaque monkeys which are by nature quite unfriendly, but it is even more striking when the same operation is performed on a lynx. Even that naturally ferocious predator becomes tame. And finally, temporal lobe ablation leads to excessive sexual activity, impelling monkeys to seek sexual contact with appropriate as well as inappropriate targets.

We have already met with the memory defect that is among the consequences of complete ablations of both temporal lobes (see Section 20.4a). This of course is due to destruction of the archicortex of the hippocampal formation and not of the neocortical association areas. It has also been thought that the diminished aggressive behavior and hypersexuality are related to the loss of the amygdala, but subsequently these behavioral changes have been linked to the combination of subcortical and cortical damage. Particularly loss of the paleocortical pyriform area and its surroundings have been implicated in these behaviors. It is possible to remove the neocortical association areas of the temporal lobe without damaging the paleocortex, the archicortex and subcortical nuclei. After such an operation the principal remaining changes consist of hyperactivity, visual exploration and diminished capacity of visual perception, without the other disturbances of behavior.

The inferotemporal cortex, on the undersurface of the temporal lobe, is now considered by many to be a principal site of the processing of visual information. This cortical area has a common border with the secondary visual receiving areas (V-II, V-III and V-IV; see Chapter 10) of the peristriate cortex, and receives part of its input from there. But signals from the retina can reach this area also by way of the superior colliculi and the pulvinar nucleus of the thalamus. Visual stimuli can excite most neurons in the inferotemporal cortex. These visually excitable cells have no sharply defined receptive fields, no optimal stimulus orientation, and no optimal direction of movement (cf. Chapter 10). Instead they respond to complex moving shapes appearing anywhere in a wide and poorly demarcated part of the contralateral visual field.

In man bilateral lesions limited to the cortex of the temporal lobes do not occur naturally. Damage to both temporal lobes would presumably destroy so much of the brain lying between these two poles that the question of specific temporal lobe signs would become moot. Unilateral disease of a temporal lobe is usually dominated by the epilepsy that it causes (see Section 4.3a). The relatively mild deficiencies of auditory function caused by limited unilateral temporal cortical lesions have been mentioned in Section 12.6, and the consequences of hippocampal disease for memory, in Section 20.4a. Since Wernicke's area lies on the superior temporal gyrus, usually on the left side, damage here causes aphasia (see Section 21.1).

There is one case report from the mid-1950s, entitled "Klüver-Bucy syndrome in man," of a patient who had undergone rather wide excision of both temporal lobes for the treatment of epilepsy. Unlike the other patients in whom ablation was more limited and whose syndromes were dominated by the memory defects already described (Section 20.4a), this man developed severe behavioral changes. Before the operation he was prone to outbursts of rage, which ceased thereafter. He also lost, however, social inhibitions of sexual behavior. Moreover, he could no longer recognize people, even close relatives he had known all his life. This case was different from the amnestic syndrome of Korsakoff patients who retain the recognition of old acquaintances, even though they cannot learn to recognize new ones.

21.2c. PARIETAL LOBES

If damage to temporal and frontal association cortex makes monkeys hyperactive, similar bilateral lesions of the parietal association areas cause them to become withdrawn and passive. If the lesion affects one side only, the animal tends to sit with his side contralateral to the lesion turned toward the wall, presenting only his healthy side for contact. When the affected hand is touched, it is moved away: the *instinctive avoidance response.* When the monkey's gaze meets a person or another animal, he averts his eyes. There seems to be differentiation within parts of the parietal association cortex itself: more rostral lesions cause tactile avoidance; those limited to the posterior part of the parietal association area produce visual avoidance.

Also typical of parietal lesions are deficiencies of orientation in space, and of purposeful movements executed in space. This has been interpreted as a specific form of agnosia, namely, an inability to discern spatial order by integrating visual and tactile sensory information. The consequence of this perceptual disintegration is a specific apraxia.

In human patients a typical sign of one-sided parietal lobe damage is a dress apraxia, limited to the side contralateral to the lesion. The patient might "forget" to put his arm through the sleeve of his coat on the affected side, or he might not put on one shoe. This is a manifestation of a more general malfunction called *unilateral neglect.* This term describes the tendency not to take notice of the affected side of the body, nor of objects in the visual field of that side. If the neglected hand is touched, human patients, like monkeys with parietal lobe lesions, often instinctively withdraw it apparently without knowing that they do so. Another method to demonstrate unilateral neglect is to instruct the patient to draw a house, or a person. The typical parietal-lobe-damaged patient draws one side of the picture well, but either "forgets" the other half or omits some of its important details. Neglect due to parietal lobe lesion must be differentiated from hemianopia and from disorders of somatic sensation; parietal lobe apraxia must be differentiated from paresis and ataxia. Neglect can transiently be overcome by calling the patient's attention to the error he is making.

Left-sided parietal cortex lesions in humans are dominated by aphasia, alexia or agraphia, as discussed earlier (Section 21.1). The defects of spatial orientation and unilateral neglect are more pronounced after right-sided lesion, but they can be present to various degrees after damage to the left parietal cortex as well. One way to bring out latent parietal lobe signs is by the demonstration of what sometimes is called *bilateral rivalry* and sometimes *cortical extinction.* On ordinary sensory examination, with the patient's attention being directed to the affected side, the cutaneous sensibility of the affected side may seem normal; but when both hands are touched simultaneously, the patient reports being touched only on the healthy side.

The firing of impulses by neurons in parietal association areas has been recorded in unanesthetized and relatively freely moving monkeys trained to perform certain standardized tasks. Several distinct patterns of firing were described, and the responses of the various cell types were related to the monkeys' behavior. Some of the neurons responded to visual input. Like the cells in inferotemporal cortex, those in the parietal association areas do not have well-defined visual receptive fields or specific optimal stimulus orientation. Here, as in inferotemporal cortex, information from many functional cell columns of the visual receptive areas seems to converge in some meaningfully integrated fashion. Some of the cells in parietal cortex are quite special in that they are excited only when an object appears in the visual field to which the monkey is paying special attention. Other objects, to which the monkey has not specifically been trained to attach some meaning, do not evoke a response of these cells. Other neurons in parietal cortex fire each time the monkey shifts his gaze in a saccade; and yet others fire only when he follows a moving object with his eyes in smooth pursuit. Other neurons discharge when the monkey reaches to grasp an object. These cells differ from those in motor cortex in that they do not fire when the muscles of the hand contract during any other type of movement.

When the results of these electrophysiological observations are combined with observations of brain-damaged subjects, a picture emerges of the several functions of parietal association cortex. Among them are: integrating visual with tactile information; directing attention to selected objects in visual space; orienting in space; and organizing movements required to explore and to manipulate objects in nearby space.

21.3. A Theory of Reciprocal Antagonism of Cortical Functions

Many clinical and laboratory investigations have contributed to our current views of the consequences of cortical damage, but the work of Denny-Brown and collaborators, performed in the 1950s and 1960s, stands out. This team removed parts of the cerebral cortex, avoiding as far as possible damage to the pial circulation and to adjoining cortical and subcortical tissue. In an extended series of observations they have removed different parts of the cortex of monkeys and compared the results with observations made on brain-damaged human patients.

From these observations Denny-Brown has derived certain hypothetical principles of cortical function following in the tradition of the schools of thought of Hughlings Jackson and Sherrington. According to his view, much of an animal's behavior consists of either exploring the environment or withdrawing from it. Both exploration and withdrawal can be construed as reflexive acts: the adequate stimuli for exploration being objects that seem attractive to the animal, those for avoidance stimuli that seem threatening. Normally these behaviors are called into action in ways that are appropriate for the well-being of the animal. Approach and exploration are supposed to be controlled by brain circuits that are in reciprocally inhibitory relationship with the circuits that control avoidance and withdrawal. While one circuit is active, the other is restrained. Each of these elementary behaviors would be laid down in a crude subcortical program which would be adjusted and refined by superimposed cortical control. Thus forced grasping and the traction reflex (Section 18.4.c.) are subcortical responses of which instinctive grasping is the cortically controlled refined counterpart. Similarly the flexor reflex (Section 15.4) may be considered to be the spinal subordinate of the cortically mediated tactile avoidance response.

If we accept the premises of this theory, then it would seem that the parietal association cortex controls exploration, its rostral half being more concerned with tactile and the posterior part with visual exploration. To frontal association cortex falls the task of withdrawal from or avoidance of tactile stimuli, to temporal cortex the avoidance of visually identified stimuli. Destruction of any of these areas results in hyperactivity due to release of its antagonist; this explains why frontal lesions cause compulsive tactile exploration and instinctive grasping, temporal lesions visual exploration, and parietal lesions withdrawal and avoidance.

Denny-Brown's theory is not universally accepted among neurologists. It has been introduced here because it provides a theoretical framework for otherwise disjointed clinical observations.

21.4. Electrophysiological Signs of Cognitive Processes

Figure 21.1 illustrates a typical experiment of a psychoelectrophysiological laboratory. A subject is wired for the recording of the electric potential from the scalp at the top of his head (the vertex); he is being presented with visual and auditory stimuli. The visual stimulus is the warning (W), and the auditory stimulus the signal (S). The auditory stimulus (S) sometimes is and sometimes is not given after the presentation of the warning flash (W). The electric potential is recorded in two ways. Above is shown the "raw" electroencephalogram (EEG), with variable frequency low-amplitude wave activity typical of an alert subject. Upon this ongoing EEG are superimposed the responses evoked by the stimuli. In order to see the details of these evoked potentials clearly, the intercurrent EEG waves must be eliminated from the tracing: in electrophysiology one man's signal is another man's noise. The responses evoked by the stimuli can be enhanced by electrically computing the averages of the electric waves of many tracings. Since the EEG waves appear at random in relation to the stimulus, they are canceled when several superimposed traces are averaged, whereas the responses which are locked in time in relation to the stimulus are enhanced. In the experiment illustrated here, the computer averaged responses to stimulus W by itself separately from those resulting from the combined presentation of $W + S$. The tracing of Figure 21.1 shows the averaged response to $W + S$.

On the averaged trace of Figure 21.1 we can detect the biphasic visual evoked potential labeled N_1 and P_2 following stimulus W, and the series of auditory evoked potentials labeled I to VI with which we are already

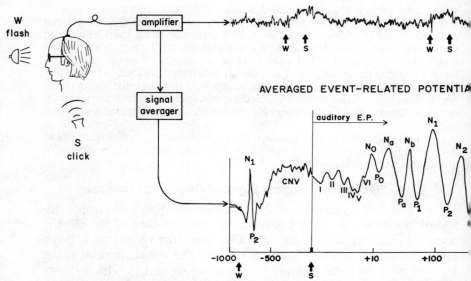

Figure 21.1. Evoked potentials and event-related potentials. A subject is presented with a flash of light, which is the warning stimulus (*W*), followed by a click, which is the signal (*S*) to which he has to attend. The *upper tracing* shows the EEG waves and two responses to such paired stimulus presentations. *Below* is the response averaged by computer. Note that the time scale of the averaged response before the stimulus *S* is linear; thereafter it is logarithmic. The numbers indicate milliseconds. For interpretation of the waves, see text. (Reprinted with permission from R. Galambos and S. A. Hillyard: *Neurosciences Research Program Bulletin* 20:140–265, 1981.

familiar (Fig. 12.3) following stimulus *S*. Of interest to our present discussion are, however, the later waves. These are not believed to reflect sensory processing, but to be related to the integration of sensory signals and to the decisions preceding action.

The wave labeled *CNV* is called the *contingent negative variation*. It is a slow negative potential shift, which appears when a subject expects that shortly he will have to make a decision. If the same flash would be seen by a subject neither instructed to pay attention nor to do anything, then only the visual evoked potential (N_1 and P_2) without the *CNV* would appear. A potential wave similar to the *CNV* was described as the *readyness potential* (or *Bereitschaftspotential* in the German original, or expectancy wave); and the debate whether the two are identical or distinct has not yet been resolved. The late waves N_o, P_o and N_b that follow the auditory evoked potentials (*I-VI*) are believed related to paying active attention to the signal, and the latest deflections, especially N_2 and P_3, to the making of a decision, whether and what to do about it. The P_3 wave is designated in another system of labeling as the *P-300 wave* because it is a positive deflection occurring about 300 msec after the stimulus. It is of interest because it seems to appear only if the stimulus is not predictable by the subject. Thus if S would follow each time W has been presented, P_3 wave would rapidly diminish in amplitude and it could disappear altogether. If the S stimulus is given after the W stimulus only sometimes, on occasions that the subject cannot foresee, then the P_3 wave becomes large. The neuronal activity that controls voluntary movement can also be detected from the scalp in the form of a negative wave that is maximal over the parietal cortex of the side contralateral to the limb moved. This so-called *motor potential* appears a fraction of a second before a movement is made.

These various electric signs of so-called higher brain functions are sometimes together called *event-related potentials.* For the present they are mainly of interest to psychophysiologists. Some investigators hope however that they will eventually become diagnostic tools for cerebral disorders.

21.5. The Limbic System

The concept of a "limbic lobe" was introduced by French neurologists toward the end of the last century to designate the anatomical border areas between telencephalon and "lower" parts of the neuraxis. The currently used anatomical definition of the limbic system was given by Papez in the 1930s. Figure 21.2 illustrates the parts of the brain included in the *Papez circuit.* Retaining an earlier term some investigators call this system the rhinencephalon, but only some parts of it actually serve the sense of smell.

Papez and many others attributed to the limbic system the control of *motivation, instinctive* behavior and *emotional* and *affective* responses. It was also thought that the limbic circuit integrates the higher mental functions of the forebrain with the autonomic responses controlled in the diencephalon and brain stem.

In discussions of limbic functions, the significance of the sense of smell for instinctive behavior is often emphasized. This relationship

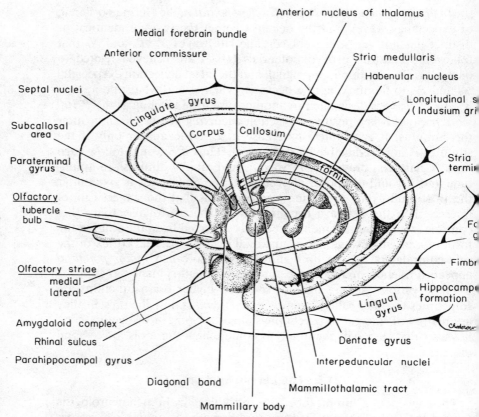

Figure 21.2. Diagram of the limbic system, also known as the Papez circuit or rhinencephalon. Some authors include the hypothalamus in the limbic system. (Reprinted with permission from M. B. Carpenter: *Core Text of Neuroanatomy*, ed. 2. Baltimore, Williams & Wilkins, 1978.)

justifies the profuse connections of regions with truly olfactory function to the remainder of the limbic structures. The anomalous instinctive and affective responses seen after lesions of amygdala and septal nuclei, or of the pathways that connect these structures to the frontal lobes, also illustrate the importance of these structures in the motivation of certain behaviors (see Section 21.2a). Furthermore, the limbic circuit has strong afferent and efferent connections with the hypothalamus. The significance of that region for the control of aggression, sexual behavior, and visceral functions is already familiar to the reader. Some authors actually include the hypothalamus among the limbic structures. Less clear is the relationship of the hippocampus to the general notions of limbic system function. For while the hippocampal formation is customarily included in the limbic system, there is no evidence that it is in any direct way involved with the control of instinctive behavior (cf. Sections 19.3b and 20.4). Its anatomical position and its connections with the other components of the limbic system may, however, perhaps be understood if one considers that learning is powerfully influenced by motivation.

An important method of studying limbic functions is the experimental arrangement that enables animals to stimulate their own brains, which is our next topic.

21.6. Intracranial Self-Stimulation

If rats are provided with electrodes implanted in certain selected points in the brain and are given the means of turning on an electric stimulating current by pushing a lever, they will stimulate their own brains for hours on end, as though they liked what they felt when the current was on. Among the most favored brain sites for self-stimulation are the lateral hypothalamic area and the septal nuclei, but several others, mostly either in the limbic system of the forebrain, or in the brain stem, are also effective. Sometimes rats prefer to push the lever that gives them the electric stimulus over another lever that provides food, even if they are hungry. Sometimes they are willing to cross an electrified grid and to accept painful foot shocks in order to reach the lever that will give them the brain stimulus. It is as though they become addicted to the pleasures of self-stimulation. These startling discoveries were first reported by Olds and Milner in 1954, and the phenomenon has been studied intensively ever since.

Besides rats, other species of animals can be induced to stimulate their own brains, although rats are apparently the favored subjects in these experiments. A small group of psychotic patients have been provided with electrodes implanted into brain areas homologous to the rats' self-stimulating points. The purpose of the procedure was to alleviate the psychotic state. When the stimulation was applied these individuals reported pleasurable feelings, sometimes of an explicitly sexual nature. In some cases, however, they reported no pleasure at all, but still continued to use the stimulator when allowed to control it. The scientific value of the reports of their subjective experiences is diminished by the severely psychotic state of these subjects. In recent years no additional similar human experiments have been reported.

Stimulation of certain other points in the brain evokes aversive responses. Given the means to do so, rats will always turn such stimulation off. The strongest aversive responses were obtained when the electrode was lodged in the dorsal midbrain tegmentum, close to the border with the tectum.

It will be recalled that the lateral hypothalamic area, one of the "reward" sites (or positive self-stimulating sites), is also implicated in generating the feeling of satiety after food intake (see Section 17.5). It was natural to link the satisfaction apparently provided by electric stimulation of this region with the good feeling that comes after a meal. Experiments designed to show that the two are indeed related gave, however, ambiguous results.

More recently attention was focused on the fact that the medial forebrain bundle also passes through the lateral hypothalamic area. The medial forebrain bundle is the one tract where all ascending monoamine systems are represented. Survey of all the sites in the brain where stimulation appeared to be positively reinforcing (i.e. rewarding), revealed one common aspect: they all contain either monoaminergic fibers or they are the targets of monoaminergic input. The rule cannot be reversed: not all monoaminergic fiber tracts are substrates for self-stimulation. Specifically, those descending into the spinal cord and those addressed to the cerebellum are not.

Pharmacological experiments seemed to confirm that excitation of monoaminergic neurons may be the "reward" sought in self-stimulation; drugs that block central noradrenergic transmission seem to block it. Some authors single out noradrenaline as being the specific rewarding brain chemical, others emphasize the role of dopamine and of serotonin as well. Some authors ascribe different but important roles to each of the three monoamines.

Some, but not all, self-stimulation sites also provide electroanalgesia (see Section 7.9b). These particular sites also contain opiate receptors and enkephalin as well (see Section 7.9c). It may be assumed that the reward provided by stimulating the enkephalin system is different from that evoked by the monoamine systems. Because of the dense packing of elements in the rat's brain stem, multiple systems are sometimes inevitably stimulated, and it is often difficult to separate the several coincident effects. For this reason it has not been possible to prove beyond a doubt that the effect of the electrical self-stimulation at these sites is the release of enkephalin from neuronal storage sites, in other words an intracerebral "morphine fix."

21.7. Chapter Summary

1. In the majority of people all functions relating to the understanding and the production of language, including reading and writing, are predominantly controlled by the left hemisphere. In a very small minority of right-handed individuals and in a larger percentage, but still a minority, of left-handers, language dominance either resides in the right hemisphere or it is shared by left and right.

2. Functions relating to spatial orientation are predominantly controlled by the right hemisphere. Certain other faculties, among them artistic and musical talent, have been attributed with lesser certainty to right hemisphere function. These asymmetric hemispheric specializations are not absolute.

3. After bilateral ablation of the association area (homotypical cortex) of the frontal lobes monkeys become restless and hyperactive, and they compulsively explore their environment by touch. Such animals lose the ability to solve tasks requiring a delayed response.

4. Human patients whose frontal lobes are damaged are usually unable to plan for the future and cannot organize a timetable. Their affect is usually impoverished and flat.

5. Bilateral experimental ablation of the temporal association areas of monkeys causes hyperactivity and compulsive exploration of visually located objects which the animal does not appear to recognize. If the amygdala and adjacent paleocortex are also damaged, the animals become tame and sexually hyperactive.

6. In human patients bilateral lesion limited to temporal association cortex does not occur naturally. One-sided lesion results either in aphasia or mild hearing defect, depending on its location. Damage to the hippocampal formation leads to memory defect (see Chapter 20). Temporal lobe lesions tend to cause complex partial seizures especially if gliosis of the damaged area ensues.

7. Experimental ablation of the parietal association cortex of monkeys causes the animal to withdraw from and to avoid contact with objects and with other animals. If the lesion is one-sided, then only the contralateral body half and objects in the contralateral visual field are involved.

8. In human patients parietal disease of the dominant hemisphere disturbs language functions. Parietal disease of the non-dominant side results in a disorder of spatial orientation, dress apraxia and unilateral neglect affecting the contralateral side only. The avoidance response and cortical extinction of sensation can usually be demonstrated in cases of parietal lobe lesions of either left or right hemisphere.

9. Among the electrophysiological accompaniments of cortical cognitive processes are the event-related potentials known as the contingent negative variation and the P-300 (or P_3) potential.

10. The anatomically defined limbic system includes several structures concerned with olfactory function, also the amygdala and septal nuclei, the hippocampus and a number of structures, the functional significance of which are obscure. This system has manifold connections with the hypo-

thalamus as well as with cortical areas, especially frontal association cortex, and some of the thalamic nuclei.

11. Given the means to do so, rats and other experimental animals will electrically stimulate their own brains, if the stimulating electrode is placed in the lateral hypothalamus, the septal nuclei, or certain other sites. These "positive self-stimulating sites" all contain monoaminergic neurons or their axons, or enkephalin-containing cells.

12. Negative self-stimulating sites (aversive points) are concentrated near the border of the tectum in the midbrain.

Further Reading

Books and Reviews

Fuster JM: *The Prefrontal Cortex*. New York, Raven Press, 1980.

Gazzaniga MS: *The Bisected Brain*. New York, Appleton-Century-Crofts, 1970.

Goodglass H: Disorders of naming following brain injury. *Am Sci* 68:647–655, 1980.

Hemispheric Specialization in Man. Excerpta Medica International Congress Series No. 568, Proceedings of the 12th International Congress of Neurology, pp. 3–82, 1982.

Isaacson RL: *The Limbic System*, ed 2. New York, Plenum Press, 1982.

Langworthy OR: *The Sensory Control of Posture and Movement: A Review of the Studies of Derek Denny-Brown*. Baltimore, Williams & Wilkins, 1970.

Lynch JC (with 34 commentaries): The functional organization of the posterior parietal cortex. *Behav Brain Sci* 3:485–534, 1980.

Mountcastle VB: Brain mechanisms for directed attention. *J R Soc Med* 71:14–28, 1978.

Olds J: *Drives and Reinforcements*. New York, Raven Press, 1977.

Springer SP, Deutsch G: *Left Brain, Right Brain*. San Francisco, W.H. Freeman, 1981.

Weiskrantz L: Varieties of residual experience. *Q J Exp Psychol* 32:365–386, 1980.

Articles

Papez JW: A proposed mechanism of emotion. *Arch Neurol Psychiatry* 38:725–744, 1937.

Index

Page numbers in *italics* denote figures; those followed by "t" denote tables.

539